Current Clinical Strategies

Outpatient and Primary Care Medicine

New Guidelines

2010 Edition

Paul D. Chan, MD
David M. Thomas, MD
Elizabeth K. Stanford, MD

Current Clinical Strategies Publishing

www.ccspublishing.com/ccs

Current Clinical Strategies Publishing
PO Box 1753
Blue Jay, CA 92317
Phone: 800-331-8227
Fax: 800-965-9420
Internet: www.ccspublishing.com/ccs
E-mail: info@ccspublishing.com

Printed in USA

ISBN 978-1-934323-23-6

Contents

Cardiovascular Disorders

Stable Angina Pectoris

Stable angina pectoris is responsible for 11 percent of chest pain episodes; unstable angina or myocardial infarction occur in only 1.5 percent. Musculoskeletal chest pain accounts for 36 percent of all diagnoses (of which costochondritis accounted for 13 percent) followed by reflux esophagitis (13 percent).

I. **Assessment and management of chest pain in the office**
   A. Myocardial infarction, pulmonary embolus, aortic dissection, or tension pneumothorax may cause chest pain and sudden death. Any patient with a recent onset of chest pain who may be potentially unstable should be transported immediately to an emergency department in an ambulance equipped with a defibrillator. Stabilization includes supplemental oxygen, intravenous access, and placement of a cardiac monitor. A 12-lead electrocardiogram and a blood sample for cardiac enzymes should be obtained.
   B. Patients who with possible myocardial infarction should chew a 325 mg aspirin tablet.
   C. Sublingual nitroglycerin should be given unless the patient has relatively low blood pressure or has recently taken a phosphodiesterase inhibitor such as sildenafil (Viagra).

II. **Clinical evaluation**
   A. **Quality of the pain.** The patient with myocardial ischemia may describe the pain as squeezing, tightness, pressure, constriction, strangling, burning, heart burn, fullness in the chest, a band-like sensation, knot in the center of the chest, lump in the throat, ache, weight on chest, and toothache. In some cases, the patient may place his fist in the center of the chest ("Levine sign").
   B. **Region or location of pain.** Ischemic pain is a diffuse discomfort that may be difficult to localize. Pain that localizes to a small area on the chest is more likely of chest wall or pleural origin.
   C. **Radiation.** The pain of myocardial ischemia may radiate to the neck, throat, lower jaw, teeth, upper extremity, or shoulder. Chest pain radiation increases the probability of myocardial infarction. Pain radiating to either arm is indicative of coronary ischemia.
   D. **Acute cholecystitis** can present with right shoulder pain and right upper quadrant pain. Chest pain that radiates between the scapulae suggests aortic dissection.
   E. **Temporal elements**
      1. The pain with a pneumothorax or an aortic dissection or acute pulmonary embolism typically has an abrupt onset.
      2. Ischemic pain usually has gradual onset with an increasing intensity over time.
      3. "Functional" or nontraumatic musculoskeletal chest pain has a vague onset.
   F. **Duration of pain**
      1. Chest discomfort that lasts only for seconds or pain that is constant over weeks is not due to ischemia. A span of years without progression makes it more likely that the origin of pain is functional. The pain from myocardial ischemia generally lasts for a few minutes.
      2. Myocardial ischemia is more likely to occur in the morning, correlating with an increase in sympathetic tone.
   G. **Provocative factors**
      1. Discomfort that reliably occurs with eating is suggestive of upper gastrointestinal disease.

2. Chest discomfort provoked by exertion is a classic symptom of angina.
3. Other factors that may provoke ischemic pain include cold, emotional stress, meals, or sexual intercourse.
4. Pain made worse by swallowing is usually of esophageal origin.
5. Body position or movement, as well as deep breathing, may exacerbate chest pain of musculoskeletal origin.
6. Pleuritic chest pain is worsened by respiration. Causes of pleuritic chest pain include pulmonary embolism, pneumothorax, viral or idiopathic pleurisy, pneumonia, and pleuropericarditis.

H. Palliation

1. Pain that is palliated by antacids or food is likely of gastroesophageal origin.
2. Pain that responds to sublingual nitroglycerin usually has a cardiac etiology or to be due to esophageal spasm. Pain relief with nitroglycerin not helpful in distinguishing cardiac from noncardiac chest pain.
3. Pain that abates with cessation of activity suggests an ischemic origin.
4. Pericarditis pain improves with sitting up and leaning forward.

I. Severity of pain is not a useful predictor of CHD. One-third of myocardial infarctions may go unnoticed by the patient.

J. Associated symptoms

1. Belching, a bad taste in the mouth, and difficult or painful swallowing are suggestive of esophageal disease, although belching and indigestion also may be seen with myocardial ischemia.
2. Vomiting may occur with myocardial ischemia (particularly transmural myocardial infarction) or with peptic ulcer disease, cholecystitis, and pancreatitis.
3. Diaphoresis is more frequently associated with myocardial infarction than esophageal disease.
4. Exertional dyspnea is common when chest pain is due to myocardial ischemia or a pulmonary disorders.
5. Cough may be caused by congestive heart failure, pulmonary embolus, neoplasm, or pneumonia.

K. Syncope. The patient with myocardial ischemia may describe presyncope. Syncope should raise a concern for aortic dissection, pulmonary embolus, a ruptured abdominal aortic aneurysm, or critical aortic stenosis.

L. Palpitations. Patients with ischemia can feel palpitations resulting from ventricular ectopy. Atrial fibrillation is associated with chronic CHD.

M. Risk factors

1. Hyperlipidemia, left ventricular hypertrophy, or a family history of premature CHD increase the risk for myocardial ischemia.
2. Hypertension is a risk factor for both CHD and aortic dissection.
3. Cigarette smoking is a nonspecific risk factor for CHD, thromboembolism, aortic dissection, pneumothorax, and pneumonia
4. Cocaine use may be suggestive of myocardial infarction.
5. Viral infection may precede pericarditis or myocarditis. Other risk factors for pericarditis include chest trauma, autoimmune disease, recent myocardial infarction or cardiac surgery, and the use of procainamide, hydralazine, or isoniazid.

N. Age. Among patients older than age 40, chest pain resulting from CHD or an acute coronary syndrome (unstable angina or myocardial infarction) becomes increasingly common.

1. Men older than age 60 are most likely to suffer aortic dissection, while young men are at highest risk for primary spontaneous pneumothorax. Young adults of both sexes are diagnosed with viral pleurisy more often than are older patients.
2. A past history of CHD, symptomatic gastroesophageal reflux, peptic ulcer disease, gallstones, panic disorder, bronchospasm, or cancer is very helpful. Diabetics often have nonclassic presentation of CHD.

O. Physical examination

1. General appearance of the patient suggests the severity and the

seriousness of the symptoms.

2. **Vital signs** can provide clues to the clinical significance of the pain.

3. **Palpation of the chest wall** may evoke pain. Hyperesthesia, particularly when associated with a rash, is often caused by herpes zoster.

4. **Cardiac examination** should include auscultation and palpation in a sitting and supine position to establish the presence of a pericardial rub or signs of acute aortic insufficiency or aortic stenosis. Ischemia may result in a mitral insufficiency murmur or an S4 or S3 gallop.

5. Asymmetric breath sounds and wheezes, crackles or evidence of consolidation should be assessed.

6. Abdominal examination should assess the right upper quadrant, epigastrium, and the abdominal aorta.

P. Ancillary studies

1. **Normal electrocardiogram.** A normal ECG markedly reduces the probability that chest pain is due to acute myocardial infarction, but it does not exclude a serious cardiac etiology (particularly unstable angina). 1 to 4 percent of patients with normal ECGs will have an acute infarction. A normal ECG in a patient with the recent onset of chest pain suggests stable angina. Aortic dissection should be considered in patients with ongoing pain and a normal ECG.

2. **Abnormal electrocardiogram.** ST segment elevation, ST segment depression or new Q waves are indications of acute myocardial infarction or unstable angina.

3. **Chest radiograph** may assist in the diagnosis of chest pain if a cardiac, pulmonary, or neoplastic etiology is being considered. Aortic dissection, pneumothorax, and pneumomediastinum may be diagnosed.

4. **Exercise stress testing** is indicated for patients with suspected ischemic heart disease who do not have an unstable coronary syndrome (eg, acute myocardial infarction or unstable angina).

5. **Transthoracic echocardiography** can identify regional wall motion abnormalities within seconds of acute coronary artery occlusion. TTE is also appropriate to assist in the identification of pericarditis with effusion, aortic dissection, and possibly pulmonary embolism.

6. **Myocardial perfusion imaging (MPI)** is a sensitive test for detecting acute myocardial infarction, particularly if the chest pain is ongoing at the time of the study. It can be used to assist in emergency department triage of patients with chest pain. The specificity of acute rest MPI is limited in patients with a previous myocardial infarction.

III. Medical therapy of stable angina pectoris

A. Nitrates are a first-line therapy for the treatment of acute anginal symptoms. The primary antiischemic effect of nitrates is to decrease myocardial oxygen demand by producing systemic vasodilation more than coronary vasodilation.

B. **Sublingual nitroglycerin** is the therapy of choice for acute anginal episodes and prophylactically for activities known to elicit angina. The onset of action is within several minutes and the duration of action is 40 minutes. The initial dose is 0.3 mg; one-half the dose (0.15 mg) can be used if the patient becomes hypotensive.

C. **The patient should contact EMS** if chest pain is unimproved or worsening five minutes after one nitroglycerin dose has been taken.

D. **Chronic nitrate therapy** in the form of an oral or transdermal preparation (isosorbide dinitrate, isosorbide mononitrate, or transdermal nitroglycerin) can prevent or reduce the frequency of recurrent anginal episodes and improve exercise tolerance. However, tolerance to long-acting nitrates can develop and has limited their use as first-line therapy. A 12 to 14 hour nitrate-free interval must be observed in order to avoid tolerance. As a result, chronic nitrate therapy is reserved for second-line antianginal therapy.

1. **Dosing for isosorbide dinitrate** begins with a dose of 10 mg at 8 AM, 1 PM, and 6 PM, which results in a 14 hour nitrate dose-free interval. The dose is increased to 40 mg three times daily as needed. Alternatively,

isosorbide dinitrate can be taken twice daily at 8 AM and 4 PM.

  a. The extended release preparation of isosorbide mononitrate, which is administered once per day, may be preferable to improve compliance. The starting dose is 30 mg once daily and can be titrated to 120 mg once daily as needed. This preparation is particularly useful in patients who have effort-induced angina. However, since the effect lasts only about 12 hours, some patients may develop nocturnal or rebound angina. Such patients require twice daily dosing or additional antianginal therapy.

  b. Transdermal nitroglycerin patch is a convenient way to administer nitroglycerin. The patient must remove the patch for 12 to 14 hours. Since most patients have angina with activity, the patch should be applied at 8 AM and removed at 8 PM. The occasional patient with significant nocturnal angina can be treated with a patch-on period from 8 PM to 8 AM. Initial dose is 0.2 mg per hour; the dose can be increased to 0.8 mg per hour as needed.

  c. Side effects associated with nitrate use are headache, lightheadedness, and flushing which are due to the vasodilatation. These symptoms tend to improve with time.

Dosages of Nitroglycerine Preparations

Preparation	Route of administration	Onset of action, minutes	Duration of action	Dose
Nitroglycerin	Sublingual tablet	2-5	15-30 min	0.15-0.9 mg
	Sublingual spray	2-5	15-30 min	0.4 mg
	Ointment	2-5	Up to 7 hours	2 percent, 15x15 cm
	Transdermal	30	8-14 hours	0.2-0.8 mg/hour q12h
	Oral sustained release	30	4-8 hours	
	Intravenous	2-5	During infusion, tolerance in 7-8 hours	2.5-13 mg 5-200 ug/min
Isosorbide dinitrate	Sublingual	2-5	Up to 60 min	2.5-15 mg
	Oral	30	Up to 8 hours	5-80 mg BID or TID
	Spray	2-5	2-3 min	1.25 mg/day
	Chewable	2-5	2-2.25 hours	5 mg
	Oral slow release	30	Up to 8 hours	40 mg QD or BID
	Intravenous	2-5	During infusion, tolerance in 7-8 hours	1.25-5 mg/hour
Isosorbide mononitrate, extended release	Oral	30	12-24 hours	20-40 mg BID 60-240 mg/day
Isosorbide mononitrate, extended release	Oral	30-60	12 hours	30-120 mg once daily

  E. **Beta blockers** relieve anginal symptoms by competitively inhibiting sympathetic stimulation of the heart, reducing both heart rate and contractility.

1. **Choice of agent.** Lower doses of the cardioselective beta blockers (atenolol and metoprolol) have the advantage of blocking beta-1-receptor mediated stimulation of the heart with lesser inhibition of the peripheral vasodilation and bronchodilation induced by the beta-2 receptors.

   a. Long-acting cardioselective agents (atenolol or metoprolol) are preferred for stable angina. There are no advantages of a nonselective agent, other than the low cost of propranolol, and there are disadvantages in obstructive lung disease, asthma, peripheral vascular disease, diabetes, and depression.

   b. **Atenolol (Tenormin)** starting dose is 25 mg once daily which can be increased as tolerated to a maximum of 200 mg once a day until the resting heart rate is 50 to 60 beats/min and does not exceed 100 beats/min with ordinary activity.

   c. **Metoprolol (Lopressor)** starting dose is 25 mg BID, which can be increased to 200 mg BID as tolerated. An extended release form of metoprolol, given once per day, can be substituted once an effective dose has been established.

   d. Beta blockers are well tolerated and extremely effective in reducing anginal episodes and improving exercise tolerance. Beta blockers are the only antianginal drugs proven to prevent reinfarction and to improve survival after an MI.

2. **Achieving adequate beta blockade.** Reasonable goals when titrating the dose include:

   a. Resting heart rate between 50 and 60 beats/min. The target heart rate for some patients with more severe angina can be <50 beats/min, as long as the bradycardia is asymptomatic and heart block does not develop.

3. Patients with resting bradycardia prior to therapy can be treated with a calcium channel blocker (such as diltiazem or nifedipine), nitrates, or a drug with intrinsic sympathomimetic activity if a beta blocker is necessary.

4. **Beta-blocker side effects.** Bradycardia, conduction disturbances, bronchoconstriction, worsening of symptoms of peripheral vascular disease, fatigue, central nervous system side effects, and impotence. As a result, beta blockers should be used with caution in patients with obstructive airways disease or peripheral vascular disease and, initially at very low doses in patients with heart failure.

5. Beta blockers should not be used in patients with vasospastic or variant (Prinzmetal) angina. In such patients, they are ineffective and may increase the tendency to induce coronary vasospasm from unopposed alpha-receptor activity.

Adverse Effects of Beta-blockers

Bradycardia, decreased contractility, AV node conduction delay

Bronchoconstriction can be induced by nonselective agents and high doses of cardioselective agents.

Worsening of symptoms of peripheral vascular disease or Raynaud's phenomenon.

Fatigue may be due to the reduction in cardiac output or to direct effects on the central nervous system.

Central side effects include depression, nightmares, insomnia, and hallucinations.

Impotence is often a problem.

Beta-blockers			
Class	**Drug name**	**Starting dose**	**Maximal dose**
Cardioselective	Atenolol (Tenormin)	25 mg QD	100 mg QD
Cardioselective	Metoprolol (Lopressor)	25 mg BID	100 mg BID
	Metoprolol extended release (Toprol XL)	50 mg qd	200 mg qd
Nonselective	Nadolol (Corgard)	25 mg QD	240 mg QD
Nonselective	Propranolol (Inderal)	40 mg BID	120 mg BID
Intrinsic sympathomimetic	Pindolol (Visken)	5 mg BID	30 mg BID
Alpha blocker	Labetalol (Normodyne)	100 mg BID	600 mg BID

F. **Calcium channel blockers** prevent calcium entry into vascular smooth muscle cells and myocytes, which leads to coronary and peripheral vasodilatation, decreased atrioventricular (AV) conduction, and reduced contractility. In patients with angina, these effects result in decreased coronary vascular resistance and increased coronary blood flow. Calcium blockers also decrease myocardial oxygen demand by reducing systemic vascular resistance and arterial pressure and a negative inotropic effect.

1. **Choice of agent**
   a. Verapamil is a negative inotrope that also slows sinus rate and decreases AV conduction (negative chronotrope). It is a much less potent vasodilator than the dihydropyridines.
   b. The dihydropyridines (eg, nifedipine, nicardipine, felodipine, amlodipine) have a greater selectivity for vascular smooth muscle than for the myocardium. They are potent vasodilators with less effect on contractility and AV conduction.
   c. Diltiazem (Cardizem) is a modest negative inotropic and chronotropic agent and vasodilator and has intermediate effects between the dihydropyridines and verapamil.
   d. If a calcium channel blocker is used, long-acting diltiazem or verapamil or a second generation dihydropyridine (amlodipine or felodipine) should be selected. Short-acting dihydropyridines, especially nifedipine, should be avoided unless used in conjunction with a beta blocker in the management of CHD because of evidence of an increase in mortality after an MI and an increase in acute MI in hypertensive patients.
   e. **When to use.** All of the calcium channel blockers reduce anginal symptoms and increase exercise tolerance and exercise time before the onset of angina or ischemia. They should be used in combination with beta blockers when initial treatment with beta blockers is not successful. They may be a substitute for a beta blocker when beta blockers are contraindicated or cause side effects. Calcium channel

blockers (eg, diltiazem at a dose of 240 to 360 mg per day) are effective in patients with vasospastic or variant (Prinzmetal) angina; they are the preferred agents in this setting.

    f. **Side effects** include symptomatic bradycardia, heart block, worsening heart failure, constipation, flushing, headache, dizziness, and pedal edema.

G. **General measures.** Treatment of any underlying medical conditions that might aggravate myocardial ischemia, such as hypertension, fever, tachyarrhythmias (eg, atrial fibrillation), thyrotoxicosis, anemia or polycythemia, hypoxemia, or valvular heart disease should be undertaken. Asymptomatic low grade arrhythmias are not treated routinely.

H. **Aspirin** should be given unless contraindicated (81 to 325 mg/day). Patients who have a gastrointestinal bleed on low dose aspirin should be treated with aspirin (81 mg/day) plus a proton pump inhibitor. Clopidogrel (Plavix)is an alternative in patients who are allergic to aspirin.

I. **Risk factor reduction** includes treatment of hypertension, cessation of smoking, lipid lowering with a regimen that includes statin therapy, weight reduction, and glycemic control in diabetics.

J. **Measurement of left ventricular systolic function.** Most patients with chronic stable angina do not need measurement of LV systolic function. Measurement of LV systolic function is recommended in patients with the following:

    1. History of prior MI, pathologic Q waves, or symptoms or signs of heart failure.

    2. A systolic murmur suggesting mitral regurgitation.

    3. Complex ventricular arrhythmias.

K. **Exercise testing.** A stress test should be performed in patients with stable angina to evaluate the efficacy of the antiischemic program and for prognostic information.

    1. A standard exercise ECG is preferred as the initial test in patients with a normal resting ECG who are able to exercise and are not taking digoxin.

    2. Exercise testing can identify a subset of high-risk patients who have an annual mortality of more than 3 per cent. In comparison, low-risk patients, with an annual mortality below one per cent, are able to exercise into stage 3 of a Bruce protocol with a normal ECG.

    3. Low- and intermediate-risk patients are generally treated medically, while high-risk patients or those with angina refractory to medical therapy undergo coronary angiography and revascularization with either PCI or CABG.

L. **Coronary angiography and revascularization.** There are two primary indications for coronary angiography followed by revascularization of appropriate lesions:

    1. Angina that significantly interferes with a patient's lifestyle despite maximal tolerable medical therapy.

    2. Patients with high-risk criteria and selected patients with intermediate-risk criteria on noninvasive testing, regardless of anginal severity.

    3. Revascularization is performed in appropriate patients in whom angiography reveals anatomy for which revascularization has a proven benefit.

    4. The choice between PCI and CABG is based upon anatomy and other factors such as left ventricular function and the presence or absence of diabetes. PCI is increasingly performed for most lesions because of the availability of drug-eluting stents.

References: See page 294.

Heart Failure

Heart failure (HF) has a mortality rate of 50 percent at two years and 60 to 70 percent at three years. Heart failure can result from any structural or functional cardiac disorder that impairs the ability of the ventricle to fill with or eject blood.

I. New York Heart Association (NYHA) classification of heart failure severity:

Class I - symptoms of HF only at activity levels that would limit normal individuals

Class II - symptoms of HF with ordinary exertion

Class III - symptoms of HF with less than ordinary exertion

Class IV - symptoms of HF at rest

Stages of heart failure:

Stage A. High risk for HF, without structural heart disease or symptoms

Stage B. Heart disease with asymptomatic left ventricular dysfunction

Stage C. Prior or current symptoms of HF

Stage D. Advanced heart disease and severely symptomatic or refractory HF

II. Etiology

A. Systolic dysfunction is most commonly caused by coronary heart disease, idiopathic dilated cardiomyopathy, hypertension, and valvular disease.

B. Diastolic dysfunction can be caused by hypertension, ischemic heart disease, hypertrophic obstructive cardiomyopathy, and restrictive cardiomyopathy.

III. Clinical evaluation of heart failure

A. History. There are two major classes of symptoms in HF: those due to excess fluid accumulation (dyspnea, edema, hepatic congestion, and ascites) and those due to a reduction in cardiac output (fatigue, weakness). Fluid retention in HF is initiated by the fall in cardiac output.

B. The acuity of HF is suggested by the presenting symptoms:

1. **Acute and subacute presentations** (days to weeks) are characterized by shortness of breath, at rest and/or with exertion. Also common are orthopnea, paroxysmal nocturnal dyspnea, and, with right HF, right upper quadrant discomfort due to hepatic congestion. Atrial and/or ventricular tachyarrhythmias may cause palpitations and lightheadedness.

2. **Chronic presentations** (months) differ in that fatigue, anorexia, bowel distension, and peripheral edema may be more pronounced than dyspnea.

3. The absence of dyspnea on exertion makes the diagnosis of HF unlikely, while a history of myocardial infarction and a displaced apical impulse, or S3 on physical examination, strongly suggest the diagnosis.

C. Clues to the cause of heart failure

1. **Exertional angina** usually indicates ischemic heart disease.

2. **Flu-like illness** before acute HF suggests viral myocarditis.

3. **Hypertension or alcohol** use suggests hypertensive or alcoholic cardiomyopathy.

4. **Amyloidosis** should be excluded in patients who also have a history of heavy proteinuria.

5. **Primary valvular dysfunction** should be considered in a patient with a history of murmurs.

6. **Antiarrhythmic agents** may provoke HF. Antiarrhythmics include disopyramide and flecainide; calcium channel blockers, particularly verapamil; beta blockers. Nonsteroidal antiinflammatory drugs (NSAIDs) may provoke HF.

7. **Acute pulmonary edema** occurring during, or shortly after, infusion of blood products suggests transfusional volume overload.

Factors Associated with Worsening Heart Failure
Cardiovascular factors
Superimposed ischemia or infarction Hypertension Primary valvular disease Worsening secondary mitral regurgitation Atrial fibrillation Excessive tachycardia Pulmonary embolism
Systemic factors
Inappropriate medications Superimposed infection Anemia Uncontrolled diabetes Thyroid dysfunction Electrolyte disorders Pregnancy
Patient-related factors
Medication noncompliance Dietary indiscretion Alcohol consumption Substance abuse

IV. Physical examination

A. **Heart sounds.** An S3 gallop indicates left atrial pressures exceeding 20 mmHg.

B. **Decreased cardiac output.** Decreased tissue perfusion, results in shunting of the cardiac output to vital organs, leading to sinus tachycardia, diaphoresis, and peripheral vasoconstriction (cool, pale or cyanotic extremities).

C. **Manifestations of volume overload in HF** include pulmonary congestion, peripheral edema, and elevated jugular venous pressure.

D. **Rales** are often absent even though the pulmonary capillary pressure is still elevated.

E. **Peripheral edema** is manifested by swelling of the legs, ascites, hepatomegaly, and splenomegaly. Manual compression of the right upper quadrant may elevate the central venous pressure (hepatojugular reflux).

F. **Elevated jugular venous pressure** is usually present if peripheral edema is due to HF. Jugular venous pressure can be estimated with the patient sitting at 45° either from the height above the left atrium of venous pulsations in the internal jugular vein.

G. **Ventricular chamber size** can be estimated by precordial palpation. An apical impulse that is laterally displaced past the midclavicular line is usually indicative of left ventricular enlargement. Left ventricular dysfunction can also lead to sustained apical impulse which may be accompanied by a parasternal heave.

H. **Blood tests for patients with signs or symptoms of heart failure:**
   1. **Complete blood count** since anemia can exacerbate preexisting HF.
   2. **Serum electrolytes and creatinine**
   3. **Liver function tests**, which may be affected by hepatic congestion.

      4. Fasting blood glucose to detect underlying diabetes mellitus.

I. If it is determined that dilated cardiomyopathy is responsible for HF and the cause is not apparent, several other blood tests may be warranted:
1. **Thyroid function tests**, particularly in patients over the age of 65 or in patients with atrial fibrillation. Thyrotoxicosis is associated with atrial fibrillation, and hypothyroidism may present as HF.
2. **Iron studies** (ferritin and TIBC) to screen for hereditary hemochromatosis (HH).

J. **Other studies that may be undertaken:**
1. ANA and other serologic tests for lupus
2. Viral serologies and antimyosin antibody if myocarditis is suspected
3. Evaluation for pheochromocytoma
4. Thiamine, carnitine, and selenium levels
5. Genetic testing and counseling (in patients suspected of familial cardiomyopathy

K. **Plasma brain natriuretic peptide**
1. In chronic HF, atrial myocytes secrete increased amounts of atrial natriuretic peptide (ANP) and ventricular myocytes secrete ANP and brain natriuretic peptide (BNP) in response to the high atrial and ventricular filling pressures. Both hormones are increased in patients with left ventricular dysfunction.
2. Rapid bedside measurement of plasma BNP is useful for distinguishing between HF and a pulmonary cause of dyspnea.
3. Plasma concentrations of BNP are markedly higher in patients with HF. Intermediate values were found in the patients with baseline left ventricular dysfunction without an acute exacerbation (346 pg/mL).
4. A value >100 pg/mL has a sensitivity, specificity, and predictive accuracy of 90, 76, and 83 percent, respectively. A low BNP concentrations has a high negative predictive value, and is useful in ruling out HF.
5. **Plasma N-pro-BNP.** The active BNP hormone is cleaved from prohormone, pro-BNP. The N-terminal fragment, N-pro-BNP, is also released into the circulation. In normal subjects, the plasma concentrations of BNP and N-pro-BNP are similar (10 pmol/L). However, in LV dysfunction, plasma N-pro-BNP concentrations are four-fold higher than BNP concentrations.
6. An elevated plasma BNP suggests the diagnosis of HF, while a low plasma BNP may be particularly valuable in ruling out HF.

L. **Chest x-ray** is useful to differentiate HF from primary pulmonary disease.
1. Findings suggestive of HF include cardiomegaly (cardiac-to-thoracic width ratio above 50 percent), cephalization of the pulmonary vessels, Kerley B-lines, and pleural effusions.
2. The presence of pulmonary vascular congestion and cardiomegaly on chest x-ray support the diagnosis of HF.

M. **Electrocardiogram** detects arrhythmias such as asymptomatic ventricular premature beats, runs of nonsustained ventricular tachycardia, or atrial fibrillation, which may be the cause of HF.
1. Dilated cardiomyopathy is frequently associated with first degree AV block, left bundle branch block, left anterior fascicular block, or a nonspecific intraventricular conduction abnormality. Potential findings on ECG include:
   a. Signs of ischemic heart disease.
   b. Left ventricular hypertrophy due to hypertension.
   c. Low limb lead voltage on the surface ECG with a pseudo-infarction pattern (loss of precordial R wave progression in leads V1-V6) suggest an infiltrative process such as amyloidosis.
   d. Low limb lead voltage with precordial criteria for left ventricular hypertrophy is most suggestive of idiopathic dilated cardiomyopathy. A widened QRS complex and/or a left bundle branch block pattern is also consistent with this diagnosis.

      e. Most patients with HF due to systolic dysfunction have a significant abnormality on ECG. A normal ECG makes systolic dysfunction extremely unlikely.

N. Echocardiography should be performed in all patients with new onset HF and can provide information about ventricular size and function. The following findings can be detected:

1. Regional wall motion abnormalities are compatible with coronary heart disease.
2. Pericardial thickening in constrictive pericarditis.
3. Mitral or aortic valve disease, as well as interatrial and interventricular shunts.
4. Abnormal myocardial texture in infiltrative cardiomyopathies.
5. Right ventricular size and function in right HF.
6. Estimation of pulmonary artery wedge pressure.
7. Right atrial and pulmonary artery pressures can be used to assess left ventricular filling pressures.
8. Cardiac output can be measured.
9. Echocardiography, especially with the use of dobutamine, is also useful in predicting recovery of cardiac function.
10. Echocardiography should be performed in all patients with new onset HF. Echocardiography has a high sensitivity and specificity for the diagnosis of myocardial dysfunction, and may determine the etiology of HF.

O. Detection of coronary heart disease

1. Heart failure resulting from coronary disease is usually irreversible due to myocardial infarction and ventricular remodeling. However, revascularization may be of benefit in the appreciable number of patients with hibernating myocardium.
2. Exercise testing should be part of the initial evaluation of any patient with HF.
3. With severe heart failure, measurement of the maximal oxygen uptake (VO_2max) provides an objective estimate of the severity of the myocardial dysfunction. VO_2max is one of the best indices of prognosis in patients with symptomatic HF and can aid in the determination of the necessity and timing of cardiac transplantation.
4. **Coronary arteriography**
   a. **Recommendations for coronary arteriography**: Coronary arteriography should be performed in patients with angina and in patients with known or suspected coronary artery disease who do not have angina.
   b. Patients with unexplained HF should be evaluated for coronary heart disease. If the exercise test is normal and HF is unexplained, cardiac catheterization should be strongly considered.

Laboratory Workup for Suspected Heart Failure

Blood urea nitrogen	Thyroid-stimulating hormone
Cardiac enzymes (CK-MB, troponin)	Urinalysis
Complete blood cell count	Echocardiogram
Creatinine	Electrocardiography
Electrolytes	Atrial natriuretic peptide (ANP)
Liver function tests	Brain natriuretic peptide (BNP)
Magnesium	

V. Treatment of heart failure due to systolic dysfunction

A. Treatment of the underlying cardiac disease

1. **Hypertension** is the primary cause of HF in many patients. Angiotensin converting enzyme (ACE) inhibitors, beta blockers, and angiotensin II receptor blockers (ARBs) are the preferred antihypertensive agents because they improve survival in HF. Beta blockers can also

provide anginal relief in ischemic heart disease and rate control in with atrial fibrillation.

2. **Renovascular disease.** Testing for renovascular disease is indicated if there is severe or refractory hypertension, a sudden rise in blood pressure, or repeated episodes of flash pulmonary edema.

3. **Ischemic heart disease.** Coronary atherosclerosis is the most common cause of cardiomyopathy, comprising 50 to 75 percent of patients with HF.

   a. All patients with documented ischemic heart disease should be treated medically for relief of angina and with risk factor reduction, such as control of serum lipids.

   b. Myocardial revascularization with angioplasty or bypass surgery may improve exercise capacity and prognosis in patients with hibernating myocardium. Revascularization should also be considered for repeated episodes of acute left ventricular dysfunction and flash pulmonary edema.

4. **Valvular disease** is the primary cause of HF 10 to 12 percent.

5. **Other causes of heart failure:** Alcohol abuse, cocaine abuse, obstructive sleep apnea, nutritional deficiencies, myocarditis, hemochromatosis, sarcoidosis, thyroid disease, and rheumatologic disorders such as systemic lupus erythematosus.

B. **Pharmacologic therapy of heart failure**

1. **Improvement in symptoms** can be achieved by digoxin, diuretics, beta blockers, ACE inhibitors, and angiotensin II receptor blockers (ARBs).

2. **Prolongation of survival** has been documented with ACE inhibitors, beta blockers, ARBs, hydralazine/nitrates, and spironolactone and eplerenone.

3. **Order of therapy:**

   a. **Loop diuretics** are used first for fluid control in overt HF. The goal is relief of dyspnea and peripheral edema.

   b. **ACE inhibitors,** or if not tolerated, angiotensin II receptor blockers (ARBs) are initiated during or after the optimization of diuretic therapy. These drugs are usually started at low doses and then titrated.

   c. **Beta blockers** are initiated after the patient is stable on ACE inhibitors, beginning at low doses with titration to goals.

   d. **Digoxin** is initiated in patients who continue to have symptoms of HF despite the above regimen; and, in atrial fibrillation, digoxin may be used for rate control.

   e. An ARB, aldosterone antagonist, or, particularly in black patients, the combination of hydralazine and a nitrate may be added in patients who are persistently symptomatic.

C. **ACE inhibitors and beta blockers.** Begin with a low dose of an ACE inhibitor (eg, lisinopril 5 mg/day), increase to a moderate dose (eg, lisinopril 15 to 20 mg/day) at one to two week intervals, and then begin a beta blocker, gradually increasing toward the target dose or the highest tolerated dose. When the beta blocker titration is completed, the ACE inhibitor titration is completed.

1. All patients with asymptomatic or symptomatic left ventricular dysfunction should be started on an ACE inhibitor. Beginning therapy with low doses (eg, 2.5 mg of enalapril (Vasotec) twice daily, 6.25 mg of captopril (Capotin) three times daily, or 5 mg of lisinopril (Prinivil) once daily) will reduce the likelihood of hypotension and azotemia.

2. If initial therapy is tolerated, the dose is then gradually increased at one to two week intervals to a target dose of 20 mg twice daily of enalapril, 50 mg three times daily of captopril, or up to 40 mg/day of lisinopril or quinapril. Plasma potassium and creatinine should be assessed one to two weeks after starting or changing a dose and periodically.

3. An ARB should be administered in patients who cannot tolerate ACE inhibitors. An ARB should be added to HF therapy in patients who are still symptomatic on ACE inhibitors and beta blockers or are hypertensive. In patients with renal dysfunction or hyperkalemia, the addition of an ARB must be done with caution. An ARB should not be added to an ACE inhibitor in the immediate post-MI setting.

D. **Beta blockers.** Carvedilol, metoprolol, and bisoprolol, improve survival in patients with New York Heart Association (NYHA) class II to III HF and probably in class IV HF. Beta blockers with intrinsic sympathomimetic activity (such as pindolol and acebutolol) should be avoided.

1. Carvedilol (Coreg), metoprolol (Toprol-XL), or bisoprolol (Ziac) is recommended for all patients with symptomatic HF, unless contraindicated. Relative contraindications to beta blocker therapy in patients with HF include:
   a. Heart rate <60 bpm
   b. Symptomatic hypotension
   c. Signs of peripheral hypoperfusion
   d. PR interval >0.24 sec
   e. Second- or third-degree atrioventricular block
   f. Severe chronic obstructive pulmonary disease
   g. Asthma

2. **Choice of agent.** Metoprolol has a high degree of specificity for the beta-1 adrenergic receptor, while carvedilol blocks beta-1, beta-2, and alpha-1 adrenergic receptors. Patients with low blood pressure may tolerate metoprolol better than carvedilol. Those with high blood pressure may have a greater lowering of blood pressure with carvedilol.

3. **Initiation of therapy.** Prior to initiation of therapy, the patient should have no fluid retention and should not have required recent intravenous inotropic therapy. Therapy should be begun at very low doses and the dose doubled every two weeks until the target dose is reached or symptoms become limiting. Initial and target doses are:
   a. **Carvedilol (Coreg),** 3.125 mg BID initially and 25 to 50 mg BID ultimately (the higher dose being used in subjects over 85 kg)
   b. **Extended-release metoprolol (Toprol-XL),** 12.5 mg daily in patients with NYHA class III or IV or 25 mg daily in patients with NYHA II, and ultimately 200 mg/day. If patients receive short acting metoprolol for cost reasons, the dosage is 6.25 mg BID initially and 50 to 100 mg BID ultimately.
   c. **Bisoprolol (Ziac),** 1.25 mg QD initially and 5 to 10 mg QD ultimately.

E. The patient should weigh himself daily and call the physician if there has been a 1 to 1.5 kg weight gain. Weight gain may be treated with diuretics.

F. **Digoxin** is given to patients with HF and systolic dysfunction to control symptoms and, in atrial fibrillation, to control the ventricular rate. Digoxin therapy is associated with a significant reduction in hospitalization for HF but no benefit in overall mortality.

1. Digoxin should be started in patients with left ventricular systolic dysfunction (left ventricular ejection fraction [LVEF] <40 percent) who continue to have NYHA functional class II, III, and IV symptoms despite therapy including an ACE inhibitor, beta blocker, and a diuretic. The usual daily dose is 0.125 mg or less, based upon renal function. The serum digoxin concentration should be maintained between 0.5 and 0.8 ng/mL.

G. **Diuretics**

1. A loop diuretic should be given to control pulmonary and/or peripheral edema. The most commonly used loop diuretic for the treatment of HF is furosemide, but some patients respond better to bumetanide or torsemide because of superior absorption.

    2. The usual starting dose is 20 to 40 mg of furosemide. In patients who are volume overloaded, a reasonable goal is weight reduction of 1.0 kg/day.

  H. Aldosterone antagonists. Spironolactone and eplerenone, which compete with aldosterone for the mineralocorticoid receptor, prolong survival in selected patients with HF.

    1. Treatment should begin with spironolactone (Aldactone, 25 to 50 mg/day), and switched to eplerenone (Inspra, 25 and after four weeks 50 mg/day) if endocrine side effects occur.

    2. Serum potassium and creatinine should be checked one to two weeks after starting spironolactone or eplerenone and periodically thereafter. Patients with poor renal function are at risk for hyperkalemia.

Treatment Classification of Patients with Heart Failure Caused by Left Ventricular Systolic Dysfunction

Symptoms	Pharmacology
Asymptomatic	ACE inhibitor or angiotensin-receptor blocker Beta blocker
Symptomatic	ACE inhibitor or angiotensin-receptor blocker Beta blocker Diuretic If symptoms persist: digoxin (Lanoxin)
Symptomatic with recent history of dyspnea at rest	Diuretic ACE inhibitor or angiotensin-receptor blocker Spironolactone (Aldactone) Beta blocker Digoxin
Symptomatic with dyspnea at rest	Diuretic ACE inhibitor or angiotensin-receptor blocker Spironolactone (Aldactone) Digoxin

Dosages of Primary Drugs Used in the Treatment of Heart Failure

Drug	Starting Dosage	Target Dosage
Drugs that decrease mortality and improve symptoms		
ACE inhibitors		
Captopril (Capoten)	6.25 mg three times daily (one-half tablet)	12.5 to 50 mg three times daily
Enalapril (Vasotec)	2.5 mg twice daily	10 mg twice daily
Lisinopril (Zestril)	5 mg daily	10 to 20 mg daily
Ramipril (Altace)	1.25 mg twice daily	5 mg twice daily
Trandolapril (Mavik)	1 mg daily	4 mg daily
Angiotensin-Receptor Blockers (ARBs)		
Candesartan (Atacand)	4 mg bid	16 mg bid
Irbesartan (Avapro)	75 mg qd	300 mg qd
Losartan (Cozaar)	12.5 mg bid	50 mg bid
Valsartan (Diovan)	40 mg bid	160 mg bid

Drug	Starting Dosage	Target Dosage
Telmisartan (Micardis)	20 mg qd	80 mg qd
Aldosterone antagonists		
Spironolactone (Aldactone)	25 mg daily	25 mg daily
Eplerenone (Inspra)	25 mg daily	25 mg daily
Beta blockers		
Bisoprolol (Zebeta)	1.25 mg daily (one-fourth tablet)	10 mg daily
Carvedilol (Coreg)	3.125 mg twice daily	25 to 50 mg twice daily
Metoprolol tartrate (Lopressor)	12.5 mg twice daily (one-fourth tablet)	50 to 75 mg twice daily
Metoprolol succinate (Toprol-XL)	12.5 mg daily (one-half tablet)	200 mg daily
Drugs that treat symptoms		
Thiazide diuretics		
Hydrochlorothiazide (Esidrex)	25 mg daily	25 to 100 mg daily
Metolazone (Zaroxolyn)	2.5 mg daily	2.5 to 10 mg daily
Loop diuretics		
Bumetanide (Bumex)	1 mg daily	1 to 10 mg once to three times daily
Ethacrynic acid (Edecrin)	25 mg daily	25 to 200 mg once or twice daily
Furosemide (Lasix)	40mg daily	40 to 400 mg once to three times daily
Torsemide (Demadex)	20 mg daily	20 to 200 mg once or twice daily
Inotrope		
Digoxin (Lanoxin)	0.125 mg daily	0.125 to 0.375 mg daily

VI. Lifestyle modification
- **A.** Cessation of smoking.
- **B.** Restriction of alcohol consumption.
- **C.** Salt restriction to 2 to 3 g (or less) of sodium per day to minimize fluid accumulation.
- **D.** Daily weight monitoring to detect fluid accumulation before it becomes symptomatic.
- **E.** Weight reduction in obese subjects with a goal of being within 10 percent of ideal body weight.
- **F.** A cardiac rehabilitation program for all stable patients.

References: See page 294.

Hypertension

The prevalence of hypertension (systolic >140 and/or diastolic >90 mm Hg) is 32 percent in the non-Hispanic black population and 23 percent in the non-Hispanic white and Mexican-American populations.

I. Definitions. The following definitions have been suggested by the seventh report of the Joint National Committee (JNC 7). Based upon the average of two or more readings at each of two or more visits after an initial screen, the following classification is used.

  A. The prehypertension category recognizes that the correlation between the risk of adverse outcomes (including stroke and death) and blood pressure level is a continuous variable in which there is an increased incidence of poor outcomes as the blood pressure rises, even within the previously delineated "normal" range.

II. Etiology/risk factors

  A. Essential hypertension has been associated with a number of risk factors:

    1. Hypertension is about twice as common in subjects who have one or two hypertensive parents.

    2. Increased salt intake is a necessary but not a sufficient cause for hypertension.

    3. There is a clear association between excess alcohol intake and hypertension.

    4. Obesity and weight gain appears to be a main determinant of the rise in blood pressure (BP).

  B. Secondary hypertension

    1. Primary renal disease. Hypertension is a frequent finding in renal disease, particularly with glomerular or vascular disorders.

    2. Oral contraceptives can induce hypertension.

    3. Pheochromocytoma. About one-half of patients with pheochromocytoma have paroxysmal hypertension, most of the rest have what appears to be essential hypertension.

Classification and Management of Blood Pressure for Adults Aged 18 Years or Older					
				Initial drug therapy	
BP classi-fication	Systolic BP	Diastolic BP	Lifestyle Modifi-cation	Without com-pelling indi-cation	With compel-ling indica-tions
Normal	<120 and	<80	Encour-age		
Prehyper-tension	120-139 or	80-89	Yes	No antihyper-tensive drug indicated	Drug(s) for the compelling indi-cations
Stage 1 hyperten-sion	140-159 or	90-99	Yes	Thiazide-type diuretics for most, may consider ACE inhibitor, ARB, beta blocker, CCB, or com-bination	Drug(s) for the compelling indi-cations Other anti-hypertensive drugs (diuretics, ACE inhibitor, ARB, beta blocker, CCB) as needed
Stage 2 hyperten-sion	$\geq$160 or	$\geq$100	Yes	2-drug combi-nation for most (usually thiazide-type diuretic and ACE inhibitor or ARB or beta blocker, CCB)	Drug(s) for the compelling indi-cations Other anti-hypertensive drugs (diuretics, ACE inhibitor, ARB, beta blocker, CCB) as needed

4. **Primary hyperaldosteronism.** The presence of primary mineralo-corticoid excess, primarily aldosterone, should be suspected in any patient with the triad of hypertension, unexplained hypokalemia and metabolic alkalosis. Some patients have a normal plasma potassium concentration.
5. **Cushing's syndrome.** Moderate diastolic hypertension is a major cause of morbidity and death in patients with Cushing's syndrome.
6. **Other endocrine disorders.** Hypertension may be induced by hypothyroidism, hyperthyroidism, and hyperparathyroidism.
7. **Sleep apnea syndrome.** Disordered breathing during sleep is an independent risk factor for awake systemic hypertension.
8. **Coarctation of the aorta** is one of the major causes of hypertension in young children.

III. **Complications of hypertension**
   A. Hypertension is the major risk factor for premature cardiovascular dis-ease, being more common than cigarette smoking, dyslipidemia, and diabetes, the other major risk factors.
   B. Hypertension increases the risk of heart failure.
   C. Left ventricular hypertrophy is a common problem in patients with hyper-tension, and is associated with an enhanced incidence of heart failure, ventricular arrhythmias, death following myocardial infarction, and sudden cardiac death.
   D. Hypertension is the most common and most important risk factor for stroke.

     E. Hypertension is the most important risk factor for intracerebral hemor-
rhage.

     F. Hypertension is a risk factor for chronic renal insufficiency.

IV. **Diagnosis**

     A. Blood pressure should be measured at each office visit for patients over
the age of 21.

     B. In the absence of end-organ damage, the diagnosis of mild hypertension
should not be made until the blood pressure has been measured on at
least three to six visits, spaced over a period of weeks to months.

     C. **White-coat hypertension and ambulatory monitoring.** 20 to 25 percent
of patients with mild office hypertension (diastolic pressure 90 to 104 mm
Hg) have "white-coat" or isolated office hypertension in that their blood
pressure is repeatedly normal when measured at home, at work, or by
ambulatory blood pressure monitoring. Ambulatory monitoring can be
used to confirm the presence of white-coat hypertension.

V. **Evaluation**

     A. **History.** The history should search for the presence of precipitating or
aggravating factors, the natural course of the blood pressure, the extent
of target organ damage, and the presence of other risk factors for cardiovascular disease.

     B. **Physical examination** should evaluate for signs of end-organ damage
(such as retinopathy) and for evidence of a cause of secondary hypertension.

     C. **Laboratory testing**

          1. Hematocrit, urinalysis, and routine blood chemistries (glucose,
creatinine, electrolytes).

          2. Fasting (9 to 12 hours) lipid profile (total and HDL-cholesterol, triglycer-
ides).

          3. Electrocardiogram.

History in the Patient with Hypertension

Duration of hypertension
  Last known normal blood pressure
  Course of the blood pressure
Prior treatment of hypertension
  Drugs: doses, side effects
Intake of agents that may cause hy-
pertension
  Estrogens, sympathomimetics, adre-
  nal steroids, excessive sodium
Family history
  Hypertension
  Premature cardiovascular disease or
  death
  Familial diseases:
  pheochromocytoma, renal disease,
  diabetes, gout
Symptoms of secondary cause
  Muscle weakness
  Spells of tachycardia, sweating,
  tremor
  Thinning of the skin
  Flank pain
	Symptoms of target organ damage
	  Headaches
	  Transient weakness or blindness
	  Loss of visual acuity
	  Chest pain
	  Dyspnea
	  Claudication
	Other risk factors
	  Smoking
	  Diabetes
	  Dyslipidemias
	  Physical inactivity
	Dietary history
	  Sodium
	  Alcohol
	  Saturated fats

Physical Examination in the Patient with Hypertension

Accurate measurement of blood pressure
General appearance: distribution of body fat, skin lesions, muscle strength, alertness
Funduscope
Neck: palpation and auscultation of carotids, thyroid
Heart: size, rhythm, sounds Lungs: rhonchi, rales
Abdomen: renal masses, bruits over aorta or renal arteries, femoral pulses
Extremities: peripheral pulses, edema
Neurologic assessment

D. **Testing for renovascular hypertension.** Renovascular hypertension is
   the most common correctable cause of secondary hypertension. It occurs
   in less than one percent of patients with mild hypertension. In comparison, between 10 and 45 percent of white patients with severe or malignant hypertension have renal artery stenosis.
   1. Signs suggesting renovascular hypertension or other cause of second-
      ary hypertension:
      a. Severe or refractory hypertension, including retinal hemorrhages or
         papilledema; bilateral renovascular disease may be present in
         patients who also have a plasma creatinine above 1.5 mg/dL (132
         µmol/L).
      b. An acute rise in blood pressure over a previously stable baseline.
      c. Age of onset before puberty or above 50.
      d. An acute elevation in the plasma creatinine concentration that is
         either unexplained or occurs after the institution of an angiotensin
         converting enzyme inhibitor or angiotensin II receptor blocker (in the
         absence of an excessive reduction in blood pressure).
      e. Moderate-to-severe hypertension in a patient with diffuse athero-
         sclerosis or an incidentally discovered asymmetry in renal disease.
         A unilateral small kidney (<9 cm) has a 75 percent correlation with
         the presence of large vessel occlusive disease.
      f. A systolic-diastolic abdominal bruit that lateralizes to one side.
      g. Negative family history for hypertension.
      h. Moderate-to-severe hypertension in patients with recurrent epi-
         sodes of acute (flash) pulmonary edema or otherwise unexplained
         congestive heart failure.
   2. Spiral CT scanning or 3D time-of-flight MR angiography are minimally
      invasive diagnostic methods. Duplex Doppler ultrasonography may be
      useful both for diagnosis and for predicting the outcome of therapy.
E. **Testing for other causes of secondary hypertension**
   1. The presence of primary renal disease is suggested by an elevated
      plasma creatinine concentration and/or an abnormal urinalysis.
   2. **Pheochromocytoma** should be suspected if there are paroxysmal
      elevations in blood pressure, particularly if associated with the triad of
      headache (usually pounding), palpitations, and sweating.
   3. **Plasma renin activity** is usually performed only in patients with
      possible low-renin forms of hypertension, such as primary
      hyperaldosteronism. Otherwise unexplained hypokalemia is the
      primary clinical clue to the latter disorder in which the plasma
      aldosterone to plasma renin activity ratio is a screening test.
   4. **Cushing's syndrome** (including that due to corticosteroid administra-
      tion) is usually suggested by cushingoid facies, central obesity,
      ecchymoses, and muscle weakness.
   5. **Sleep apnea syndrome** should be suspected in obese individuals
      who snore loudly while asleep, awake with headache, and fall asleep
      inappropriately during the day.
   6. Coarctation of the aorta is characterized by decreased or lagging
      peripheral pulses and a vascular bruit over the back.

7. Hypertension may be induced by both hypothyroidism and primary hyperparathyroidism, suspected because of hypercalcemia.

Evaluation of Secondary Hypertension	
Renovascular Hypertension	Captopril test: Plasma renin level before and 1 hr after captopril 25 mg. A greater than 150% increase in renin is positive Captopril renography: Renal scan before and after 25 mg MRI angiography Arteriography (DSA)
Hyperaldosteronism	Serum potassium Serum aldosterone and plasma renin activity CT scan of adrenals
Pheochromocytoma	24 hr urine catecholamines CT scan Nuclear MIBG scan
Cushing's Syndrome	Plasma cortisol Dexamethasone suppression test
Hyperparathyroidism	Serum calcium Serum parathyroid hormone

VI. Treatment of essential hypertension

A. **Benefits of blood pressure control.** Antihypertensive therapy is associated with 35 to 40 percent reduction in stroke incidence; 20 to 25 percent in myocardial infarction; and more than 50 percent in heart failure. Optimal control to below 130/80 mm Hg could prevent 37 and 56 percent of coronary heart disease events.

B. **All patients should undergo lifestyle modification.** A patient should not be labeled as having hypertension unless the blood pressure is persistently elevated after three to six visits over a several-month period.

Lifestyle Modifications in the Management of Hypertension		
Modification	**Recommendation**	**Approximate systolic BP reduction, range***
Weight reduction	Maintain normal body weight (BMI), 18.5 to 24.9 kg/m^2	5 to 20 mm Hg per 10-kg weight loss
DASH eating plan	Consume a diet rich in fruits, vegetables, and low-fat dairy products, with a reduced content of saturated and total fat	8 to 14 mm Hg
Dietary sodium reduction	Reduce dietary sodium intake to no more than 100 meq/day (2.4 sodium or 6 g sodium chloride)	2 to 8 mm Hg

Modification	Recommendation	Approximate systolic BP reduction, range*
Physical activity	Regular aerobic physical activity, such as brisk walking (at least 30 minutes per day, most days of the week)	4 to 9 mm Hg
Moderate consumption of alcohol consumption	Limit consumption to no more than 2 drinks per day in most men and no more than 1 drink per day in women	2 to 4 mm Hg

C. Antihypertensive medications should be begun if the systolic pressure is persistently ≥140 mm Hg and/or the diastolic pressure is persistently ≥90 mm Hg in the office and at home despite attempted nonpharmacologic therapy. Starting with two drugs may be considered in patients with a baseline blood pressure more than 20/10 mm Hg above goal.

D. In patients with diabetes or chronic renal failure, antihypertensive therapy is indicated when the systolic pressure is persistently above 130 mm Hg and/or the diastolic pressure is above 80 mm Hg.

E. Patients with office hypertension, normal values at home, and no evidence of end-organ damage should undergo ambulatory blood pressure monitoring.

F. **Lifestyle modifications**
   1. Treatment of hypertension generally begins with nonpharmacologic therapy, including dietary sodium restriction, weight reduction in the obese, avoidance of excess alcohol, and regular aerobic exercise.
   2. A low-sodium diet will usually lower high blood pressure and may prevent the onset of hypertension. The overall impact of moderate sodium reduction is a fall in blood pressure of 4.8/2.5 mm Hg. Dietary intake should be reduced to 2.3 g of sodium or 6 g of salt.
   3. Weight loss in obese individuals can lead to a significant fall in blood pressure.
   4. **Goal blood pressure**
      a. The goal of antihypertensive therapy in patients with uncomplicated combined systolic and diastolic hypertension is a blood pressure of below 140/90 mm Hg.
      b. For individuals over age 65 with isolated systolic hypertension (eg, a diastolic blood pressure below 90 mm Hg), caution is needed not to inadvertently lower the diastolic blood pressure to below 65 mm Hg to attain a goal systolic pressure <140 mm Hg, since this level of diastolic pressure has been associated with an increased risk of stroke.
      c. A goal blood pressure of less than 130/80 mm Hg is recommended in patients with diabetes mellitus; and patients with slowly progressive chronic renal failure, particularly those excreting more than 1 g of protein per day.

VII. **Drug therapy in essential hypertension**
   A. Each of the antihypertensive agents is roughly equally effective, producing a good antihypertensive response in 30 to 50 percent of cases.
   B. A thiazide diuretic is recommended as initial drug therapy in most patients. African American patients generally responding better to monotherapy with a thiazide diuretic or calcium channel blocker and relatively poorly to an ACE inhibitor or beta-blocker.

C. **Initial therapy**
   1. The seventh Joint National Committee (JNC 7) report recommends initiating therapy in uncomplicated hypertensives with a thiazide diuretic (eg, 12.5 to 25 mg of hydrochlorothiazide or chlorthalidone). This regimen is associated with a low rate of metabolic complications, such as hypokalemia, glucose intolerance, and hyperuricemia.
   2. If low-dose thiazide monotherapy fails to attain goal blood pressure in uncomplicated hypertensives, an ACE inhibitor/ARB, beta-blocker, or calcium channel blocker can be sequentially added or substituted. Most often an ACE inhibitor/ARB, which acts synergistically with a diuretic, is used.

Considerations for Individualizing Antihypertensive Therapy	
Indication	**Antihypertensive drugs**
Compelling indications (major improvement in outcome independent of blood pressure)	
Systolic heart failure	ACE inhibitor or ARB, beta blocker, diuretic, aldosterone antagonist
Post-myocardial infarction	beta blocker, ACE inhibitor, aldosterone antagonist
Proteinuric chronic renal failure	ACE inhibitor and/or ARB
High coronary disease risk	Diuretic, perhaps ACE inhibitor
Diabetes mellitus (no proteinuria)	Diuretic, perhaps ACE inhibitor
Angina pectoris	Beta blocker, calcium channel blocker
Atrial fibrillation rate control	Beta blocker, nondihydropyridine calcium channel blocker
Atrial flutter rate control	Beta blocker, nondihydropyridine calcium channel blocker
Likely to have a favorable effect on symptoms in comorbid conditions	
Essential tremor	Beta blocker (noncardioselective)
Hyperthyroidism	Beta blocker
Migraine	Beta blocker, calcium channel blocker
Osteoporosis	Thiazide diuretic
Raynaud's syndrome	Dihydropyridine calcium channel blocker

Contraindications to Specific Antihypertensive Agents	
Indication	Antihypertensive drugs
Bronchospastic disease	Beta blocker
Pregnancy	ACE inhibitor, ARB (includes women likely to become pregnant)
Second or third degree heart block	Beta blocker, nondihydropyridine calcium channel blocker
May have adverse effect on comorbid conditions	
Depression	Beta blocker, central alpha agonist
Gout	Diuretic
Hyperkalemia	Aldosterone antagonist, ACE inhibitor, ARB
Hyponatremia	Thiazide diuretic
Renovascular disease	ACE inhibitor or ARB

D. Diuretics
1. A low-dose thiazide diuretic provides better cardioprotection than an ACE inhibitor or a calcium channel blocker in patients with risk factors for coronary artery disease, including left ventricular hypertrophy, type 2 diabetes, previous myocardial infarction or stroke, current cigarette smoking habits, hyperlipidemia, or atherosclerotic cardiovascular disease.
2. Diuretics should also be given for fluid control in patients with heart failure or nephrotic syndrome; these settings usually require loop diuretics. In addition, an aldosterone antagonist is indicated in patients with advanced HF who have relatively preserved renal function and for the treatment of hypokalemia.

Thiazide Diuretics	
Drug	Usual dose
Hydrochlorothiazide (HCTZ, Hydrodiuril)	12.5-25 mg qd
Chlorthalidone (Hygroton)	12.5-25 mg qd
Chlorothiazide (Diuril)	125-500 mg qd
Indapamide (Lozol)	1.25 mg qd
Metolazone (Zaroxolyn)	1.25-5 mg qd

E. ACE inhibitors provide survival benefits in heart failure and myocardial infarction (particularly ST elevation) and renal benefits in proteinuric chronic renal failure. Thus, an ACE inhibitor should be used in heart failure, prior myocardial infarction, asymptomatic left ventricular dysfunction, type 1 diabetics with nephropathy, and nondiabetic proteinuric chronic renal failure. The use of ACE inhibitors in these settings is independent of the need for BP control.

Angiotensin-converting enzyme inhibitors		
Drug	Usual doses	Maximum dose
Benazepril (Lotensin)	10-40 mg qd or divided bid	80 mg/d
Captopril (Capoten)	50 mg bid-qid	450 mg/d
Enalapril (Vasotec, Vasotec IV)	10-40 mg qd or divided bid	40 mg/d
Fosinopril (Monopril)	20-40 mg qd or divided bid	80 mg/d
Lisinopril (Prinivil, Zestril)	20-40 mg qd	40 mg/d
Moexipril (Univasc)	15-30 mg qd	30 mg/d
Quinapril (Accupril)	20-80 mg qd or divided bid	80 mg/d
Ramipril (Altace)	5-20 mg qd or divided bid	20 mg/d
Trandolapril (Mavik)	1-4 mg qd	8 mg/d
Perindopril (Aceon)	4-8 mg qd-bid	8 mg/d

F. ARBs. The indications for and efficacy of ARBs are the same as those with ACE inhibitors. An ARB is particularly indicated in patients who do not tolerate ACE inhibitors (mostly because of cough).

Angiotensin II Receptor Blockers		
Drug	Usual dose	Maximum dose
Losartan (Cozaar)	50 mg qd	100 mg/d
Candesartan (Atacand)	4-8 mg qd	16 mg/d
Eprosartan (Teveten)	400-800 mg qd	800 mg/d
Irbesartan (Avapro)	150-300 mg qd	300 mg/d
Telmisartan (Micardis)	40-80 mg qd	80 mg/d
Valsartan (Diovan)	80 mg qd	320 mg/d

G. Beta-blockers. A beta-blocker without intrinsic sympathomimetic activity should be given after an acute myocardial infarction and to stable patients with heart failure or asymptomatic left ventricular dysfunction (beginning with very low doses). The use of beta-blockers in these settings is in addition to the recommendations for ACE inhibitors in these disorders.

Beta-blockers are also given for rate control in atrial fibrillation and for angina.

Beta-blockers		
Drug	Usual dose	Maximum dose
Acebutolol (Sectral)	200-800 mg/d (qd or bid)	1.2 g/d (bid)
Atenolol (Tenormin)	50-100 mg qd	100 mg qd
Betaxolol (Kerlone)	10 mg qd	20 mg qd
Bisoprolol (Zebeta)	5 mg qd	20 mg qd
Carteolol (Cartrol)	2.5 mg qd	10 mg qd
Carvedilol (Coreg)	6.26-25 mg bid	100 mg/d
Labetalol (Normodyne, Trandate)	100-600 mg bid	1200 mg/d
Metoprolol (Toprol XL)	100-200 mg qd	400 mg qd
Metoprolol (Lopressor)	100-200 mg/d (qd or bid)	450 mg/d (qd or bid)
Nadolol (Corgard)	40 mg qd	320 mg/d
Penbutolol(Levatol)	20 mg qd	NA
Pindolol (Visken)	5 mg bid	60 mg/d
Propranolol (Inderal, Inderal LA)	120-160 mg qd (LA 640 mg/d)	
Timolol (Blocadren)	10-20 mg bid	60 mg/d (bid)

H. Calcium channel blockers. Like beta-blockers, they can be given for rate control in patients with atrial fibrillation or for control of angina. Calcium channel blockers may be preferred in obstructive airways disease.

Calcium channel blockers	
Drug	Dosage
Diltiazem extended-release (Cardizem SR)	120-360 mg in 2 doses
Diltiazem CD (Cardizem CD)	120-360 mg in 1 dose
Diltiazem XR (Dilacor XR)	120-480 mg in 1 dose
Verapamil (Calan)	120-480 mg in 2 or 3 doses
Verapamil extended-release (Calan SR)	120-480 mg in 1 or 2 doses
Verapamil HS (Covera-HS)	180-480 mg in 1 dose

Drug	Dosage
Dihydropyridines	
Amlodipine (Norvasc)	2.5-10 mg in 1 dose
Felodipine (Plendil)	2.5-10 mg in 1 dose
Isradipine (DynaCirc)	5-10 mg in 2 doses
Isradipine extended-release (DynaCirc CR)	5-10 mg in 1 dose
Nicardipine (Cardene)	60-120 mg in 3 doses
Nicardipine extended-release (Cardene SR)	60-120 mg in 2 doses
Nifedipine extended-release (Adalat CC, Procardia XL)	30-90 mg in 1 dose
Nisoldipine (Sular)	10-60 mg in 1 dose

I. **Combination therapy**
  1. If two drugs are required, use of a low dose of a thiazide diuretic as one of the drugs increases the response rate to all other agents. By minimizing volume expansion, diuretics increase the antihypertensive effect of all other antihypertensive drugs.
  2. The combination of a thiazide diuretic with a beta-blocker, an ACE inhibitor, or an ARB has a synergistic effect, controlling the BP in up to 85 percent of patients.
  3. **Fixed-dose combination.** A wide variety of (low) dose combination preparations are available, including low doses of a diuretic with a beta-blocker, ACE inhibitor, or ARB. Combination preparations include:
    a. Sustained-release verapamil (180 mg) - trandolapril (2 mg).
    b. Atenolol (100 mg) - chlorthalidone (25 mg).
    c. Lisinopril (20 mg) - hydrochlorothiazide (12.5 mg).
    d. The three combinations were equally effective, normalizing the blood pressure or lowering the diastolic pressure by more than 10 mm Hg in 69 to 76 percent of patients. All are well tolerated.

Combination Agents for Hypertension		
Drug	**Initial dose**	**Comments**
Beta-Blocker/Diuretic		
Atenolol/chlorthalidone (Tenoretic)	50 mg/25 mg, 1 tab qd	Additive vasodilation
Bisoprolol/HCTZ (Ziac)	2.5 mg/6.25 mg, 1 tab qd	
Metoprolol/HCTZ (Lopressor HCTZ)	100 mg/25 mg, 1 tab qd	
Nadolol/HCTZ (Corzide)	40 mg/5 mg, 1 tab qd	
Propranolol/HCTZ (Inderide LA)	80 mg/50 mg, 1 tab qd	

Drug	Initial dose	Comments
Timolol/HCTZ (Timolide)	10 mg/25 mg, 1 tab qd	
ACE inhibitor/Diuretic		
Benazepril/HCTZ (Lotensin HCT)	5 mg/6.25 mg, 1 tab qd	ACE inhibitor conserves potassium and magnesium; combination beneficial for CHF patients with HTN
Captopril/HCTZ (Capozide)	25 mg/15 mg, 1 tab qd	
Enalapril/HCTZ (Vaseretic)	5 mg/12.5 mg, 1 tab qd	
Lisinopril/HCTZ (Zestoretic, Prinzide)	10 mg/12.5 mg, 1 tab qd	
Moexipril/HCTZ (Uniretic)	7.5 mg/12.5 mg, 1 tab qd	
ACE inhibitor/Calcium-channel blocker		
Benazepril/amlodipine (Lotrel)	2.5 mg/10 mg, 1 tab qd	
Enalapril/felodipine (Lexxel)	5 mg/5 mg, 1 tab qd	
Enalapril/diltiazem (Teczem)	5 mg/180 mg, 1 tab qd	
Trandolapril/verapamil (Tarka)	2 mg/180 mg, 1 tab qd	
Angiotensin II receptor blocker/Diuretic		
Losartan/HCTZ (Hyzaar)	50 mg/12.5 mg, 1 tab qd	
Valsartan/HCTZ (Diovan HCT)	80 mg/12.5 mg, 1 tab qd	
Alpha-1-Blocker/Diuretic		
Prazosin/polythiazide (Minizide)	1 mg/0.5 mg, 1 cap bid	Synergistic vasodilation
K$^+$-sparing diuretic/Thiazide		
Amiloride/HCTZ (Moduretic)	5 mg/50 mg, 1 tab qd	Electrolyte-sparing effect
Triamterene/HCTZ (Dyazide, Maxzide)	37.5 mg/25 mg, 1/2 tab qd	

References: See page 294.

Atrial Fibrillation

Atrial fibrillation (AF) is more prevalent in men and with increasing age. AF can have adverse consequences related to a reduction in cardiac output and to atrial thrombus formation that can lead to systemic embolization.

I. Classification
A. Atrial fibrillation occurs in the normal heart and in the presence of organic heart disease. Classification of Atrial fibrillation:
   1. **Paroxysmal (ie, self-terminating) AF** in which the episodes of AF generally last less than seven days (usually less than 24 hours) and may be recurrent.
   2. **Persistent AF** fails to self-terminate and lasts for longer than seven days. Persistent AF may also be paroxysmal if it recurs after reversion. AF is considered recurrent when the patient experiences two or more episodes.
   3. **Permanent AF** is considered to be present if the arrhythmia lasts for more than one year and cardioversion either has not been attempted or has failed.
   4. **"Lone" AF** describes paroxysmal, persistent, or permanent AF in individuals without structural heart disease.
B. If the AF is secondary to cardiac surgery, pericarditis, myocardial infarction (MI), hyperthyroidism, pulmonary embolism, pulmonary disease, or other reversible causes, therapy is directed toward the underlying disease as well as the AF.
C. Some of the causes not involving the heart include hyperthyroidism, alcohol use, pulmonary embolism, pneumonia. Most commonly, atrial fibrillation occurs as a result of some other cardiac condition (secondary atrial fibrillation), such as valvular heart disease, left ventricular hypertrophy, coronary artery disease, hypertension, cardiomyopathy, sick sinus syndrome, or pericarditis.

II. Clinical evaluation
A. **History and physical examination.** Associated symptoms with AF should be sought; the clinical type or "pattern" should be defined; the onset or date of discovery of the AF; the frequency and duration of AF episodes; any precipitating causes and modes of termination of AF; the response to drug therapy; and the presence of heart disease or potentially reversible causes (eg, hyperthyroidism).
B. The frequency and duration of AF episodes are determined from the history. Symptoms include palpitations, weakness, dizziness, and dyspnea. However, among patients with paroxysmal AF, up to 90% of episodes are not recognized by the patient.
C. **Electrocardiogram** is used to verify the presence of AF; identify left ventricular hypertrophy, pre-excitation, bundle branch block, or prior MI; define P-wave duration and morphology.
D. **Chest x-ray** is useful in assessing the lungs, vasculature, and cardiac outline.
E. **Transthoracic echocardiography** is required to evaluate the size of the right and left atria and the size and function of the right and left ventricles; to detect possible valvular heart disease, left ventricular hypertrophy, and pericardial disease; and to assess peak right ventricular pressure. It may also identify a left atrial thrombus, although the sensitivity is low. Transesophageal echocardiography is much more sensitive for atrial thrombi and can be used to determine the need for three to four weeks of anticoagulation prior to cardioversion.
F. **Assessment for hyperthyroidism.** A low-serum thyroid-stimulating hormone (TSH) value is found in 5.4% of patients with AF; only 1% have clinical hyperthyroidism. Measurement of serum TSH and free T4 is indicated in all patients with a first episode of AF, when the ventricular response to AF is difficult to control, or when AF recurs unexpectedly after cardioversion. Patients with low TSH values (<0.5 mU/L) and normal serum free T4 probably have subclinical hyperthyroidism.
G. Additional testing
   1. **Exercise testing** is often used to assess the adequacy of rate control in permanent AF, to reproduce exercise-induced AF, and to evaluate for ischemic heart disease.

2. **Holter monitoring** or event recorders are used to identify the arrhythmia if it is intermittent and not captured on routine electrocardiography.
3. **Electrophysiologic studies** may be required with wide QRS complex tachycardia or a possible predisposing arrhythmia, such as atrial flutter or a paroxysmal supraventricular tachycardia.

III. **General treatment issues**

Risk-based Approach to Antithrombotic Therapy in Atrial Fibrillation	
Patient features	**Antithrombotic therapy**
Age <60 years No heart disease (line AF)	Aspirin (325 mg per day) or no therapy
Age <60 years Hear disease by no risk factors*	Aspirin (325 mg per day)
Age ≥60 years No risk factors*	Aspirin (325 mg per day)
Age ≥60 years With diabetes mellitus or CAD	Oral anticoagulation (INR 2 to 3) Addition of aspirin, 81 to 162 mg/day is optional
Age ≥75 years, especially women	Oral anticoagulation (INR ≈ 2.0)
Heart failure (HF) LVEF ≤0.35 Thyrotoxicosis Hypertension	Oral anticoagulation (INR 2 to 3)
Rheumatic heart disease (mitral stenosis) Prosthetic heart valves Prior thromboembolism Persistent atrial thrombus on TEE	Oral anticoagulation (INR 2.5 to 3.5 or higher may be apropriate)
*Risk factors for thromboembolism include heart failure, left ventricular ejection fraction (LVEF) less than 0.35, and hypertension.	

A. Rate control with chronic anticoagulation is recommended for the majority of patients with AF.
B. Beta-blockers (eg, atenolol or metoprolol), diltiazem, and verapamil are recommended for rate control at both rest and exercise; digoxin is not effective during exercise and should be used in patients with heart failure or as a second-line agent.
C. Anticoagulation should be achieved with adjusted-dose warfarin unless the patient is considered at low embolic risk or has a contraindication. Aspirin may be used in such patients.
D. When rhythm control is chosen, both DC and pharmacologic cardioversion are appropriate options. To prevent dislodgment of pre-existing thrombi, warfarin therapy should be given for three to four weeks prior to cardioversion unless transesophageal echocardiography demonstrates no left atrial thrombi. Anticoagulation is continued for at least one month after cardioversion to prevent de novo thrombus formation.

E. After cardioversion, antiarrhythmic drugs to maintain sinus rhythm are not recommended, since the risks outweigh the benefits, except for patients with persistent symptoms during rate control that interfere with the patient's quality of life. Recommended drugs are amiodarone, disopyramide, propafenone, and sotalol.

IV. Rhythm control

A. Reversion to NSR. Patients with AF of more than 48 hours duration or unknown duration may have atrial thrombi that can embolize. In such patients, cardioversion should be delayed until the patient has been anticoagulated at appropriate levels for three to four weeks or transesophageal echocardiography has excluded atrial thrombi.

1. DC cardioversion is indicated in patients who are hemodynamically unstable. In stable patients in whom spontaneous reversion due to correction of an underlying disease is not likely, either DC or pharmacologic cardioversion can be performed. Electrical cardioversion is usually preferred because of greater efficacy and a low risk of proarrhythmia. The overall success rate of electrical cardioversion for AF is 75 to 93 percent and is related inversely both to the duration of AF and to left atrial size.

2. Antiarrhythmic drugs will convert 30 to 60 percent of patients.

3. Rate control with an atrioventricular (AV) nodal blocker (beta-blocker, diltiazem, or verapamil), or (if the patient has heart failure or hypotension) digoxin should be attained before instituting a class IA drug.

B. Maintenance of NSR. Only 20 to 30 percent of patients who are successfully cardioverted maintain NSR for more than one year without chronic antiarrhythmic therapy. This is more likely to occur in patients with AF for less than one year, no enlargement of the left atrium (ie, <4.0 cm), and a reversible cause of AF such as hyperthyroidism, pericarditis, pulmonary embolism, or cardiac surgery.

1. Prophylactic antiarrhythmic drug therapy is indicated only in patients who have a moderate-to-high risk for recurrence.

2. Evidence of efficacy is best for amiodarone, propafenone, disopyramide, sotalol, flecainide, and quinidine. Flecainide may be preferred in patients with no or minimal heart disease, while amiodarone is preferred in patients with a reduced left ventricular (LV) ejection fraction or heart failure and sotalol in patients with coronary heart disease. Concurrent administration of an AV nodal blocker is indicated in patients who have demonstrated a moderate-to-rapid ventricular response to AF.

3. Amiodarone is significantly more effective for maintenance of sinus rhythm than other antiarrhythmic drugs. Amiodarone should be used as first-line therapy in patients without heart failure.

V. Rate control in chronic AF. Rapid ventricular rate in patients with AF should be prevented because of hemodynamic instability and/or symptoms.

A. Rate control in AF is usually achieved by slowing AV nodal conduction with a beta-blocker, diltiazem, verapamil, or, in patients with heart failure or hypotension, digoxin. Amiodarone is also effective in patients who are not cardioverted to NSR.

B. Heart rate control include:

1. Rest heart rate ≤80 beats/min.

2. 24-hour Holter average ≤100 beats/min and no heart rate >110% of the age-predicted maximum.

3. Heart rate ≤110 beats/min in six minute walk.

C. Nonpharmacologic approaches. The medical approaches to either rate or rhythm control described above are not always effective.

1. **Rhythm control.** Alternative methods to maintain NSR in patients who are refractory to conventional therapy include surgery, radiofrequency catheter ablation, and pacemakers.

2. **Rate control.** Radio-frequency AV nodal-His bundle ablation with permanent pacemaker placement or AV nodal conduction modification are nonpharmacologic therapies for achieving rate control in patients who do not respond to pharmacologic therapy.

Intravenous Agents for Heart Rate Control in Atrial Fibrillation

Drug	Loading Dose	Onset	Maintenance Dose	Major Side Effects
Diltiazem	0.25 mg/kg IV over 2 min	2–7 min	5–15 mg per hour infusion	Hypotension, heart block, HF
Esmolol	0.5 mg/kg over 1 min	1 min	0.05–0.2 mg/kg/min	Hypotension, heart block, bradycardia, asthma, HF
Metoprolol	2.5–5 mg IV bolus over 2 min up to 3 doses	5 min	5 mg IV q6h	Hypotension, heart block, bradycardia, asthma, HF
Verapamil	0.075–0.15 mg/kg IV over 2 min	3–5 min	5-10 mg IV q6h	Hypotension, heart block, HF
Digoxin	0.25 mg IV q2h, up to 1.5 mg	2 h	0.125–0.25 mg daily	Digitalis toxicity, heart block, bradycardia

Oral Agents for Heart Rate Control

Drug	Loading Dose	Usual Maintenance Dose	Major Side Effects
Digoxin	0.25 mg PO q2h up to 1.5 mg	0.125–0.375 mg daily	Digitalis toxicity, heart block, bradycardia
Diltiazem Extended Release	NA	120–360 mg daily	Hypotension, heart block, HF
Metoprolol	NA	25–100 mg BID	Hypotension, heart block, bradycardia, asthma, HF
Propranolol Extended Release	NA	80–240 mg daily	Hypotension, heart block, bradycardia, asthma, HF
Verapamil Extended Release	NA	120–360 mg daily	Hypotension, heart block, HF, digoxin interaction

Drug	Loading Dose	Usual Mainte-nance Dose	Major Side Effects
Amiodarone	800 mg daily for 1 wk 600 mg daily for 1 wk 400 mg daily for 4–6 wk	200 mg daily	Pulmonary toxicity, skin discoloration, hypo or hyperthyroidism, corneal deposits, optic neuropathy, warfarin interaction, proarrhythmia (QT prolongation)

VI. Prevention of systemic embolization

A. Anticoagulation during restoration of NSR

1. **AF for more than 48 hours or unknown duration.** Outpatients without a contraindication to warfarin who have been in AF for more than 48 hours should receive three to four weeks of warfarin prior to and after cardioversion. This approach is also recommended for patients with AF who have valvular disease, evidence of left ventricular dysfunction, recent thromboembolism, or when AF is of unknown duration, as in an asymptomatic patient.
   a. The recommended target INR is 2.5 (range 2.0 to 3.0). The INR should be ≥2.0 in the weeks before cardioversion.
   b. An alternative approach that eliminates the need for prolonged anticoagulation prior to cardioversion is the use of transesophageal echocardiography-guided cardioversion.
   c. Thus, the long-term recommendations for patients who have been cardioverted to NSR but are at high risk for thromboembolism are similar to those in patients with chronic AF, even though the patients are in sinus rhythm.

2. **Atrial fibrillation for less than 48 hours.** A different approach with respect to anticoagulation can be used in low-risk patients (no mitral valve disease, severe left ventricular dysfunction, or history of recent thromboembolism) in whom there is reasonable certainty that AF has been present for less than 48 hours. Such patients have a low risk of clinical thromboembolism if converted early (0.8%), even without a screening TEE.

3. Long-term anticoagulation prior to cardioversion is not recommended in such patients, but heparin use is recommended at presentation and during the pericardioversion period.

Antithrombotic Therapy in Cardioversion for Atrial Fibrillation	
Timing of cardioversion	**Anticoagulation**
Early cardioversion in patients with atrial fibrillation for less than 48 hours	Heparin during cardioversion period to achieve PTT of 50-70 seconds. Heparin 70 U/kg load, 15 U/kg/hr drip.
Early cardioversion in patients with atrial fibrillation for more than 48 hours or an unknown duration, but with documented absence of atrial thrombi	Heparin during cardioversion period to achieve PTT of 50-70 seconds. Warfarin (Coumadin) for 4 weeks after cardioversion to achieve target INR of 2.0 to 3.0.
Elective cardioversion in patients with atrial fibrillation for more than 48 hours or an unknown duration	Warfarin for 3 weeks before and 4 weeks after cardioversion to achieve target INR of of 2.0 to 3.0.

4. Current practice is to administer aspirin for a first episode of AF that converts spontaneously and warfarin for at least four weeks to all other patients.

5. Aspirin should not be considered in patients with AF of less than 48 hours duration if there is associated rheumatic mitral valve disease, severe left ventricular dysfunction, or recent thromboembolism. Such patients should be treated the same as patients with AF of longer duration: one month of oral anticoagulation with warfarin or shorter-term anticoagulation with screening TEE prior to elective electrical or pharmacologic cardioversion followed by prolonged warfarin therapy after cardioversion.

B. **Anticoagulation in chronic AF**

1. The incidence of stroke associated with AF is 3 to 5 percent per year in the absence of anticoagulation; compared with the general population, AF significantly increases the risk of stroke (relative risk 2.4 in men and 3.0 in women).

2. The incidence of stroke is relatively low in patients with AF who are under age 65 and have no risk factors. The prevalence of stroke associated with AF increases strikingly with age and with other risk factors including diabetes, hypertension, previous stroke as clinical risk factors, and left ventricular dysfunction.

3. **Choice of antiembolism therapy**

   a. Patients with a CHADS2 score of 0 are at low risk of embolization (0.5% per year) and can be managed with aspirin.

   b. Patients with a CHADS2 score ≥ 3 are at high risk (5.3 to 6.9 percent per year) and should, in the absence of a contraindication, be treated with warfarin.

   c. Patients with a CHADS2 score of 1 or 2 are at intermediate risk of embolization (1.5 to 2.5 percent per year). In this group, the choice between warfarin therapy and aspirin will depend upon many factors, including patient preference.

4. An INR between 2.0 and 3.0 is recommended for most patients with AF who receive warfarin therapy. A higher goal (INR between 2.5 and 3.5) is reasonable for patients at particularly high risk for embolization (eg, prior thromboembolism, rheumatic heart disease, prosthetic heart valves). An exception to the latter recommendation occurs in patients over the age of 75 who are at increased risk for major bleeding. A target INR of 1.8 to 2.5 is recommended for this age group.

C. **Anticoagulation in paroxysmal AF.** The stroke risk appears to be equivalent in paroxysmal and chronic AF. The factors governing the choice between warfarin and aspirin therapy and the intensity of warfarin therapy are similar to patients with chronic AF.

VII. **Presentation and management of recent onset AF**

A. **Indications for hospitalization**

1. For the treatment of an associated medical problem, which is often the reason for the arrhythmia.

2. For elderly patients who are more safely treated for AF in hospital.

3. For patients with underlying heart disease who have hemodynamic consequences from the AF or who are at risk for a complication resulting from therapy of the arrhythmia.

B. **Search for an underlying cause,** such as heart failure (HF), pulmonary problems, hypertension, or hyperthyroidism.

C. Serum should be obtained for measurement of thyroid stimulating hormone (TSH) and free T4. This should be done even if there are no symptoms suggestive of hyperthyroidism, since the risk of AF is increased up to threefold in patients with subclinical hyperthyroidism. The latter disorder is characterized by low serum TSH (<0.5 mU/L) and normal serum free T4.

D. If AF appears to have been precipitated by a reversible medical problem, cardioversion should be postponed until the condition has been successfully treated, which will often lead to spontaneous reversion. If this treatment is to be initiated as an outpatient, anticoagulation with warfarin should be begun with cardioversion performed, if necessary, after three to four weeks of adequate anticoagulation. If the patient is to be admitted to the hospital for treatment of the underlying disease, it is prudent to begin heparin therapy and then institute oral warfarin. Cardioversion is again performed after anticoagulation if the patient does not revert to NSR. In either case, three to four weeks of anticoagulation is not necessary if TEE shows no left atrial thrombus.

E. **Indications for urgent cardioversion**
  1. Active ischemia.
  2. Significant hypotension, to which poor LV systolic function, diastolic dysfunction, or associated mitral or aortic valve disease may contribute.
  3. Severe manifestations of HF.
  4. The presence of a pre-excitation syndrome, which may lead to an extremely rapid ventricular rate.
  5. In a patient who has truly urgent indications for cardioversion, the need for restoration of NSR takes precedence over the need for protection from thromboembolic risk. If feasible, the patient should still be heparinized for the cardioversion procedure.

F. **Initial rate control with mild-to-moderate symptoms** Initial treatment directed at slowing the ventricular rate will usually result in improvement of the associated symptoms. This can be achieved with beta-blockers, calcium channel blockers (verapamil and diltiazem), or digoxin.
  1. Digoxin is the preferred drug only in patients with AF due to HF. Digoxin can also be used in patients who cannot take or who respond inadequately to beta-blockers or calcium channel blockers. The effect of digoxin is additive to both of these drugs.
  2. A beta-blocker, diltiazem, or verapamil is the preferred drug in the absence of HF. Beta-blockers are particularly useful when the ventricular response increases to inappropriately high rates during exercise, after an acute MI, and when exercise-induced angina pectoris is also present. A calcium channel blocker is preferred in patients with chronic lung disease.

G. **Elective cardioversion.** In some patients, antiarrhythmic drugs are administered prior to cardioversion to increase the chance of successful reversion and to prevent recurrence. Patients who are successfully cardioverted generally require antiarrhythmic drugs to increase the likelihood of maintaining sinus rhythm.

H. **Immediate cardioversion.** There is a low risk of systemic embolization if the duration of the arrhythmia is 48 hours or less and there are no associated cardiac abnormalities (mitral valve disease or LV enlargement). In such patients, electrical or pharmacologic cardioversion can be attempted after systemic heparinization. Aspirin should be administered for a first episode of AF that converts spontaneously and warfarin for at least four weeks to all other patients.

I. **Delayed cardioversion.** It is preferable to anticoagulate with warfarin for three to four weeks before attempted cardioversion to allow any left atrial thrombi to resolve if:
  1. The duration of AF is more than 48 hours or of unknown duration.
  2. There is associated mitral valve disease or cardiomyopathy or HF.
  3. The patient has a prior history of a thromboembolic event.
  4. During this time, rate control should be maintained with an oral AV nodal blocker. The recommended target INR is 2.5 (range 2.0 to 3.0). The INR should be consistently ≥ 2.0 in the weeks before cardioversion.

J. **Trans-esophageal echocardiogram** immediately prior to elective cardioversion should be considered for those patients at increased risk for left atrial thrombi (eg, rheumatic mitral valve disease, recent thromboembolism, severe LV systolic dysfunction). Among patients with AF of recent onset (but more than 48 hours) who are not being anticoagulated, an alternative approach to three to four weeks of warfarin therapy before cardioversion is TEE-based screening with cardioversion performed if no thrombi are seen.

References: See page 294.

Hypercholesterolemia

There is a direct relation between the plasma levels of total and low density lipoprotein (LDL) plasma cholesterol and the risk of CHD and coronary mortality. LDL cholesterol lowering in moderate to high-risk patients leads to a reduction in cardiovascular events.

I. Pathophysiology
A. CHD remains the leading cause of death for both men and women of all races. In men over the age of 65, nearly one-half of all deaths are attributed to CHD, compared to less than 25 percent for all cancers and less than 2 percent for all infections. An even higher proportion of deaths are due to CHD in older women (56 percent), with less than 20 percent due to cancer.
B. The optimal value for LDL cholesterol in both men and women is <100 mg/dL; a one standard deviation (38.5 mg/dL) LDL increase above the mean of 118 mg/dL was associated with relative risk for CHD of 1.42 for men and 1.37 for women.
C. A one standard deviation increase in HDL (15.5 mg/dL) above the mean of 40 mg/dL in men and 51 mg/dL in women was associated with relative risk of 0.64 and 0.69, respectively.
D. Triglycerides were an independent predictor of CHD only in women in whom a one standard deviation increase (62 mg/dL) above the mean of 115 mg/dL was associated with a relative risk of 1.31.
E. When used in combination with blood pressure, smoking, and diabetes, LDL, HDL, Lp(a) and triglycerides (in women) provided a relative risk for CHD.

II. Lipoprotein measurement.
A standard serum lipid profile consists of total cholesterol, triglycerides, and HDL-cholesterol. Lipoprotein analysis should be performed after 12 to 14 hours of fasting to minimize the influence of postprandial hyperlipidemia.

III. Risk stratification:
A. Obtain a fasting lipid profile
B. Identify the presence of CHD equivalents
C. Identify the presence of other major CHD risk factors
D. If two or more risk factors other than LDL (as defined in step 3) are present in a patient without CHD or a CHD equivalent (as defined in step 2), the 10-year risk of CHD is assessed using the ATP III modification of the Framingham risk tables.
E. National Cholesterol Education Program guidelines. Screening should be performed at least once every five years for all persons age 20 and over. A fasting lipid profile is recommended for screening, although if the testing opportunity is nonfasting, the total and HDL-cholesterol should be measured. In the latter circumstance, a total cholesterol >200 mg/dL or HDL cholesterol <40 mg/dL suggests the need for a follow-up fasting lipid profile.
F. Individuals without known CHD who have a desirable serum LDL cholesterol concentration (<160 mg/dL for 0 to one risk factor and <130 mg/dL for two or more risk factors) can be rescreened in five years. Patients with borderline-high cholesterol and less than two risk factors should be rescreened within one to two years.
G. The desirable LDL cholesterol level for those with CHD or CHD equivalent is <100 mg/dL; CHD equivalents include:
1. Symptomatic carotid artery disease
2. Peripheral arterial disease
3. Abdominal aortic aneurysm
4. Diabetes mellitus

H. Elderly. Screening and primary preventive drug therapy is recommended in some elderly subjects who are at very high risk, such as those with a serum LDL-cholesterol of 160 mg/dL or greater despite attempts at dietary modification plus two or more cardiac risk factors — cigarette smoking, hypertension, diabetes mellitus, or an HDL-cholesterol level below 35 mg/dL.

IV. **Treatment of hypercholesterolemia**

A. **Identification of patients at risk**

Step 1 — The first step in determining patient risk is to obtain a fasting lipid profile.

Classification of LDL, Total, and HDL Cholesterol (mg/dL)	
LDL Cholesterol	
<100	Optimal
100-129	Near optimal/above optimal
130-159	Borderline high
160-189	High
$\geq$190	Very high
Total Cholesterol	
<200	Desirable
200-239	Borderline high
$\geq$240	High
HDL Cholesterol	
<40	Low
$\geq$60	High

Step 2 — CHD equivalents, that is, risk factors that place the patient at similar risk for CHD events as a history of CHD itself, are identified:
  a. Diabetes mellitus
  b. Symptomatic carotid artery disease
  c. Peripheral arterial disease
  d. Abdominal aortic aneurysm
  e. Multiple risk factors that confer a 10-year risk of CHD >20 percent.

B. In addition to the conditions identified as CHD equivalents, chronic renal insufficiency (defined by a plasma creatinine concentration that exceeds 1.5 mg/dL or an estimated glomerular filtration rate that is less than 60 mL/min per 1.73 m^2) to be a CHD equivalent.

Step 3 — Major CHD factors other than LDL are identified:
  Cigarette smoking
  Hypertension (BP $\geq$140/90 or antihypertensive medication)
  Low HDL-cholesterol (HDL-C) (<40 mg/dL)
  Family history of premature CHD (in male first degree relatives <55 years, in female first degree relative <65 years)
  Age (men $\geq$45 years, women $\geq$55 years)

HDL-C >60 mg/dL counts as a "negative" risk factor; its presence removes one risk factor from the total count.

Step 4 — If two or more risk factors other than LDL (as defined in step 3) are present in a patient without CHD or a CHD equivalent, the 10-year risk of CHD is assessed using the ATP III modification of the Framingham risk tables.

Step 5 — The last step in risk assessment is to determine the risk category that establishes the LDL goal, when to initiate therapeutic lifestyle changes, and when to consider drug therapy.

LDL Cholesterol Goals for Therapeutic Lifestyle Changes and Drug Therapy in Different Risk Categories

Risk Category	LDL-C Goal	LDL Level at Which to Initiate Therapeutic Lifestyle Changes	LDL Level at Which to Consider Drug Therapy
CHD	<100 mg/dL	≥100 mg/dL	≥130 mg/dL (100-129 mg/dL: drug optional)
2+ Risk Factors	≤130 mg/dL	≥130 mg/dL	10-year risk 10-20%:>130 mg/dL 10-year risk <10%:≥160 mg/dL
0-1 Risk Factor	≤160 mg/dL	≥160 mg/dL	≥190 mg/dL (160-189 mg/dL: LDL-lowering drug optional)

V. Summary and recommendations

A. All patients with an LDL-C above goal should undergo lifestyle modifications in an effort to reduce the serum cholesterol. These modifications include diet and exercise.

B. In patients with CHD or a CHD equivalent (diabetes mellitus, symptomatic carotid artery disease, peripheral arterial disease, abdominal aortic aneurysm, chronic renal insufficiency, or multiple risk factors that confer a 10-year risk of CHD greater than 20 percent) who are significantly above the goal LDL-C, drug therapy should not be delayed while waiting to see if lifestyle modifications are effective.

C. Patients who require drug therapy should almost always be treated with a statin.

D. **Secondary prevention goals and therapy.** Goals for LDL-C in patients with CHD or CHD equivalents being treated for secondary prevention:

1. **Statin therapy with atorvastatin (Lipitor)** 80 mg daily reduces mortality in patients with an acute coronary syndrome and is recommended as initial therapy. Given that benefit occurs earlier than the first cholesterol measurement on therapy would normally be obtained, patients be started on atorvastatin 80 mg daily early in their hospital course.

2. Patients at very high risk for CHD events might also be expected to benefit from more intensive lipid lowering therapy. We suggest that such patients be treated with the lowest dose of a statin that reduces their LDL-C below 80 mg/dL. If such patients cannot achieve an LDL-C below 100 mg/dL with a statin alone, a second lipid-lowering agent should be added.

E. **Primary prevention goals and therapy**

1. Patients without CHD or a CHD equivalent should be assessed for major non-LDL risk factors (cigarette smoking, hypertension [BP ≥140/90 or antihypertensive medication], HDL-C <40 mg/dL, family

history of premature CHD [male first degree relative <55 years; female first degree relative <65 years], age (men >45, women >55).

2. Count the number of risk factors, subtracting one risk factor if the HDL-C is >60 mg/dL. In patients with two or more risk factors, assess the 10-year risk of CHD using the ATP III modification of the Framingham risk tables.

3. Patients with no or one risk factor have a goal LDL-C of less than 160 mg/dL. Patients with two or more risk factors have a goal LDL-C of less than 130 mg/dL. Patients with a 10-year CHD risk of greater than 20 percent should be considered to have a CHD equivalent.

4. Drug therapy with a statin should be considered if after an adequate trial of lifestyle modification the LDL-C remains above 190 mg/dL in patients with no or one risk factor or above 160 mg/dL in patients with two or more risk factors.

Dose, Side Effects, and Drug Interactions of Lipid-Lowering Drugs

Drug class	Dose	Dosing	Major side effects and drug interactions
HMG CoA reductase inhibitors			
Atorvastatin (Lipitor) Lovastatin (generic, Mevacor) Extended-release lovastatin (Altocor) Pravastatin (Pravachol) Simvastatin (Zocor) Fluvastatin (Lescol, Lescol XL) Rosuvastatin (Crestor)	10-40 mg/day 20-80 mg/day 10-60 mg/day 10-40 mg/day 5-40 mg/day 10-40 mg/day 10-40 mg/day	Take at bed-time. Take BID if dose >20 mg/day.	Headache; nausea; sleep disturbance; elevations in liver enzymes and alkaline phosphatase. Myositis and rhabdomyolysis. Lovastatin and simvastatin potentiate warfarin and increase digoxin levels
Cholesterol absorption inhibitors			
Ezetimibe (Zetia)	10 mg/day	10 mg qd	Increased transaminases in combination with statins
Bile acid sequestrants			
Cholestyramine (Questran, Questran Lite) Colestipol (Colestid) Colesevelam (WelChol)	4-24 g/day 5-30 g/day 3.75 gm once or divided BID	Take within 30 min of meal. A double dose with dinner produces same effect as BID dosing	Nausea, bloating, cramping, constipation; elevations in hepatic transaminases and alkaline phosphatase. Impaired absorption of fat soluble vitamins, digoxin, warfarin, thiazides, beta-blockers, thyroxine, phenobarbital.
Nicotinic acid	1-12 g/day	Given with meals. Start with 100 mg BID and titrate to 500 mg TID. After 6 weeks, check lipids, glucose, liver function, and uric acid.	Prostaglandin-mediated cutaneous flushing, headache, pruritus; hyperpigmentation; acanthosis nigricans; dry skin; nausea; diarrhea; myositis.

Drug class	Dose	Dosing	Major side effects and drug interactions
Fibrates			
Gemfibrozil (Lopid)	600 mg BID	50 to 60 min before meals.	Potentiates warfarin. Absorption of gemfibrozil diminished by bile acid sequestrants.
Fenofibrate (Lofibra, micronized)	200 mg qd	Take with breakfast. Use lower dosage with renal insufficiency.	Skin rash, nausea, bloating, cramping, myalgia; lowers cyclosporin levels; nephrotoxic in cyclosporin-treated patients.
Fenofibrate (TriCor)	160 mg qd		
Probucol	500 mg BID		Loose stools; eosinophilia; QT prolongation; angioneurotic edema.
Extended-release niacin plus (immediate-release) lovastatin (Advicor)	1000 mg/40 mg/day	1000 mg + 40 mg h.s.3	markedly lowers LDL and triglycerides and raises HDL

VI. **Approach to the patient with hypertriglyceridemia**
  A. **Normal serum triglyceride concentration.** The serum triglyceride concentration can be stratified in terms of coronary risk:
  Normal <150 mg/dL
  Borderline high — 150 to 199 mg/dL
  High — 200 to 499 mg/dL
  Very high ≥500 mg/dL).
  B. **General treatment guidelines**
    1. Nonpharmacologic therapy is recommended for serum triglyceride values above 200 mg/dL. Although the risk is enhanced at these levels, CHD risk begins to increase at a fasting triglyceride concentration of 160 to 190 mg/dL and, among patients with CHD, may begin to increase at values above 100 mg/dL.

Treatment of Hypertriglyceridemia*		
Review medications	**Laboratory studies**	**Diet**
Change to lipid neutral or favorable agents (eg, alpha-blockers, biguanides, thiazolidinedione) Lower doses of drugs that increase triglycerides, such as beta-blockers, glucocorticoids, diuretics (thiazide and loop), ticlopidine, estrogens.	Exclude secondary disorders of lipid metabolism Fasting blood glucose Serum creatinine Thyroid function studies	Weight loss Avoid concentrated sugars Increase omega-3 fatty acid intake through fish consumption Exercise Aerobic exercise minimum of 3 hours weekly

*Hypertriglyceridemia is defined as a serum triglyceride concentration above 200 mg/dL

2. The National Cholesterol Education Program (Adult Treatment Panel [ATP] III) recommended that in all patients with borderline high or high triglycerides, the primary goal of therapy is to achieve the targets for LDL cholesterol. In addition, the following recommendations were made for various levels of elevated triglycerides:

   a. When triglycerides are borderline high (150 to 199 mg/dL), emphasis should be upon weight reduction and increased physical activity.

   b. When triglycerides are high (200 to 499 mg/dL), non-HDL cholesterol becomes a secondary target of therapy after LDL cholesterol. Drug therapy can be considered in high-risk patients, including those who have had an acute myocardial infarction, to reach the non-HDL cholesterol goals. These goals may be achieved by intensifying therapy with an LDL cholesterol lowering drug, or by adding nicotinic acid or a fibrate.

   c. When triglycerides are very high (≥500 mg/dL), the initial goal is to prevent pancreatitis by lowering triglycerides with a fibrate or nicotinic acid. Once triglycerides are below 500 mg/dL, LDL cholesterol goals should be addressed.

References: See page 294.

Pulmonary Disorders

Acute Bronchitis

Acute bronchitis is one of the most common diagnoses in ambulatory care medicine, accounting for 2.5 million physician visits per year. Viruses are the most common cause of acute bronchitis in otherwise healthy adults. Only a small portion of acute bronchitis infections are caused by nonviral agents, with the most common organisms being *Mycoplasma pneumoniae and Chlamydia pneumoniae*.

I. **Diagnosis**
   A. The cough in acute bronchitis may produce either clear or purulent sputum. This cough generally lasts seven to 10 days. Approximately 50 percent of patients with acute bronchitis have a cough that lasts up to three weeks, and 25 percent of patients have a cough that persists for over a month.
   B. **Physical examination.** Wheezing, rhonchi, or a prolonged expiratory phase may be present.
   C. **Diagnostic studies**
      1. The appearance of sputum is not predictive of bacterial infection. Purulent sputum is most often caused by viral infections. Microscopic examination or culture of sputum is not helpful. Since most cases of acute bronchitis are caused by viruses, cultures are usually negative or exhibit normal respiratory flora. M. pneumoniae or C. pneumoniae infection are not detectable on routine sputum culture.
      2. When pneumonia is suspected, chest radiographs and pulse oximetry may be helpful.
II. **Pathophysiology**

Selected Triggers of Acute Bronchitis

Viruses: adenovirus, coronavirus, coxsackievirus, enterovirus, influenza virus, parainfluenza virus, respiratory syncytial virus, rhinovirus
Bacteria: *Bordetella pertussis, Bordetella parapertussis, Branhamella catarrhalis, Haemophilus influenzae, Streptococcus pneumoniae*, atypical bacteria (eg, *Mycoplasma pneumoniae, Chlamydia pneumoniae*, Legionella species)
Yeast and fungi: *Blastomyces dermatitidis, Candida albicans, Candida tropicalis, Coccidioides immitis, Cryptococcus neoformans, Histoplasma capsulatum*
Noninfectious triggers: asthma, air pollutants, ammonia, cannabis, tobacco, trace metals, others

---

   A. Acute bronchitis is usually caused by a viral infection. In patients younger than one year, respiratory syncytial virus, parainfluenza virus, and coronavirus are the most common isolates. In patients one to 10 years of age, parainfluenza virus, enterovirus, respiratory syncytial virus, and rhinovirus predominate. In patients older than 10 years, influenza virus, respiratory syncytial virus, and adenovirus are most frequent.
   B. Parainfluenza virus, enterovirus, and rhinovirus infections most commonly occur in the fall. Influenza virus, respiratory syncytial virus, and coronavirus infections are most frequent in the winter and spring.
III. **Signs and symptoms**
   A. Cough is the most commonly observed symptom of acute bronchitis. Most patients have a cough for less than two weeks; however, 26 percent are still coughing after two weeks, and a few cough for six to eight weeks.
   B. Other signs and symptoms include sputum production, dyspnea, wheezing, chest pain, fever, hoarseness, malaise, rhonchi, and rales. Sputum

may be clear, white, yellow, green, or tinged with blood. Color alone should not be considered indicative of bacterial infection.

IV. **Physical examination and diagnostic studies**
  A. **Fever, tachypnea, wheezing, rhonchi**, and prolonged expiration are comon. Consolidation is absent. High fever should prompt consideration of pneumonia or influenza.
  B. **Chest radiography** should be reserved for patients with possible pneumonia, heart failure, advanced age, chronic obstructive pulmonary disease, malignancy, tuberculosis, or immunocompromised or debilitated status.

V. **Differential diagnosis**
  A. Acute bronchitis or pneumonia can present with fever, constitutional symptoms and a productive cough. Patients with pneumonia often have rales. When pneumonia is suspected on the basis of the presence of a high fever, constitutional symptoms or severe dyspnea, a chest radiograph should be obtained.

Differential Diagnosis of Acute Bronchitis	
Disease process	**Signs and symptoms**
Asthma	Evidence of reversible airway obstruction even when not infected
Allergic aspergillosis	Transient pulmonary infiltrates Eosinophilia in sputum and peripheral blood smear
Occupational exposures	Symptoms worse during the work week but tend to improve during weekends, holidays and vacations
Chronic bronchitis	Chronic cough with sputum production on a daily basis for a minimum of three months Typically occurs in smokers
Sinusitis	Tenderness over the sinuses, postnasal drainage
Common cold	Upper airway inflammation and no evidence of bronchial wheezing
Pneumonia	Evidence of infiltrate on the chest radiograph
Congestive heart failure	Basilar rales, orthopnea Cardiomegaly Evidence of increased interstitial or alveolar fluid on the chest radiograph S_3 gallop, tachycardia
Reflux esophagitis	Intermittent symptoms worse when lying down Heartburn
Bronchogenic tumor	Constitutional signs often present Cough chronic, sometimes with hemoptysis
Aspiration syndromes	Usually related to a precipitating event, such as smoke inhalation Vomiting Decreased level of consciousness

  B. **Asthma** should be considered in patients with repetitive episodes of acute bronchitis. Patients who repeatedly present with cough and wheezing can be given spirometric testing with bronchodilation to help differentiate asthma from recurrent bronchitis.
  C. **Congestive heart failure** may cause cough, shortness of breath and wheezing in older patients. Reflux esophagitis with chronic aspiration can

cause bronchial inflammation with cough and wheezing. Bronchogenic tumors may produce a cough and obstructive symptoms.

VI. **Treatment**
  A. **Protussives and antitussives**
  1. Because acute bronchitis is most often caused by a viral infection, usually only symptomatic treatment is required. Treatment can focus on preventing or controlling the cough (antitussive therapy).
  2. Antitussive therapy is indicated if cough is creating significant discomfort. Studies have reported success rates ranging from 68 to 98 percent. Nonspecific antitussives, such as hydrocodone (Hycodan), dextromethorphan (Delsym), codeine (Robitussin A-C), carbetapentane (Rynatuss), and benzonatate (Tessalon), simply suppress cough.

Selected Nonspecific Antitussive Agents		
Preparation	**Dosage**	**Side effects**
Hydromorphone-guaifenesin (Hycotuss)	5 mg per 100 mg per 5 mL (one teaspoon)	Sedation, nausea, vomiting, respiratory depression
Dextromethorphan (Delsym)	30 mg every 12 hours	Rarely, gastrointestinal upset or sedation
Hydrocodone (Hycodan syrup or tablets)	5 mg every 4 to 6 hours	Gastrointestinal upset, nausea, drowsiness, constipation
Codeine (Robitussin A-C)	10 to 20 mg every 4 to 6 hours	Gastrointestinal upset, nausea, drowsiness, constipation
Carbetapentane (Rynatuss)	60 to 120 mg every 12 hours	Drowsiness, gastrointestinal upset
Benzonatate (Tessalon)	100 to 200 mg three times daily	Hypersensitivity, gastrointestinal upset, sedation

  B. **Bronchodilators.** Patients with acute bronchitis who used an albuterol metered-dose inhaler are less likely to be coughing at one week, compared with those who received placebo.
  C. **Antibiotics.** Physicians often treat acute bronchitis with antibiotics, even though scant evidence exists that antibiotics offer any significant advantage over placebo. Antibiotic therapy is beneficial in patients with exacerbations of chronic bronchitis.

Oral Antibiotic Regimens for Bronchitis	
Drug	**Recommended regimen**
Azithromycin (Zithromax)	500 mg; then 250 mg qd
Erythromycin	250-500 mg q6h
Clarithromycin (Biaxin)	500 mg bid

Drug	Recommended regimen
Levofloxacin (Levaquin)	500 mg qd
Trovafloxacin (Trovan)	200 mg qd
Trimethoprim/sulfamethoxazole (Bactrim, Septra)	1 DS tablet bid
Doxycycline	100 mg bid

    D. Bronchodilators. Significant relief of symptoms occurs with inhaled albuterol (two puffs four times daily). When productive cough and wheezing are present, bronchodilator therapy may be useful.

References: See page 294.

Asthma

Asthma is the most common chronic disease among children. Asthma triggers include viral infections; environmental pollutants, such as tobacco smoke; aspirin, nonsteroidal anti-inflammatory drugs, and sustained exercise, particularly in cold environments.

I. Diagnosis
    A. Symptoms of asthma may include episodic complaints of breathing difficulties, seasonal or nighttime cough, prolonged shortness of breath after a respiratory infection, or difficulty sustaining exercise.
    B. Wheezing does not always represent asthma. Wheezing may persist for weeks after an acute bronchitis episode. Patients with chronic obstructive pulmonary disease may have a reversible component superimposed on their fixed obstruction. Etiologic clues include a personal history of allergic disease, such as rhinitis or atopic dermatitis, and a family history of allergic disease.
    C. The frequency of daytime and nighttime symptoms, duration of exacerbations and asthma triggers should be assessed.
    D. Physical examination. Hyperventilation, use of accessory muscles of respiration, audible wheezing, and a prolonged expiratory phase are common. Increased nasal secretions or congestion, polyps, and eczema may be present.
    E. Measurement of lung function. An increase in the forced expiratory volume in one second (FEV_1) of 12% after treatment with an inhaled beta$_2$ agonist is sufficient to make the diagnosis of asthma. A 12% change in peak expiratory flow rate (PEFR) measured on a peak-flow meter is also diagnostic.

II. Treatment of asthma
    A. Beta$_2$ agonists
        1. Inhaled short-acting beta$_2$-adrenergic agonists are the most effective drugs available for treatment of acute bronchospasm and for prevention of exercise-induced asthma. Levalbuterol (Xopenex), the R-isomer of racemic albuterol, offers no significant advantage over racemic albuterol.
        2. Salmeterol (Serevent), a long-acting beta$_2$ agonist, has a relatively slow onset of action and a prolonged effect.
            a. Salmeterol should not be used in the treatment of acute bronchospasm. Patients taking salmeterol should use a short-acting beta$_2$ agonist as needed to control acute symptoms. Twice-daily inhalation of salmeterol has been effective for maintenance treatment in combination with inhaled corticosteroids.

b. **Fluticasone/Salmeterol (Advair Diskus)** is a long-acting beta agonist and corticosteroid combination; dry-powder inhaler [100, 250 or 500 g/puff],1 puff q12h.

3. **Formoterol (Foradil)** is a long-acting beta2 agonist. It should only be used in patients who already take an inhaled corticosteroid. Patients taking formoterol should use a short-acting beta$_2$ agonist as needed to control acute symptoms. For maintenance treatment of asthma in adults and children at least 5 years old, the dosage is 1 puff bid.

4. **Adverse effects of beta$_2$ agonists.** Tachycardia, palpitations, tremor and paradoxical bronchospasm can occur. High doses can cause hypokalemia.

Drugs for Asthma		
Drug	**Formulation**	**Dosage**
Inhaled beta$_2$-adrenergic agonists, short-acting		
Albuterol *Proventil* *Proventil-HFA* *Ventolin* *Ventolin Rotacaps*	metered-dose inhaler (90 µg/puff) dry-powder inhaler (200 µg/inhalation)	2 puffs q4-6h PRN 1-2 capsules q4-6h PRN
Albuterol *Proventil* multi-dose vials *Ventolin Nebules* *Ventolin*	nebulized	2.5 mg q4-6h PRN
Levalbuterol - *Xopenex*	nebulized	0.63-1.25 mg q6-8h PRN
Inhaled beta2-adrenergic agonist, long-acting		
Formoterol - *Foradil*	oral inhaler (12 µg/capsule)	1 cap q12h via inhaler
Salmeterol *Serevent* *Serevent Diskus*	metered-dose inhaler (21 µg/puff) dry-powder inhaler (50 µg/inhalation)	2 puffs q12h 1 inhalation q12h
Fluticasone/Salmeterol *Advair Diskus*	dry-powder inhaler (100, 250 or 500 µg/puff)	1 puff q12h
Inhaled Corticosteroids		
Beclomethasone dipropionate *Beclovent* *Vanceril* Vanceril Double-Strength	metered-dose inhaler (42 µg/puff) (84 µg/puff)	4-8 puffs bid 2-4 puffs bid
Budesonide *Pulmicort Turbuhaler*	dry-powder inhaler (200 µg/inhalation)	1-2 inhalations bid
Flunisolide - *AeroBid*	metered-dose inhaler (250 µg/puff)	2-4 puffs bid

Drug	Formulation	Dosage
Fluticasone Flovent *Flovent Rotadisk*	metered-dose inhaler (44, 110 or 220 µg/puff) dry-powder inhaler (50, 100 or 250 µg/inhalation)	2-4 puffs bid (44 µg/puff) 1 inhalation bid (100 µg/inhalation)
Triamcinolone acetonide *Azmacort*	metered-dose inhaler (100 µg/puff)	2 puffs tid-qid or 4 puffs bid
Leukotriene Modifiers		
Montelukast - *Singulair*	tablets	10 mg qhs
Zafirlukast - *Accolate*	tablets	20 mg bid
Zileuton - *Zyflo*	tablets	600 mg qid
Mast Cell Stabilizers		
Cromolyn *Intal*	metered-dose inhaler (800 µg/puff)	2-4 puffs tid-qid
Nedocromil *Tilade*	metered-dose inhaler (1.75 mg/puff)	2-4 puffs bid-qid
Phosphodiesterase Inhibitor		
Theophylline *Slo-Bid Gyrocaps, Theo-Dur, Unidur*	extended-release capsules or tablets	100-300 mg bid

B. **Inhaled corticosteroids**
 1. Regular use of an inhaled corticosteroid can suppress inflammation and bronchial hyperresponsiveness. Inhaled corticosteroids are recommended for most patients.
 2. **Adverse effects.** Inhaled corticosteroids are usually free of toxicity. Slowing of linear growth may occur within 6-12 weeks in some children. Decreased bone density, glaucoma and cataract formation have been reported. Churg-Strauss vasculitis is rare. Dysphonia and oral candidiasis can occur. A spacer device and rinsing the mouth after inhalation decreases the incidence of candidiasis.

C. **Leukotriene modifiers**
 1. Leukotrienes increase production of mucus and edema of the airway and cause bronchoconstriction. Montelukast and zafirlukast are leukotriene receptor antagonists. Zileuton inhibits synthesis of leukotrienes.
 2. **Montelukast (Singulair)** is modestly effective for maintenance treatment. It is taken once daily in the evening. It is less effective than inhaled corticosteroids, but addition of montelukast may permit a reduction in corticosteroid dosage.
 3. **Zafirlukast (Accolate)** is modestly effective for mild-to-moderate asthma It is less effective than inhaled corticosteroids. Taking zafirlukast with food markedly decreases its bioavailability. Theophylline can decrease its effect. Zafirlukast increases serum concentrations of oral anticoagulants. Infrequent adverse effects include headache, gastrointestinal disturbances and increased serum aminotransferase activity. Lupus and Churg-Strauss vasculitis have been reported.

4. **Zileuton (Zyflo)** is modestly effective, but it is taken four times a day and patients must be monitored for hepatic toxicity.

D. **Cromolyn (Intal) and nedocromil (Tilade)**
1. Cromolyn sodium, an inhibitor of mast cell degranulation, can decrease airway hyperresponsiveness in some patients. The drug has no bronchodilating activity and is useful only for prophylaxis. Cromolyn has virtually no systemic toxicity.
2. Nedocromil (Tilade) has similar effects as cromolyn. Both cromolyn and nedocromil are much less effective than inhaled corticosteroids.

E. **Theophylline**
1. Oral theophylline has a slower onset of action than inhaled beta$_2$ agonists and has limited usefulness for treatment of acute symptoms. It can, however, reduce the frequency and severity of symptoms, especially in nocturnal asthma, and can decrease inhaled corticosteroid requirements.
2. When theophylline is used alone, serum concentrations between 8-12 mcg/mL provide a modest improvement is FEV$_1$. Serum levels of 15-20 mcg/mL are only minimally more effective and are associated with a higher incidence of cardiovascular adverse events.

F. **Oral corticosteroids** are the most effective drugs available for acute exacerbations of asthma unresponsive to bronchodilators.
1. Oral corticosteroids decrease symptoms and may prevent an early relapse. Chronic use of oral corticosteroids can cause glucose intolerance, weight gain, increased blood pressure, osteoporosis, cataracts, immunosuppression and decreased growth in children. Alternate-day use of corticosteroids can decrease the incidence of adverse effects, but not of osteoporosis.
2. **Prednisone, prednisolone or methylprednisolone** (Solu-Medrol), 40-60 mg qd; for children, 1-2 mg/kg/day to a maximum of 60 mg/day. Therapy is continued for 3-10 days. The oral steroid dosage does not need to be tapered after short-course "burst" therapy if the patient is receiving inhaled steroid therapy.

Pharmacotherapy for Asthma Based on Disease Classification		
Classification	**Long-term control medications**	**Quick-relief medications**
Mild intermittent		Short-acting beta$_2$ agonist as needed
Mild persistent	Low-dose inhaled corticosteroid or cromolyn sodium (Intal) or nedocromil (Tilade)	Short-acting beta$_2$ agonist as needed
Moderate persistent	Medium-dose inhaled corticosteroid plus a long-acting bronchodilator (long-acting beta$_2$ agonist)	Short-acting beta$_2$ agonist as needed
Severe persistent	High-dose inhaled corticosteroid plus a long-acting bronchodilator and systemic corticosteroid	Short-acting beta$_2$ agonist as needed

III. **Management of acute exacerbations**
A. High-dose, short-acting beta$_2$ agonists delivered by a metered-dose inhaler with a volume spacer or via a nebulizer remains the mainstay of urgent treatment.
B. Most patients require therapy with systemic corticosteroids to resolve symptoms and prevent relapse. Hospitalization should be considered if the PEFR remains less than 70% of predicted. Patients with a PEFR less

than 50% of predicted who exhibit an increasing pCO_2 level and declining mental status are candidates for intubation.

C. Non-invasive ventilation with bilevel positive airway pressure (BIPAP) may be used to relieve the work-of-breathing while awaiting the effects of acute treatment, provided that consciousness and the ability to protect the airway have not been compromised.

References: See page 294.

Chronic Obstructive Pulmonary Disease

Chronic obstructive pulmonary disease (COPD) is the fourth-ranked cause of death. Chronic obstructive pulmonary disease is defined as "disease state characterized by airflow limitation that is not fully reversible. Airflow limitation is usually progressive and associated with an abnormal inflammatory response of the lungs to noxious particles or gases."

I. **Pathophysiology**
   A. Airflow obstruction is the result of both small airway disease (obstructive bronchiolitis) and parenchymal destruction (emphysema). The relative contributions of each vary from person to person, and can be accompanied by partially reversible airways hyperreactivity.
   B. Chronic bronchitis is defined by the presence of chronic productive cough for three months in each of two successive years.
   C. Emphysema is the abnormal permanent enlargement of airspaces distal to the terminal bronchioles, accompanied by destruction of their walls without obvious fibrosis. Emphysema is frequently present in patients with moderate and severe COPD.
   D. Asthma is defined as an inflammatory disease of the airways characterized by an increased responsiveness of the trachea and bronchi to various stimuli, and manifested by a widespread narrowing of the airways.
   E. Cigarette smoking is the major cause of COPD. However, only about 15 to 20 percent of smokers develop COPD suggesting that host factors (most likely genetic) also contribute to pathogenesis of the disease.
   F. **Alpha-1 antitrypsin deficiency.** The only established genetic abnormality that predisposes to lung disease clinically and pathologically similar to COPD is alpha-1 antitrypsin [AAT] deficiency. Severe AAT deficiency has a frequency of about 1 in 3,000 live births. Persons with known COPD, or asthma with non-remittent airflow obstruction, should be screened for AAT deficiency.

II. **Clinical features**
   A. **History.** Patients with COPD have usually been smoking at least 20 cigarettes per day for 20 or more years before symptoms develop. Chronic productive cough, sometimes with wheezing, often begins when patients are in their forties.
   B. Dyspnea on effort does not usually begin until the mid sixties or early seventies. Sputum production is insidious, initially occurring only in the morning; the daily volume rarely exceeds 60 mL. Sputum is usually mucoid but becomes purulent with an exacerbation.
   C. Acute chest illnesses occur intermittently, and are characterized by increased cough, purulent sputum, wheezing, dyspnea, and occasionally fever.
   D. With disease progression, the intervals between acute exacerbations shorten. Late in the course of the illness, an exacerbation may give rise to hypoxemia with cyanosis. Associated findings also include:
      1. **Weight loss** - Approximately 20 percent of patients with moderate and severe disease experience weight loss and loss.
      2. **Hypercapnia with more severe hypoxemia** in the setting of end-stage disease.
      3. **Morning headache**, which suggests hypercapnia.
      4. **Cor pulmonale** with right heart failure and edema.

5. **Hemoptysis.** Since bronchogenic carcinoma occurs with increased frequency in smokers with COPD, an episode of hemoptysis raises the possibility that carcinoma has developed. However, most episodes of hemoptysis are due to bronchial mucosal erosion.

Diagnosis of chronic obstructive pulmonary disease

History
Smoking history
Age at initiation
Average amount smoked per day
Date when stopped smoking or a current smoker
Environmental history
Cough
Chronic productive cough for at least one quarter of the year for two successive years is the defining characteristic of chronic bronchitis. Sputum, blood or blood streaking in the sputum.
Wheezing
Acute chest illnesses
Frequency of episodes of increased cough and sputum with wheezing.
Dyspnea
Amount of effort required to induce uncomfortable breathing.

Physical examination
Chest
The presence of severe emphysema is indicated by: overdistention of the lungs in the stable position; decreased intensity of breath and heart sounds and prolonged expiratory phase.
Wheezes during auscultation on slow or forced breathing and prolongation of forced expiratory time.
Severe disease is indicated by pursed-lip breathing, use of accessory respiratory muscles, retraction of lower interspaces.
Other
Unusual positions to relieve dyspnea at rest.
Digital clubbing suggests the possibility of lung cancer or bronchiectasis.
Mild dependent edema may be seen in the absence of right heart failure.

Differential diagnosis of COPD

Diagnosis	Features
COPD	Onset in mid-life Symptoms slowly progressive Long smoking history Dyspnea during exercise Largely irreversible airflow limitation
Asthma	Onset in childhood Symptoms vary from day to day Symptoms at night/early morning Allergy, rhinitis, and/or eczema also present Family history of asthma Largely reversible airflow limitation

Diagnosis	Features
Heart failure	Fine basilar crackles Chest X-ray shows dilated heart, pulmonary edema Pulmonary function tests indicate volume restriction, not airflow limitation
Bronchiectasis	Large volumes of purulent sputum Commonly associated with bacterial infection Coarse crackles/clubbing on auscultation Chest X-ray/CT shows bronchial dilation, bronchial wall thickening
Tuberculosis	Onset all ages Chest X-ray shows lung infiltrate Microbiological confirmation High local prevalence of tuberculosis
Obliterative bronchiolitis	Onset in younger age, nonsmokers May have history of rheumatoid arthritis or fume exposure CT on expiration shows hypodense areas
Diffuse panbronchiolitis	Most patients are male and non-smokers. Almost all have chronic sinusitis Chest X-ray and HRCT show diffuse small centrilobular nodular opacities and hyperinflation

Classification of Severity of Chronic Obstructive Pulmonary Disease

Stage	Characteristics
0: At risk	Normal spirometry Chronic symptoms (cough, sputum production)
I: Mild COPD	FEV_1/FVC <70 percent $FEV_1 \geq 80$ percent predicted With or without chronic symptoms (cough, sputum production)
II: Moderate COPD	FEV_1/FVC <70 percent 30 percent $\leq FEV1$ <80 percent predicted IIA: 50 percent $\leq FEV1$ <80 percent predicted IIB: 30 percent $\leq FEV1$ <50 percent predicted
Severe COPD	FEV_1/FVC <70 percent FEV_1 30 percent predicted or FEV_1 <50 percent predicted plus respiratory failure or clinical signs of right heart failure

E. Physical examination

1. Early in the disease there is only prolonged expiration and wheezes on forced exhalation. As obstruction progresses, hyperinflation becomes evident, and the anteroposterior diameter of the chest increases. The diaphragm is depressed and limited in its motion. Breath sounds are

decreased and heart sounds often become distant. Coarse crackles may be heard at the lung bases. Wheezes are frequently heard.

2. If the history and chest radiograph are compatible, a clinical diagnosis of COPD may be made. However, a forced expiratory spirogram before and after bronchodilator is always necessary for confirmation and quantification of the airflow obstruction.

3. Patients with end-stage COPD may adopt positions which relieve dyspnea, such as leaning forward with arms outstretched and weight supported on the palms. Other signs in a patient with end-stage disease may include:

   a. The full use of the accessory respiratory muscles of the neck and shoulder girdle.

   b. Expiration through pursed lips.

   c. Paradoxical retraction of the lower interspaces during inspiration (Hoover's sign).

   d. Cyanosis.

   e. An enlarged, tender liver secondary to right heart failure. Neck vein distention, especially during expiration.

   f. Asterixis due to severe hypercapnia.

4. **Plain chest radiography** is insensitive for diagnosing emphysema; only about half of the instances are detected when the disease is of moderate severity.

   a. Overdistention of the lungs is indicated by a low, flat diaphragm and a long, narrow heart shadow. Flattening of the diaphragmatic contour and an increased retrosternal airspace are observed on the lateral projection. Rapid tapering of the vascular shadows accompanied by hypertransradiancy of the lungs is a sign of emphysema.

   b. Bullae, presenting as radiolucent areas larger than one centimeter in diameter and surrounded by arcuate hairline shadows, are proof of the presence of emphysema. However, bullae reflect only locally severe disease and are not necessarily indicative of widespread emphysema.

   c. Pulmonary hypertension and right ventricular hypertrophy are indicated by prominent hilar vascular shadows and encroachment of the heart shadow on the retrosternal space as the right ventricle enlarges anteriorly.

5. **Pulmonary function tests** are necessary for diagnosing and assessing the severity of airflow obstruction, and are helpful in following its progress. The FEV1 has less variability than other measurements of airways dynamics.

   a. The FVC is also readily measured, although it is dependent on the expiratory time in severe COPD. In the mildest degree of airflow obstruction, the FEV1/FVC ratio falls below 0.70 and the FEV1 percent predicted is normal. The FEV1 and the FEV1/FVC ratio fall progressively as the severity of COPD increases. Up to 30 percent of patients have an increase of 15 percent or more in their FEV1 following inhalation of a beta-agonist aerosol.

   b. Lung volume measurements reveal an increase in total lung capacity, functional residual capacity, and residual volume, and often a decrease in the vital capacity. The single breath carbon monoxide diffusing capacity is decreased in proportion to the severity of emphysema.

6. **Arterial blood gases** reveal mild or moderate hypoxemia without hypercapnia in the early stages. As the disease progresses, hypoxemia becomes more severe and hypercapnia supervenes. Hypercapnia is observed with increasing frequency as the FEV1 falls below one liter.

7. **Erythrocytosis** increases as arterial PO2 falls below 55 mmHg.

8. **Sputum examination.** In stable chronic bronchitis, sputum is mucoid and the predominant cell is the macrophage. During an exacerbation, sputum usually becomes purulent with an influx of neutrophils. The Gram stain usually shows a mixture of organisms. The most frequent

pathogens cultured from the sputum are Streptococcus pneumoniae and Haemophilus influenzae. Other oropharyngeal flora such as Moraxella catarrhalis have been shown to cause exacerbations.

III. **Management of stable chronic obstructive pulmonary disease**
   A. **Bronchodilators** can improve symptoms and reduce airflow limitation in patients with COPD.
      1. **Metered dose inhalers** (MDI) result in a bronchodilator response equivalent to that of a nebulizer. However, nebulizer therapy may still be necessary if dyspnea and severe bronchospasm during exacerbations impair proper MDI technique.
      2. **Beta agonists.** The primary pharmacologic therapy of COPD is the sympathomimetic bronchodilator. Among these, short-acting selective beta-2 agonists (eg, albuterol) are the agents of choice. Beta-2 agonists can cause tremor and reflex tachycardia due to peripheral arterial dilation. Hypokalemia can also occur in extreme cases. There is no advantage of using short-acting beta-2 agonists on a regular basis instead of as-needed.
   B. **Anticholinergics.** Inhaled anticholinergic bronchodilators (eg, ipratropium and tiotropium) are an integral component of COPD treatment. Anticholinergic drugs reduce the frequency of severe exacerbations and respiratory deaths.
      1. Tiotropium (Spiriva), a long-acting inhaled anticholinergic agent, confers longer bronchodilation than ipratropium (Atrovent) and also appears to lessen the frequency of acute exacerbations.
      2. The effects of anticholinergics and beta-2 agonists are additive. Combination therapy may be simplified by the use of a single metered dose inhaler that delivers a combination of ipratropium and albuterol.
   C. **Theophylline** provides clear benefits to some patients with COPD. Theophylline is associated with decreased dyspnea, improved arterial blood gases, improved spirometry, and improved respiratory muscle function. Theophylline also has pulmonary vasodilator and cardiac inotropic effects, resulting in improvements in right ventricular performance in cor pulmonale.
      1. Serum levels should be maintained in the 8 to 12 mcg/mL range. The use of a long-acting preparation at night may reduce the nocturnal decrements in respiratory function and the morning respiratory symptoms.
   D. **Systemic corticosteroids** have long been used to treat patients with COPD; however, chronic use can have significant adverse effects. Inhaled corticosteroids have substantially fewer adverse consequences.
      1. Chronic corticosteroid administration does not benefit most patients with COPD. However, as many as 20 percent of stable patients with COPD demonstrate objective improvement in airflow with oral corticosteroid treatment.
      2. Chronic steroid therapy should be considered only in patients who have continued symptoms or severe airflow limitation despite maximal therapy with other agents. Only patients with documented improvement in airflow should be considered for long-term therapy. Steroids should be reduced to the lowest dose possible. Alternate day or inhaled steroid usage should be considered.
      3. **Inhaled corticosteroids** may benefit patients with COPD with chronic bronchitis and frequent exacerbations.

Therapy at each stage of COPD			
Stage	**Characteristics**	**Recommended treatments**	
ALL		Avoidance of risk factor(s) Influenza vaccination	
0: At risk	Chronic symptoms (cough, sputum) Exposure to risk factor(s)		
I: Mild COPD	FEV_1/FVC <70 percent $FEV_1 \geq 80$ percent predicted with or without symptoms	Short-acting bronchodilator when needed	
II: Moderate COPD	IIA		
	FEV_1/FVC <70 percent 50 percent $\leq FEV_1$ <80 percent With or without symptoms	Regular treatment with one or more bronchodialtors Rehabilitation	Inhaled glucorticoster oids if significant symptoms and lung function response
	IIB		
	FEV_1/FVC <70 percent 50 percent $\leq FEV_1$ <50 percent With our without symptoms	Regular treatment with one or more bronchodilators Rehabilitation	Inhaled glucortico- steroids if significant symptoms and lung function response or if repeated exacerbations
III: Severe COPD	FEV_1/FVC <70 percent FEV_1 <30 percent predicted or presence of respiratory or right heart failure	Regular treatment with one or more bronchodilators Inhaled glucorticosteroids if significant symptoms and lung function response or if repeated exacerbations Treatment of complications Rehabilitation Long-term oxygen therapy if respiratory failure Surgical treatments	

E. Supplemental therapy
   1. **Oxygen.** Assessment of arterial blood gases or pulse oximetry is the only reliable method for detecting hypoxemia. Arterial blood gas analysis is also helpful in assessing the presence and severity of hypercapnia.
   2. **Surgery.** Selected patients may benefit from lung volume reduction surgery or lung transplantation. **Indications for lung transplantation**
      a. FEV1 is <25 percent of predicted, or
      b. $PaCO_2$ is >55 mmHg, or
      c. Cor pulmonale is present.

       d. Candidates must be under 65 years of age, not have dysfunction of major organs other than the lung, and not have active or recent malignancy or infection with HIV, hepatitis B, or hepatitis C viruses.

IV. **Management of acute exacerbations of chronic obstructive pulmonary disease**

  A. An acute exacerbation of chronic obstructive pulmonary disease (COPD) is characterized by an acute worsening of symptoms accompanied by an impairment of lung function.

  B. **Precipitants**. Acute exacerbations of COPD are most commonly precipitated by infection (bacterial or viral), air pollution or temperature.

  C. Other medical conditions can mimic or cause COPD exacerbation include myocardial ischemia, congestive heart failure, pulmonary embolism, or aspiration

  D. **Criteria for hospitalization:**
1. High risk comorbidities including pneumonia, cardiac arrhythmia, congestive heart failure, diabetes mellitus, renal failure, or liver failure
2. Inadequate response to outpatient management
3. Marked increase in dyspnea
4. Inability to eat or sleep due to symptoms
5. Worsening hypoxemia
6. Worsening hypercapnia
7. Changes in mental status
8. Inability to care for oneself
9. Uncertain diagnosis
10. Acute respiratory acidemia

  E. **Pharmacologic treatment**
1. The major components of managing an acute exacerbation of COPD include inhaled beta adrenergic agonists, anticholinergic bronchodilators, corticosteroids, and antibiotics.
2. **Inhaled beta-2 adrenergic agonists** such as albuterol are the mainstay of therapy for an acute exacerbation of COPD. These medications may be administered via a nebulizer or a metered dose inhaler (MDI) with a spacer device. Nebulized therapy is preferred in this clinical setting.
   a. **Albuterol (Ventolin)** dosages are 180 mcg (two puffs) by metered dose inhaler, or 2.5 mg (diluted to a total of 3 mL) by nebulizer, given every one to two hours.
   b. Subcutaneous injection of beta adrenergic agonists is reserved for situations in which inhaled administration is not possible. Parenteral use may cause arrhythmias or myocardial ischemia.
3. **Anticholinergic bronchodilators**, such as ipratropium bromide and glycopyrrolate, may be used in combination with beta adrenergic agonists to produce greater bronchodilation.
   a. **Ipratropium (Atrovent)** may be administered during acute exacerbations either by nebulizer (500 mcg every two to four hours) or via MDI (two puffs [36 mcg] every two to four hours with a spacer).
4. **Corticosteroids.** Methylprednisolone (60 to 125 mg intravenously, two to four times daily) is given to inpatients. Prednisone (40 to 60 mg orally, once daily) is given to outpatients.
5. **Antibiotics** are recommended for acute exacerbations of COPD with increased secretions. Outpatients should be prescribed a ten day course of amoxicillin, doxycycline, or trimethoprim-sulfamethoxazole. Beta-lactam antibiotics with a beta-lactamase inhibitor should be administered to hospitalized patients. Hospitalized patients at risk for infection with pseudomonas aeruginosa should receive a fluoroquinolone.

Choice of empirical antibiotic therapy for COPD exacerbation	
First-line treatment	**Dosage***
Amoxicillin (Amoxil, Trimox, Wymox)	500 mg tid
Trimethoprim-sulfamethoxazole (Bactrim, Cotrim, Septra)	1 tablet (80/400 mg) bid
Doxycycline	100 mg bid
Erythromycin	250-500 mg qid
Second-line treatment**	
Amoxicillin-clavulanate (Augmentin)	500-875 mg bid
Second- or third-generation cephalosporin (eg, cefuroxime [Ceftin])	250-500 mg bid
Macrolides	
Clarithromycin (Biaxin)	250-500 mg bid
Azithromycin (Zithromax)	500 mg on day 1, then 250 mg qd X 4 days
Quinolones	
Ciprofloxacin (Cipro)	500-750 mg bid
Levofloxacin (Levaquin)***	500 mg qd

*May need adjustment in patients with renal or hepatic insufficiency.
**For patients in whom first-line therapy has failed and those with moderate to severe disease or resistant or gram-negative pathogens.
***Although the newer quinolones have better activity against Streptococcus pneumoniae, ciprofloxacin may be preferable in patients with gram-negative organisms.

6. **Methylxanthines.** Aminophylline and theophylline are not recommended for the management of acute exacerbations of COPD. Randomized controlled trials of intravenous aminophylline in this setting have failed to show efficacy.

F. **Oxygen therapy**

1. Acute hypoxemia during an acute exacerbation of COPD may cause tissue hypoxia. Supplemental oxygen should be given to achieve a target PaO2 of 60 to 65 mmHg, with a hemoglobin saturation around 90 percent.

2. **Venturi masks** are the preferred means of oxygen delivery because they permit a precise delivered fraction of inspired oxygen (FiO2). Venturi masks can deliver an FiO2 of 24, 28, 31, 35, or 40 percent.

3. During oral feedings, nasal cannulae are also more comfortable and convenient for the patient. They can provide flow rates up to 6 L/min with FiO2 of approximately 44 percent.

4. When higher inspired concentrations of oxygen are needed, simple facemasks can provide an FiO2 up to 55 percent using flow rates of 6

to 10 L/min. Non-rebreather masks with a reservoir, one-way valves, and a tight face seal can deliver an inspired oxygen concentration up to 90 percent.

   5. **Adequate oxygenation** must be assured, even if it results in acute hypercapnia due to altered ventilation-perfusion relationships, the Haldane effect of unloading CO2 from oxyhemoglobin, or decreased ventilatory drive. Hypercapnia is generally well tolerated in patients whose PaCO2 is chronically elevated; however, noninvasive positive pressure ventilation or intubation may be required when hypercapnia is associated with depressed mental status, profound acidemia, or cardiac dysrhythmias.

G. **Noninvasive positive pressure ventilation (NIPPV)** is effective and less morbid than intubation for selected patients with acute exacerbations of COPD. Early use of NIPPV is recommended when each of the following is present:

   a. Respiratory distress with moderate-to-severe dyspnea.
   b. pH less than 7.35 or $PaCO_2$ above 45 mm Hg.
   c. Respiratory rate of 25/minute or greater.

   2. NIPPV is contraindicated in the presence of cardiovascular instability (eg, hypotension, serious dysrhythmias, myocardial ischemia), craniofacial trauma or burns, inability to protect the airway, or when indications for emergent intubation are present. Approximately 26 to 31 percent of patients initially treated with NIPPV ultimately require intubation and mechanical ventilation.

H. **Surgical management**
   1. **Lung volume reduction surgery (LVRS)** is recommended in patients with upper lobe predominant disease and low exercise capacity.
   2. **Indications for lung transplantation**
      a. FEV_1 is <25 percent of predicted, **OR**
      b. $PaCO_2$ is >55 mm Hg (7.3 kPa), **OR**
      c. Cor pulmonale is present.
      d. Candidates must be under 65 years of age, not have dysfunction of major organs other than the lung, and not have active or recent malignancy or infection with HIV, hepatitis B, or hepatitis C viruses.

References: See page 294.

Infectious Diseases

Influenza

Influenza is an acute respiratory illness caused by influenza A or B viruses, occurring in outbreaks and epidemics, mainly in the winter season. Signs and symptoms of upper and/or lower respiratory tract involvement are present, along with fever, headache, myalgia, and weakness. Influenza is a self-limited infection in the general population; however, it is associated with increased morbidity and mortality in certain "high risk" populations (complicated influenza).

I. **Uncomplicated influenza**
   A. Influenza characteristically begins with the abrupt onset of fever, headache, myalgia and malaise after an incubation period of one to two days. Cough and sore throat are also present. Influenza infections can range from afebrile respiratory illnesses similar to the common cold, to illnesses in which systemic signs and symptoms predominate with relatively little clinical indication of respiratory tract involvement.
   B. **Physical findings.** The patient may appear hot and flushed; oropharyngeal abnormalities other than hyperemia are uncommon. Mild cervical lymphadenopathy may be present. Chest examination is generally unremarkable in uncomplicated influenza.
   C. Patients with uncomplicated influenza usually gradually improve over two to five days, although the illness may last for one week or more. Some patients have persistent symptoms of weakness or easy fatiguability, (postinfluenza asthenia), which may last for several weeks.

II. **Complications of influenza**
   A. Pneumonia is the most common complication of influenza. Pneumonia occurs most frequently in patients with underlying chronic illnesses.
   B. **Myositis and rhabdomyolysis**
      1. Myositis and rhabdomyolysis, have been reported most frequently in children. Although myalgias are a prominent feature of most cases of influenza, true myositis is uncommon. Evidence for the presence of influenza virus in affected muscles has been noted.
      2. The hallmark of acute myositis is extreme tenderness of the affected muscles, most commonly in the legs. In the most severe cases, swelling and bogginess of the muscles may be noted. Markedly elevated serum creatine phosphokinase (CK) concentrations are seen, and myoglobinuria with associated renal failure has been reported.
   C. **Central nervous system disease.** Influenza may cause encephalitis, transverse myelitis, aseptic meningitis, and Guillain-Barré syndrome.

III. **Diagnosis**
   A. **Clinical diagnosis.** During an influenza outbreak, acute febrile respiratory illnesses brought to the attention of physicians can be diagnosed as influenza with a high degree of certainty by clinical criteria.
   B. Rapid diagnostic tests include immunofluorescence (IF) assays, enzyme immunoassays (EIA), and polymerase chain reaction (PCR)-based testing. All are rapid (range 15 minutes to 2 days).
   C. The Quick Vue A+B and ZstatFlu tests can be used in any office setting. The Quick Vue A+B Test distinguishes between influenza A and B. The Directigen Flu A, FLU OIA, Quick-Vue Influenza Test, and ZstatFlu Test have sensitivities of 72 to 95 percent and specificities of 76 to 84 percent. The ZstatFlu test has a significantly lower sensitivity than the other tests.
   D. PCR-based testing can detect low quantities of viral RNA in specimens such as nasopharyngeal aspirates, BAL, or nasal and throat swabs. These tests are generally more sensitive than culture and specific for both influenza A and B.

E. **Viral culture.** Laboratory diagnosis is accomplished by the detection of virus or viral antigen in throat swabs, nasal washes, sputum, or bronchoalveolar lavage (BAL) specimens. In one study sputum and nasal washes were superior to throat swabs for the isolation of influenza virus. Although viral culture is the gold standard for laboratory diagnosis, it takes 48 to 72 hours.

F. **Recommendations.** Viral cultures are used mainly for epidemiological purposes. For sporadic cases of flu-like illness, rapid diagnostic tests such as EIA or PCR are appropriate.

IV. **Treatment of influenza in adults**

A. Two classes of antiviral drugs are available for the treatment and prevention of influenza:

1. The neuraminidase inhibitors, zanamivir (Relenza) and oseltamivir (Tamiflu), are active against both influenza A and influenza B.

2. Amantadine and rimantadine, are only active against influenza A. However, due to a marked increase in resistant isolates, the Centers for Disease Control and Prevention has issued an alert that these agents should not be used in the United States for treatment.

Comparison of the anti-influenza drugs				
Characteristic	Amantadine (Symmetrel)	Rimantadine (Flumadine)	Zanamivir (Relenza)	Oseltamivir (Tamiflu)
Chemical classification	Adamantamines		Neuraminidase inhibitor	
Spectrum	Influenza A only	Influenza A only	Influenza A and B	Influenza A and B
Side effects	CNS (5%-30%): drowsiness, confusion, seizures, gastrointestinal upset	CNS: <6% Gastrointestinal upset	Bronchospasm in patients with reactive airway disease	Nausea and vomiting (8%-10%)
Approved indications	Treatment and prophylaxis of adults and children >1 yr	Treatment and prophylaxis of adults Treatment of children >14 yr and prophylaxis >1 yr	Treatment of adults and children >7 yr	Treatment of adults >18 yr Prophylaxis of adults and children >13 yr
Treatment dose	200 mg/d or 100 mg PO bid		10 mg inhaled powder bid	75 mg PO bid
Prophylaxis dose	Adults: 200 mg/d or 100 mg bid		10 mg inhaled powder qd	75 mg qd
Length of therapy	5-7 or 1-2 days after symptoms resolve		5 days	5 days
Length of prophylaxis	10 days	10 days	Undetermined	7 days post-exposure, 42 days seasonal outbreak

B. **Benefits of therapy.** The benefit of treatment is greatest (two to three day shortening of the duration of symptoms) when given within the first 24 to 30 hours and in patients with fever at presentation.

C. **Neuraminidase inhibitors.** Zanamivir and oseltamivir are approved for the treatment of influenza in adults. Each drug is moderately effective, reducing the duration and severity of symptoms, particularly when treatment is initiated on the first day of illness.
   1. **Zanamivir (Relenza)** is administered by oral inhalation. The inhibitory effect begins within 10 seconds.
   2. **Oseltamivir (Temiflu)** is orally administered and is available as a capsule or powder for liquid suspension. It has good bioavailability. Since the drug in primarily excreted by the kidneys, dosing must be modified in renal insufficiency.
   3. **Side effects.** Zanamivir can cause bronchospasm in patients with asthma and other chronic respiratory conditions. Oseltamivir can cause nausea and vomiting.
D. **M2 inhibitors**, also known as adamantanes, are active against only influenza A viruses and are used for both treatment and chemoprophylaxis of influenza A infection.
   1. **Side effects.** Use of amantadine is associated with a discontinuation rate of 13 to 17 percent because of anxiety, insomnia, impaired thinking, confusion, lightheadedness, and hallucinations. Such toxicity is more common in the elderly.
   2. Rimantadine causes fewer central nervous system side effects than amantadine.
   3. **Resistance** can occur spontaneously or emerge on therapy as rapidly as two to three days following initiation of M2 inhibitor treatment.
   4. The CDC has recommended against the use of amantadine or rimantadine for treatment or prevention of influenza.
E. **Drug dosing** — The doses of zanamivir (Relenza, 10 mg [two inhalations] twice daily) and oseltamivir (Tamiflu, 75 mg twice daily) do not need to be reduced in elderly patients. The recommended duration of therapy is five days.

V. **Antiviral drugs for the prevention of influenza in adults**
   A. The neuraminidase inhibitors, zanamivir and oseltamivir, are active against both influenza A and influenza B.
   B. Amantadine and rimantadine, which are only active against influenza A. However, due to a marked increase in resistant isolates, the Centers for Disease Control and Prevention has issued an alert that these agents should not be used in the United States for preventive therapy.
   C. Antiviral drugs should not be used as a substitute for influenza vaccination. Their adjunctive application is appropriate in certain situations, particularly outbreaks in hospitals, nursing homes and other long-term care facilities.
   D. **Neuraminidase inhibitors.** Oseltamivir is the only neuraminidase inhibitor approved by the FDA for prophylaxis of influenza. However, available data suggest that the efficacy of zanamivir is comparable to that of oseltamivir.
      1. Prophylactic therapy with oseltamivir or zanamivir was associated with a relative reduction in the odds of developing influenza of 70 to 90 percent.
      2. Zanamivir recipients had significantly fewer episodes of laboratory confirmed clinical influenza (2 versus 6 percent), laboratory confirmed clinical influenza with fever (<1 versus 3 percent), or any febrile illness (6 versus 10 percent).
      3. **Side effects** of neuraminidase inhibitors have generally been mild.
      4. Zanamivir can cause bronchospasm and a decline in respiratory function in patients with asthma and other chronic respiratory disorders. The ready availability of a fast acting bronchodilator if it is used in such patients.
      5. Oseltamivir can cause nausea and vomiting but these side effects have not generally resulted in discontinuation of therapy.
   E. **Target populations.** Antiviral prophylaxis during peak influenza activity is recommended for the following populations:

   1. Persons at high risk for complications of influenza who receive the vaccine after influenza activity has begun in a community, since the development of antibodies can take two weeks
   2. To individuals who provide care to those at high risk (eg, healthcare workers) if they are unvaccinated or the outbreak is caused by a variant strain that might not be controlled by the vaccine
   3. Persons expected to mount an inadequate response to the vaccine, such as those with advanced HIV infection.
   4. Other persons at high risk for complications of influenza or who wish to avoid influenza who cannot receive the vaccine

   F. Administration of antiviral drugs for both treatment and prevention should be a central component of influenza outbreak control in nursing homes and other health care institutions. Chemoprophylaxis is recommended for all residents of an institution during an outbreak, even if they had been vaccinated during the previous fall, and should be continued for at least two weeks or for one week after the end of the outbreak. Rapid recognition of the outbreak (defined as ≥2 cases) is an important determinant of the efficacy of antiviral prophylaxis.
   G. Chemoprophylaxis can also be offered to unvaccinated health care workers who provide care to patients at high risk, and should be considered for all employees if the outbreak is known to be caused by a strain of influenza A poorly covered by the season's vaccine.

VI. **Drug dosing.** The recommended dose of oseltamivir (Tamiflu) is 75 mg/day; zanamivir has not been approved for prophylaxis.
   A. Prophylactic antiviral therapy should begin within two days after exposure to an infected individual and should be given for seven to ten days.
   B. During community outbreaks, prophylaxis in unvaccinated individuals may be given throughout the period of peak influenza activity or throughout the entire influenza season (usually six to eight weeks). The development of immunity following vaccination takes about two weeks; therefore, prophylactic therapy should be considered for high-risk patients from the time of vaccination until immunity has developed.

References: See page 294.

Community-acquired Pneumonia

Pneumonia is the sixth most common cause of death in the United States. Community-acquired pneumonia (CAP) is defined as an acute infection of the pulmonary parenchyma in a patient who has acquired the infection in the community.

I. **Clinical evaluation**
   A. Common clinical features of CAP include cough, fever, pleurisy, dyspnea and sputum production. Mucopurulent sputum production is most frequently found in association with bacterial pneumonia, while scant or watery sputum is suggestive of an atypical pathogen.
   B. Other common features are nausea, vomiting, diarrhea, and mental status changes. Chest pain occurs in 30 percent of cases, chills in 40 to 50 percent, and rigors in 15 percent.
   C. **Physical examination.** Fever is present in 80 percent, although frequently absent in older patients. A respiratory rate above 24 breaths/minute is noted in 45 to 70 percent of patients and may be the most sensitive sign in the elderly; tachycardia is also common. Chest examination reveals rales in most patients, while one-third have evidence of consolidation.
   D. The major blood test abnormality is leukocytosis (15,000 and 30,000 per mm^3) with a leftward shift. Leukopenia can occur, and generally has a poor prognosis.

II. **Radiologic evaluation.** An infiltrate on plain chest radiograph is considered the "gold standard" for diagnosing pneumonia and should be obtained in most patients. The radiographic appearances of CAP include lobar consolidation, interstitial infiltrates, and cavitation. Bacterial pneumonia and nonbacterial pneumonia can not be differentiated on the basis of the radiographic appearance.

III. **Diagnostic testing for microbial etiology**
  A. **Outpatients.** Culture and Gram's stain are usually not done in outpatients.
  B. **Hospitalized patients.** Blood cultures and sputum Gram's stain and culture should be obtained in hospitalized patients with suspected CAP.
  C. Blood cultures are positive for a pathogen in 7 to 16 percent of hospitalized patients. Streptococcus pneumoniae accounts for two-thirds of the positive blood cultures.
  D. The preferred tests for Legionella are culture on selective media and the urinary antigen assay. A new polymerase chain reaction (PCR) test that detects L. pneumophila (all serogroups) in respiratory secretions may become the preferred method to detect Legionella infection.
  E. **Urine antigen assays** are complementary methods to detect S. pneumoniae and Legionella. The advantages are:
    1. Results of urine antigen testing are immediately available.
    2. The test retains validity even after the initiation of antibiotic therapy.
    3. The test has high sensitivity compared to blood cultures and sputum studies.
  F. The pneumococcal urinary antigen assay is an acceptable test to augment blood culture and sputum Gram's stain and culture, with the potential advantage of rapid results similar to those for sputum Gram's stain.

Causes of Community-acquired Pneumonia	
Etiology	**Prevalence (percent)**
Streptococcus pneumoniae	20-60
Hemophilus influenzae	3-10
Staphylococcus aureus	3-5
Gram-negative bacilli	3-10
Aspiration	6-10
Miscellaneous	3-5
Legionella sp.	2-8
Mycoplasma pneumoniae	1-6
Chlamydia pneumoniae	4-6
Viruses	2-15

IV. **Organisms of special interest**
  A. **Streptococcus pneumoniae** accounts for about 65 percent of bacteremic pneumonia cases and is the most common identified pathogen in nearly all studies.
  B. **Staphylococcus aureus** is an infrequent pulmonary pathogen.
  C. **Influenza** is important to recognize because of the need for appropriate infection control in hospitalized patients, for public health reporting purposes, and for rapid treatment with antiviral agents. The rapid antigen assays provide results in 15 to 20 minutes.
  D. **Legionella spp** is implicated in 2 to 10 percent of CAP cases. Legionella is important to identify because of the potential to cause epidemics (usually in hospitals and hotels) and because Legionella spp infection has a relatively high mortality.
  E. **Chlamydia pneumoniae** is implicated in 10 to 30 percent of cases of CAP in adults. Diagnostic testing consists of PCR.
  F. **Mycoplasma pneumoniae** has historically been considered a pathogen primarily of children and adolescents, but there are reports of increasingly high rates of infection in adults, especially elderly adults.
  G. **Bioterrorism agents** that may be used for bioterrorism and can present as a CAP syndrome include Bacillus anthracis (inhalational anthrax),

Yersinia pestis (pneumonic plague), Francisella tularensis (tularemia), Coxiella burnetii (Q fever), Legionella spp, Influenza virus, and hantavirus.

V. Summary and recommendations

  A. The combination of sputum specimen for Gram's stain and culture plus urinary pneumococcal antigen testing is likely to be most useful for the rapid diagnosis of CAP in hospitalized patients. In addition, hospitalized patients should have pretreatment blood cultures.

  B. The blood culture positivity rate is relatively low, but when positive establishes the microbial diagnosis.

VI. Treatment of community-acquired pneumonia in adults

  A. Indications for hospitalization. Inability to maintain oral intake, history of substance abuse, cognitive impairment, and poor functional status.

  B. Initial antimicrobial therapy should provide coverage for S. pneumoniae plus atypical pathogens (particularly M. pneumoniae or C. pneumoniae, which are common causes of outpatient CAP). The macrolides, which are effective against the atypical pathogens, are therefore recommended when there are no significant risk factors for macrolide-resistant S. pneumoniae.

  C. Recommendations for outpatient therapy

  1. Patients treated with an effective drug usually improve within 72 hours. Median time to resolution is three days for fever, six days for dyspnea, and 14 days for both cough and fatigue. Patients who do not improve within 72 hours are considered nonresponders.

  2. No comorbidities or recent antibiotic use. For uncomplicated pneumonia in patients who do not require hospitalization, have no significant comorbidities, or use of antibiotics within the last three months, one of the following oral regimens is recommended:

   a. Azithromycin (Zithromax, 500 mg on day one followed by four days of 250 mg a day); 500 mg a day for three days or 2 g single dose (microsphere formulation).

   b. Clarithromycin XL (Biaxin XL, two 500 mg tablets daily) for five days or until afebrile for 48 to 72 hours.

   c. Doxycycline (100 mg twice a day) for seven to 10 days

  3. Comorbidities or recent antibiotic use. For pneumonia in patients who do not require hospitalization, but who have significant comorbidities (ie, chronic obstructive pulmonary disease, liver or renal disease, cancer, diabetes, heart disease, alcoholism, asplenia, or immunosuppression), or use of antibiotics within prior three months, one of the following oral regimens is recommended:

   a. A respiratory fluoroquinolone (gemifloxacin [Factive] 320 mg daily or levofloxacin [Levaquin] 750 mg daily or moxifloxacin [Avelox] 400 mg daily).

   b. Combination therapy with a beta-lactam effective against S. pneumoniae (high-dose amoxicillin, 1 gm three times daily or amoxicillin clavulanate [Augmentin] 2 g twice daily or cefpodoxime [Vantin] 200 mg twice daily or cefuroxime [Ceftin] 500 mg twice daily) plus either a macrolide (azithromycin [Zithromax]500 mg on day one followed by four days of 250 mg a day or clarithromycin [Biaxin]250 mg twice daily or clarithromycin XL 1000 mg once daily) or doxycycline (100 mg twice daily).

   c. These regimens are also appropriate in patients without comorbidities or recent antimicrobial use in locations where the prevalence of "high-level" macrolide-resistant S. pneumoniae is high. When choosing between fluoroquinolones, moxifloxacin and gemifloxacin in vitro are progressively more active against penicillin-resistant pneumococci strains than levofloxacin. Gemifloxacin causes a mild rash in 2.8 percent of patients, but an unexpectedly higher rate (14 percent) in women under 40 years of age.

   d. Patients should be treated for a minimum of five days, and therapy should not be stopped until patients are afebrile for 48 to 72 hours.

Longer duration of therapy is required if there is an extrapulmonary infection or for infections caused by S. aureus or Pseudomonas.

Recommended Empiric Drug Therapy for Patients with Community-Acquired Pneumonia

Clinical Situation	Primary Treatment	Alternative(s)
Younger (<60 yr) out-patients without under-lying disease	Macrolide antibiotics (azithromycin, clarithromycin, dirithromycin, or erythromycin)	Levofloxacin or doxycycline
Older (>60 yr) outpa-tients with underlying disease	Levofloxacin or cefuroxime or Trimethoprim-sulfa-methoxazole Add vancomycin in severe, life-threatening pneumonias	Beta-lactamase inhibitor (with macrolide if legionella infec-tion suspected)
Gross aspiration sus-pected	Clindamycin IV	Cefotetan, ampicillin/sulbactam

Common Antimicrobial Agents for Community-Acquired Pneumonia in Adults

Type	Agent	Dosage
Oral therapy		
Macrolides	Erythromycin Clarithromycin (Biaxin) Azithromycin (Zithromax)	500 mg PO qid 500 mg PO bid 500 mg PO on day 1, then 250 mg qd x 4 days
Beta-lactam/beta-lactamase inhibitor	Amoxicillin-clavulanate (Augmentin) Augmentin XR	500 mg tid or 875 mg PO bid 2 tabs q12h
Quinolones	Ciprofloxacin (Cipro) Levofloxacin (Levaquin) Ofloxacin (Floxin)	500 mg PO bid 500 mg PO qd 400 mg PO bid
Tetracycline	Doxycycline	100 m g PO bid
Sulfonamide	Trimethoprim-sulfamethoxazole	160 mg/800 mg (DS) PO bid

Type	Agent	Dosage
Intravenous Therapy		
Cephalosporins Second-generation	Cefuroxime (Kefurox, Zinacef)	0.75-1.5 g IV q8h
Third-generation (anti-Pseudomonas aeruginosa)	Ceftizoxime (Cefizox) Ceftazidime (Fortaz) Cefoperazone (Cefobid)	1-2 g IV q8h 1-2 g IV q8h 1-2 g IV q8h
Beta-lactam/beta-lactamase inhibitors	Ampicillin-sulbactam (Unasyn) Piperacillin/tazobactam (Zosyn) Ticarcillin-clavulanate (Timentin)	1.5 g IV q6h 3.375 g IV q6h 3.1 g IV q6h
Quinolones	Ciprofloxacin (Cipro) Levofloxacin (Levaquin) Ofloxacin (Floxin)	400 mg IV q12h 500 mg IV q24h 400 mg IV q12h
Aminoglycosides	Gentamicin Amikacin	Load 2.0 mg/kg IV, then 1.5 mg/kg q8h
Vancomycin	Vancomycin	1 gm IV q12h

A. Recommendations for hospitalized patients

1. Hospitalized patients with CAP are initially treated with empiric antibiotic therapy. When the etiology of CAP has been identified, treatment regimens may be simplified and directed to that pathogen.
2. **Not in the ICU**. For patients admitted to a general ward, one of the following regimens is recommended:
3. Combination therapy with ceftriaxone (Rocephin, 2 g IV daily; 1 g IV daily in patients >65 years of age) or cefotaxime (Claforan, 1 g IV every 8 hours) plus azithromycin (Zithromax, 500 mg IV daily) **OR**
4. Monotherapy with a respiratory fluoroquinolone given either IV or orally except as noted (levofloxacin, [Levaquin] 750 mg daily or moxifloxacin [Avelox] 400 mg daily or gemifloxacin [Factive] 320 mg daily (only available in oral formulation).
5. **Admitted to an intensive care unit.** Patients requiring admission to an ICU are more likely to have risk factors for resistant pathogens, including the possibility of community-associated MRSA. Treatment consists of an intravenous combination therapy with a potent antipneumococcal beta-lactam (ceftriaxone 2 g daily or cefotaxime 1 g every eight hours) plus either an advanced macrolide (azithromycin 500 mg daily) or a respiratory fluoroquinolone (levofloxacin 750 mg daily or moxifloxacin 400 mg daily).
6. **Patients who may be infected with Pseudomonas aeruginosa** or other resistant pathogens (particularly those with bronchiectasis or COPD with frequent antimicrobial or corticosteroid use) should be treated with agents that are effective against pneumococcus, P. aeruginosa, and Legionella spp. Regimens include the following:
   a. **Combination therapy with a beta-lactam antibiotic** such as piperacillin-tazobactam (Zosyn, 4.5 g every six hours) OR imipenem (Primaxin, 500 mg IV every six hours) OR meropenem (Merrem, 1 g every eight hours) OR cefepime (Maxipime, 2 g every eight hours) OR ceftazidime (Fortaz, 2 g every 8 hours) PLUS either ciprofloxacin (Cipro, 400 mg every 8 hours) OR levofloxacin

(Levaquin, 750 mg daily). For beta-lactam allergic patients, aztreonam (Azactam) plus levofloxacin (750 mg daily).

   b. **For severely ill patients,** early Gram's stain of respiratory secretions should be completed. If S. aureus is suspected by Gram's stain, the addition of **vancomycin** (15 mg/kg every 12 hours, adjusted for renal function) or **linezolid (Zyvox,** 600 mg every 12 hours). In addition, we suggest empiric therapy of MRSA in patients with severe CAP who have risk factors for CA-MRSA, such as, prior antimicrobial therapy or recent influenza-like illness.

7. **Response to therapy.** With appropriate antibiotic therapy, some improvement in the patient's clinical course is usually seen within 48 to 72 hours. However, fever in patients with lobar pneumonia may take 72 hours or longer to improve. With pneumococcal pneumonia, the cough usually resolves within eight days and auscultatory crackles clear within three weeks.

8. **Duration of therapy.** Among hospitalized patients who have received initial therapy with intravenous antibiotics, switching to oral therapy may occur when the patient is improving, hemodynamically stable, and able to take oral medications.

9. **Treatment of hospitalized patients** should be continued for a minimum of five days. The patient should be afebrile for 48 to 72 hours, breathing without supplemental oxygen (unless required for preexisting disease), and have no more than one clinical instability factor (defined as heart rate [HR] >100 beats/min, respiratory rate [RR] >24 breaths/min, and systolic blood pressure [SBP] of ≤90 mm Hg) before stopping therapy.

References: See page 294.

Acute Sinusitis and Rhinosinusitis

Acute sinusitis is caused by infection of one or more of the paranasal sinuses. Viral infection is the most frequent causes of acute sinusitis. Only two percent of viral rhinosinusitis is complicated by acute bacterial sinusitis. Uncomplicated viral rhinosinusitis usually resolves in seven to ten days. Complications of untreated acute bacterial sinusitis include intracranial and orbital complications, and chronic sinus disease.

I. **Microbial etiology**
   A. Viral. Rhinovirus, parainfluenza, and influenza viruses have all been recovered from sinus aspirates of patients with colds and influenza-like illnesses.
   B. Bacterial. Bacterial sinusitis can be divided into community-acquired and nosocomial infections.
   C. Community-acquired bacterial sinusitis is usually a complication of viral rhinosinusitis, occurring in 0.5 to 2 percent of cases. Other risk factors include nasal allergy, swimming, intranasal cocaine use, problems with mucociliary clearance (eg, cystic fibrosis, cilial dysfunction), and immunodeficiency states (eg, HIV). Patients with nasal obstruction due to polyps, foreign bodies or tumors are also at risk.
   D. The most common bacterial organisms are Streptococcus pneumoniae and Haemophilus influenzae. S. pneumoniae and H. influenzae are each responsible for 35 percent of cases in adults.
II. **Clinical manifestations**
   A. Symptoms of acute sinusitis include nasal congestion, purulent nasal discharge, maxillary tooth discomfort, hyposmia, and facial pain or pressure that is worse when bending forward. Headache, fever (nonacute), halitosis, fatigue, cough, ear pain, and ear fullness are symptoms of rhinosinusitis.

Microbial causes of acute sinusitis
Viral
Rhinovirus Parainfluenza virus Influenza virus Coronavirus Respiratory syncytial virus Adenovirus
Bacterial
Community-acquired Streptococcus pneumoniae Haemophilus influenzae Moraxella catarrhalis Other streptococcal species Staphylococcus aureus Anaerobic bacteria
Nosocomial Staphylococcus aureus Streptococcal species Pseudomonas species Escherichia coli Klebsiella species Other Gram negative bacteria Anaerobic bacteria Candida species
Fungal
Aspergillus species Pseudallescheria boydii Sporothrix schenckii Homobasidiomycetes Phaeohyphomycosis Zygomycetes

B. **Diagnosis**. Since rhinoviral infection typically improves in seven to ten days, a patient with a cold or influenza-like illness that has persisted without improvement or has worsened over seven to ten days may have developed bacterial sinusitis. The presence of nasal discharge, particularly if purulent, and/or maxillary pain or tenderness in the face or teeth, particularly if unilateral, is suggestive of acute bacterial sinusitis. Fever with facial pain, swelling, and erythema may develop.

C. Patients with acute bacterial sinusitis may give a history of tooth pain, foul odor to the breath, and other signs of dental infection.

D. Sinus aspirate culture is the gold standard for making a microbial diagnosis in sinus infection. However, this procedure is not appropriate for use in routine medical practice. Sinus aspirate culture should be considered if there is a suspicion of intracranial extension of the infection or other serious complications.

E. **Radiologic tests.** Imaging studies are not indicated in the usual case of acute community-acquired sinusitis, unless intracranial or orbital complications are suspected. CT scanning is the imaging procedure of choice as it provides better sensitivity than plain x-ray. However, neither test can distinguish viral from bacterial infection. One limitation of CT scanning is that it is frequently abnormal in patients with the common cold.

1. Magnetic resonance imaging (MRI) can be used to demonstrate intracranial spread of infection but is not as good as CT scanning for the diagnosis of acute sinusitis.
2. Plain films of the sinuses are not recommended. If imaging is performed, CT is the usual test of choice.

III. **Treatment of acute bacterial sinusitis**

A. Treatment for acute bacterial sinusitis should be considered in patients with persistent symptoms after seven to ten days and at least one of the following:
   1. Maxillary pain or tenderness/pressure in the face or teeth
   2. Purulent nasal discharge
   3. Postnasal discharge
   4. Cough

B. **Viral rhinosinusitis**
   1. Used in combination, chlorpheniramine (12 mg sustained release) and ibuprofen (400 mg) are effective in reducing nasal mucus and the severity of sneezing, rhinorrhea, sore throat, cough, malaise, and headache.

C. **Community-acquired bacterial sinusitis**
   1. **Choice of antibiotics.** The development of beta-lactamase production by H. influenzae and M. catarrhalis and of multiple antibiotic resistance by S. pneumoniae has limited the selection of antimicrobials that provide adequate coverage of these common bacteria in community-acquired sinusitis. Cephalexin and the macrolides generally either do not provide the necessary antibacterial spectrum or are associated with too much resistance among pneumococci.
   2. **Amoxicillin** is recommended at the higher end of the dose range (eg, 1 g three times per day). Contact in children with daycare centers or recent antibiotic use warrants broader spectrum antibiotics.
   3. Antibiotics that cover resistant S. pneumoniae, H. influenzae, and M. catarrhalis: amoxicillin-clavulanate (Augmentin, 875-125 mg every 12 hours) for 7 to 10 days, cefpodoxime (Vantin, 200 mg every 12 hours), cefdinir (Omnicef, 600 mg once daily), levofloxacin (Levaquin, 500 mg once daily) or moxifloxacin (Avelox, 400 mg once daily).

Antibiotics for acute community-acquired bacterial sinusitis	
Drug	**Dose**
Amoxicillin-clavulanate (Augmentin)	875/125 mg q12h
Cefpodoxime proxetil (Vantin)	200 mg q12h
Cefdinir (Omnicef)	600 mg qd
Levofloxacin (Levaquin)	500 mg qd
Moxifloxacin (Avelox)	400 mg qd

4. A seven to ten day course of antimicrobial treatment is recommended. This duration of therapy can be expected to provide a 90 percent or better bacterial eradication rate in cases of acute community-acquired sinusitis.
5. **Treatment failure.** One alternative is to give a second, more prolonged course of treatment with another antibiotic (particularly if a narrow spectrum antibiotic was used as first-line therapy). Another approach is to obtain a sinus CT scan and refer the patient to an otolaryngologist for sinus aspirate culture and sinus washing, followed by another course of antibiotics.
6. **Sinus surgery** should be strongly considered in patients with CT-confirmed sinus disease persisting over several months despite adequate medical management. Endoscopic sinus surgery is successful in 85 percent of cases.

7. **Nosocomial bacterial sinusitis**. Treatment should be based upon sinus aspirate culture and sensitivity data when available. If such information is not available, antimicrobial coverage should be directed at S. aureus and the Gram negative bacteria which commonly infect the respiratory tract.
8. **Complications of acute bacterial sinusitis**, which now rarely occur, include meningitis, orbital cellulitis, and osteitis of the sinus bones.

References: See page 294.

Tonsillopharyngitis

In about a quarter of patients with a sore throat, the disorder is caused by group A beta-hemolytic streptococcus. Treatment of streptococcal tonsillopharyngitis reduces the occurrence of subsequent rheumatic fever, an inflammatory disease that affects the joints and heart, skin, central nervous system, and subcutaneous tissues.

I. **Prevalence of pharyngitis**
   A. Group A beta-hemolytic streptococcus (GABHS) typically occurs in patients 5-11 years of age, and it is uncommon in children under 3 years old. Most cases of GABHS occur in late winter and early spring.
   B. **Etiologic causes of sore throat**
      1. **Viral.** Rhinoviruses, influenza, Epstein-Barr virus
      2. **Bacterial.** GABHS (Streptococcus pyogenes), Streptococcus pneumoniae, Haemophilus influenzae, Moraxella catarrhalis, Staphylococcus aureus, anaerobes, Mycoplasma pneumoniae, Candida albicans.
   C. In patients who present with pharyngitis, the major goal is to detect GABHS infection because rheumatic fever may result. Severe GABHS infections may also cause a toxic-shock-like illness (toxic strep syndrome), bacteremia, streptococcal deep tissue infections (necrotizing fasciitis), and streptococcal cellulitis.
II. **Clinical evaluation of sore throat**
   A. GABHS infection is characterized by sudden onset of sore throat, fever and tender swollen anterior cervical lymph nodes, typically in a child 5-11 years of age. Headache, nausea and vomiting may occur.
   B. Cough, rhinorrhea and hoarseness are generally absent.
III. **Physical examination**
   A. Streptococcal infection is suggested by erythema and swelling of the pharynx, enlarged and erythematous tonsils, tonsillar exudate, or palatal petechiae. The clinical diagnosis of GABHS infection is correct in only 50-75% of cases when based on clinical criteria alone.
   B. Unilateral inflammation and swelling of the pharynx suggests peritonsillar abscess. Distortion of the posterior pharyngeal wall suggests a retropharyngeal abscess. Corynebacterium diphtheriae is indicated by a dull membrane which bleeds on manipulation. Viral infections may cause oral vesicular eruptions.
   C. The tympanic membranes should be examined for erythema or a middle ear effusion.
   D. The lungs should be auscultated because viral infection occasionally causes pneumonia.
IV. **Diagnostic testing**
   A. Rapid streptococcal testing has a specificity of 90% and a sensitivity of 80%. A dry swab should be used to sample both the posterior wall and the tonsillar fossae, especially erythematous or exudative areas.
   B. **Throat culture** is the most accurate test available for the diagnosis of GABHS pharyngitis.
   C. **Clinical predictors.** Physicians are not able to reliably predict which patients will have a positive throat culture for GAS; sensitivity and speci-

ficity estimates range from 55 to 74 and 58 to 76 percent, respectively. The Centor criteria include:
1. Tonsillar exudates.
2. Tender anterior cervical adenopathy.
3. Fever by history.
4. Absence of cough.
5. If three or four of these criteria are met, the positive predictive value are 40 to 60 percent. However, the absence of three or four of the criteria has a fairly high negative predictive value of 80 percent.

D. Diagnostic tests
1. Throat cultures are the "gold standard" for diagnosing GAS pharyngitis. However, cultures take 24 to 48 hours to grow and thus cannot be used to decide which patients merit antibiotic therapy. Throat culture has a 90 percent and specificity of 95 to 99 percent.
2. **Rapid Antigen Test (RAT)** uses enzyme or acid extraction of antigen from throat swabs. The diagnostic accuracy shows a sensitivity of 80 to 90 percent and specificity of 90 to 100 percent.

E. Reasons to treat a streptococcal pharyngitis with antibiotics:
1. To prevent rheumatic fever — treatment works, but this complication has nearly disappeared in North America.
2. To prevent peritonsillar abscess — again a vanishing complication.
3. To reduce symptoms, there is a modest (approximately one day) reduction in symptoms with early treatment.
4. To prevent transmission — this is important in pediatrics due to extensive exposures.

V. Recommendations: Using the Centor criteria and the rapid antigen test (RAT):
A. Empirically treat patients who have all four clinical criteria (fever, tonsillar exudate, tender anterior cervical adenopathy, and absence of cough).
B. Do not treat with antibiotics or perform diagnostic tests on patients with zero or one criterion.
C. Perform RAT on those with two or three criteria and use antibiotic treatment only for patients with positive RAT results.
D. Another approach is to treat empirically those adults with three or four of the clinical criteria.

VI. Antibiotic therapy
A. Starting antibiotic therapy within the first 24-48 hours of illness decreases the duration of sore throat, fever and adenopathy by 12-24 hours. Treatment also minimizes risk of transmission and of rheumatic fever.
B. Penicillin VK is the antibiotic of choice for GABHS; 250 mg PO qid or 500 mg PO bid x 10 days [250, 500 mg]. A 10-day regimen is recommended. Penicillin G benzathine (Bicillin LA) may be used as one-time therapy when compliance is a concern; 1.2 million units IM x 1 dose.
C. Azithromycin (Zithromax) offers the advantage of once-a-day dosing for just 5 days; 500 mg x 1, then 250 mg qd x 4 days [6 pack].
D. Clarithromycin (Biaxin), 500 mg PO bid; bacteriologic efficacy is similar to that of penicillin VK, and it may be taken twice a day.
E. Erythromycin is also effective; 250 mg PO qid; or enteric coated delayed release tablet (PCE) 333 mg PO tid or 500 mg PO bid [250, 333, 500 mg]. **Erythromycin ethyl succinate (EES)** 400 PO qid or 800 mg PO bid [400 mg]. Gastrointestinal upset is common.

VII. Treatment of recurrent GABHS pharyngitis
A. When patient compliance is an issue, an injection of penicillin G benzathine may be appropriate. When patient compliance is not an issue, therapy should be changed to a broader spectrum agent.
1. **Cephalexin (Keflex)** 250-500 mg tid x 5 days [250, 500 mg]
2. **Cefadroxil (Duricef)** 500 mg bid x 5 days [500 mg]
3. **Loracarbef (Lorabid)** 200-400 mg bid x 5 days [200, 400 mg]
4. **Cefixime (Suprax)** 400 mg qd x 5 days [200, 400 mg]
5. **Ceftibuten (Cedax)** 400 mg qd x 5 days [400 mg]

6. **Cefuroxime axetil (Ceftin)** 250-500 mg bid x 5 days [125, 250, 500 mg]
   B. **Amoxicillin-clavulanate (Augmentin)** has demonstrated superior results in comparison with penicillin; 250-500 mg tid or 875 mg bid [250, 500, 875 mg].
   C. Sulfonamides, trimethoprim, and the tetracyclines are not effective for the treatment of GABHS pharyngitis.

References: See page 294.

Primary Care of the HIV-Infected Adult

I. **Initial evaluation**
   A. The initial evaluation of the HIV-infected adult should include an assessment of the patient's past medical history, current symptoms and treatments, a complete physical examination, and laboratory testing.
   B. **Previous conditions**
      1. Prior medical conditions related to HIV infection should be assessed. Mucocutaneous candidiasis, oral hairy leukoplakia, hepatitis, pneumonia, sexually transmitted diseases, and tuberculosis should be sought. Past episodes of varicella-zoster, herpes simplex virus lesions, and opportunistic infections should be assessed.
      2. Dates and results of earlier tuberculin skin tests should be obtained. Women should be are asked about dates and results of Pap smears. Previous immunizations and antiretroviral therapy should be documented.
   C. **Current conditions and symptoms.** Fever, night sweats, unexplained weight loss, lymphadenopathy, oral discomfort, visual changes, unusual headaches, swallowing difficulties, diarrhea, dermatologic conditions, and respiratory and neurologic symptoms are suggestive of opportunistic infections or a malignant process.
   D. **Social history** includes information on past and present drug use, sexual behavior, dietary habits, household pets, employment, and current living situation. Residence and travel history should be assessed because coccidioidomycosis and histoplasmosis are more common in certain geographic regions.

II. **Physical examination**
   A. Weight, temperature, skin, oropharynx, fundi, lymph nodes, lungs, abdominal organs, genitalia, rectum, and the nervous system should be assessed. A cervical Pap smear should be obtained from women who have not had a normal result in the past year.
   B. Screening for Neisseria gonorrhoeae and chlamydial infection should be considered for sexually active men and women.

III. **Laboratory tests**
   A. **Complete blood count, chemistry profile, and serologic studies** for syphilis (rapid plasma reagin or VDRL), Toxoplasma gondii (IgG antibody), and hepatitis B (surface antigen, core antibody) should be obtained.
   B. Patients should have a tuberculin skin test unless they have been reactive in the past or have been treated for the disease. In HIV-infected persons, a positive test is 5 mm or more of induration.
   C. **A baseline chest film** is useful because many opportunistic pulmonary infections present with very subtle radiographic findings. A chest radiograph may suggest unrecognized tuberculosis.
   D. **CD4$^+$ counts** assist in determination of the degree of immunologic damage, assess risk of opportunistic complications, and guide the use of prophylaxis against infections.
   E. **HIV RNA levels**
      1. Quantitation of plasma HIV RNA (viral load), a marker of the rate of viral replication, is useful in determining prognosis. It is used to estimate the risk of disease progression and to aid in making antiretroviral therapy decisions.

2. HIV RNA levels generally vary no more than 0.3 log in clinically stable patients. Sustained changes greater than threefold (0.5 log) are significant. A decrease occurs with successful antiretroviral therapy. Increases noted during treatment suggest antiretroviral drug failure or poor adherence.

Treatment Goals for HIV RNA Levels	
Parameter	Recommendation
Target level of HIV RNA after initiation of treatment	Undetectable; <below 50 copies of HIV RNA per mL
Minimal decrease in HIV RNA indicative of antiretroviral activity	>0.5 $\log_{10}$ decrease
Change in HIV RNA that suggests drug treatment failure	Rise in HIV RNA level Failure to achieve desired reduction in HIV RNA level
Suggested frequency of HIV RNA measurement	At baseline: 2 measurements, 2-4 wk apart. 3-4 wk after initiating or changing therapy Every 3-4 mo in conjunction with $CD4^+$ counts

3. HIV RNA levels should be obtained before the initiation or change of antiretroviral therapy. The next determination should be done a month after therapeutic intervention to assess its effect and then every 3 or 4 months.
4. Quantitative HIV RNA assays include branched DNA (bDNA) (Multiplex) and reverse transcriptase-initiated polymerase chain reaction (RT-PCR) (Amplicor HIV-1 Monitor). While both tests provide similar information, concentrations of HIV RNA obtained with the RT-PCR test are about twofold higher than those obtained by the bDNA method. For this reason, all HIV RNA determinations in a single patient should be obtained using the same assay.

IV. **Antiretroviral therapy**
   A. Antiretroviral drug regimens may suppress HIV replication almost completely in some patients. These changes are associated with improved survival and a lengthening in the time to development of AIDS-defining conditions.

Antiretroviral Therapy
Initiate therapy for patients with: Symptomatic HIV disease Asymptomatic HIV disease but $CD4^+$ count <350 cells/μL HIV RNA levels >30,000 (bDNA) or >55,000 (RT-PCR)
Consider therapy for patients with: Detectable HIV RNA levels who request it and are committed to lifelong adherence

---

Change therapy for:
  Treatment failure, as indicated by
    Rising HIV RNA level
    Failure to achieve target decrease in HIV RNA
    Declining CD4$^+$ count
    Clinical progression
  Toxicity, intolerance, or nonadherance

Recommended Antiretroviral Agents for Initial Treatment of Established HIV Infection

Antiretroviral drug regimens are comprised of one choice each from columns A and B. Drugs are listed in alphabetical order.

Column A	Column B
Efavirenz (Sustiva)	Didanosine (Videx) + Lamivudine (Epivir)
Indinavir (Crixivan)	Stavudine (Zerit) + Didanosine
Nelfinavir (Viracept)	Stavudine + Lamivudine
Ritonavir (Norvir) + Indinavir (Kaletra)	Zidovudine (Retrovir) + Didanosine
Ritonavir + Lopinavir	Zidovudine + Lamivudine
Ritonavir + Saquinavir (Fortovase or Invirase)	

V. Prevention of infections
A. Vaccinations
  1. Vaccination with pneumococcal vaccine, polyvalent (Pneumovax 23, Pnu-Immune 23) is recommended when HIV infection is diagnosed. Yearly influenza vaccination is suggested. Those who are seronegative for hepatitis B and at risk for infection should be offered hepatitis B vaccine (Recombivax HB, Engerix-B).
  2. Tetanus vaccine should be administered every 10 years, and hepatitis A vaccine (Havrix, Vaqta) should be considered for nonimmune sexually active patients.
B. Opportunistic infections
  1. **Pneumocystis carinii pneumonia** is rarely encountered in patients receiving prophylactic therapy. Indications for prophylaxis are a CD4$^+$ count below 200 cells/μL, HIV-related thrush, or unexplained fever for 2 or more weeks regardless of CD4$^+$ count. Anyone with a past history of PCP should continue suppressive therapy indefinitely because of the high risk of relapse.
  2. **Toxoplasmosis** risk increases as the CD4$^+$ count approaches 100 cells/μL, and patients who are seropositive for IgG antibody to toxoplasma should begin preventive therapy when the count nears this level. Patients who have been treated for toxoplasmosis require lifelong suppressive therapy.
C. Tuberculosis. Patients who have HIV infection and positive results on tuberculin skin tests have a 2-10% per year risk of reactivation. If active tuberculosis has been excluded, prophylaxis should be prescribed to HIV-infected patients who have a tuberculin skin test reaction of 5 mm or more, who have a history of a positive tuberculin skin test reaction but were never treated, or who have had close contact with someone with active tuberculosis.

USPHS/IDSA Guidelines for Prevention of Opportunistic Infections in HIV-Infected Patients

Pathogen	Indication for prophylaxis	First-choice drug	Selected alternative drugs
Prophylaxis Strongly Recommended			
Pneumocystis carinii	CD4$^+$ count <200 cells/µL or unexplained fever for >2 wk or oropharyngeal candidiasis	TMP-SMX (Bactrim, Septra), 1 DS tablet PO daily	Dapsone, 100 mg PO daily, or aerosolized pentamidine (NebuPent), 300 mg monthly
Mycobacterium tuberculosis	Tuberculin skin test reaction of >5 mm or prior positive test without treatment or exposure to active tuberculosis	Isoniazid, 300 mg PO, plus pyridoxine, 50 mg PO daily for 12 mo	Rifampin, 600 mg PO daily for 12 mo
Toxoplasma gondii	IgG antibody to T gondii and CD4$^+$ count <100 cells/µL	TMP-SMX, 1 DS tablet PO daily	Dapsone, 50 mg PO daily, plus pyrimethamine (Daraprim), 50 mg PO weekly, plus leucovorin (Wellcovorin), 25 mg PO weekly
Mycobacterium avium complex	CD4$^+$ <50 cells/µL	Clarithromycin (Biaxin), 500 mg PO bid, or azithromycin (Zithromax), 1,200 mg PO weekly	Rifabutin (Mycobutin), 300 mg PO daily
Streptococcus pneumoniae	All patients	Pneumococcal vaccine (Pneumovax 23, Pnu-Immune 23), 0.5 mL IM once	None
Consideration of Prophylaxis Recommended			
Hepatitis B virus	All seronegative patients	Hepatitis B vaccine (Engerix-B, 20 pg IM x 3, or Recombivax HB, 10 µg IM x 3)	None
Influenza virus	All patients, annually before influenza season	0.5 mL IM	Rimantadine (Flumadine), 100 mg PO bid, or amantadine (Symadine, Symmetrel), 100 mg PO bid

D. **Mycobacterium avium complex infection.** Prophylactic therapy is recommended for patients whose CD4$^+$ counts are less than 50 cells/µL. Azithromycin (Zithromax), 1,200 mg (2 tabs) weekly by mouth is recommended.

References: See page 294.

Colonic Diverticulitis

The prevalence colonic diverticular disease increases from less than 5 percent at age 40, to 30 percent by age 60, to 65 percent by age 85. Among all patients with diverticulosis, 70 percent remain asymptomatic, 15 to 25 percent develop diverticulitis, and 5 to 15 percent develop diverticular bleeding.

I. **Pathophysiology**
   A. Diverticulitis represents micro- or macroscopic perforation of a diverticulum. The inflammation is frequently mild. Complications may include development of an abscess, fistula, obstruction, perforation and peritonitis.
   B. **Complicated diverticulitis** refers to the presence of an abscess, fistula, obstruction, or perforation while simple diverticulitis refers to inflammation in the absence of these complications.

II. **Clinical evaluation**
   A. **Left lower quadrant pain** is the most common complaint, occurring in 70 percent of patients. Pain is often present for several days prior to admission. Up to one-half have had one or more previous episodes of similar pain. Other possible symptoms include nausea and vomiting in 20 to 62 percent, constipation in 50 percent, diarrhea in 25 to 35 percent, and urinary symptoms (eg, dysuria, urgency and frequency) in 10 to 15 percent.
   B. **Right-sided diverticulitis** occurs in only 1.5 percent of patients
   C. **Physical examination** usually reveals abdominal tenderness in the left lower quadrant. A tender mass is palpable in 20 percent and abdominal distention is common. Right lower quadrant tenderness usually results from redundant sigmoid colon or right-sided diverticulitis which is rare in the west but common in Asia. Generalized tenderness suggests free perforation and peritonitis.
   D. **Low grade fever and mild leukocytosis** are common. However, the absence of these findings does not exclude the diagnosis; a normal white count occurs in 45 percent. Liver function tests are usually normal and amylase is either normal or mildly elevated, especially in the patient with perforation and peritonitis. The urinalysis may reveal sterile pyuria; the presence of colonic flora on culture suggests a colovesical fistula.

Differential Diagnosis of Diverticulitis	
Elderly	**Middle Aged and Young**
Ischemic colitis Carcinoma Volvulus Colonic Obstruction Penetrating ulcer Nephrolithiasis/urosepsis	Appendicitis Salpingitis Inflammatory bowel disease Penetrating ulcer Urosepsis

III. **Diagnosis of diverticulitis**
   A. **Radiologic evaluation** in the acute setting. Routine abdominal and chest radiographs are commonly performed in the patient with acute abdominal pain, and are most useful in excluding other causes, such as intestinal obstruction, rather than in making the diagnosis of diverticulitis. Free air may be present in patients with a perforated diverticulum.
   B. **Computer tomographic (CT) scanning** is the optimal method of investigation in suspected acute diverticulitis. The sensitivity and specificity of helical CT (with colonic contrast) are 97 and 100 percent, respectively.
      1. **CT features of acute diverticulitis:**

        a. Increased soft tissue density within pericolic fat, secondary to inflammation — 98 percent

        b. Colonic diverticula — 84 percent

        c. Bowel wall thickening — 70 percent

        d. Soft tissue masses representing phlegmon, and pericolic fluid collections, representing abscesses — 35 percent

    2. CT can permit percutaneous drainage of abscesses, thereby downstaging complicated diverticulitis, avoiding emergent surgery, and permitting single-stage elective surgical resection.

  C. **Contrast enema** is safe in the acute phase if performed by the single contrast technique and if there is no evidence of complications. In the presence of complications, such as pneumoperitoneum or generalized peritonitis, barium is absolutely contraindicated. Water soluble contrast should be used in any patient suspected of having acute diverticulitis.

  D. **Evaluation in the elective setting.** After resolution of an episode of acute diverticulitis, the colon requires full evaluation to establish the extent of disease and to rule out coexistent lesions, such as polyps or carcinoma. This can be accomplished either with colonoscopy, or with the combination of barium enema plus flexible sigmoidoscopy.

IV. **Treatment of acute diverticulitis**

  A. **Uncomplicated diverticulitis**

    1. Conservative treatment (with bowel rest and antibiotics) is successful in 70 to 100 percent of patients with acute uncomplicated diverticulitis.

    2. Selection for outpatient management. The elderly, immunosuppressed, those with significant comorbidities, and those unable to tolerate oral intake, those with high fever or significant leukocytosis should be hospitalized.

    3. Causative bacteria are principally Gram negative rods and anaerobes (particularly E. coli and B. fragilis). Reasonable antibiotic choices include a quinolone with metronidazole, amoxicillin-clavulanate, or sulfamethoxazole-trimethoprim with metronidazole.

    4. **Outpatient treatment of diverticulitis**

        a. **Ciprofloxacin (Cipro)**, 500 mg PO twice daily plus metronidazole, 500 mg PO three times daily.

        b. An alternative is amoxicillin-clavulanate (Augmentin, 875/125 mg twice daily) is an acceptable alternative. Treatment should be continued for 7 to 10 days. Oral ciprofloxacin achieves levels similar to those with intravenous administration, has broad coverage of enteric Gram negative pathogens, and requires only twice daily dosing.

        c. Patients requiring hospitalization should receive empiric broad-spectrum intravenous antibiotics directed at colonic anaerobic and gram-negative flora. Metronidazole is the antibiotic of choice for anaerobic coverage, while gram-negative coverage can be achieved with a third-generation cephalosporin (ceftriaxone 1 to 2 g daily or cefotaxime 1 to 2 g every six hours) or a fluoroquinolone (ciprofloxacin 400 mg IV every 12 hours or levofloxacin 500 mg IV daily).

        d. Single agent coverage is also reasonable with the following alternative agents:

           (1) **Ampicillin-sulbactam (Unasyn)** (3 g every six hours), piperacillin-tazobactam (3.375 g or 4.5 g every six hours), or ticarcillin-clavulanate (3.1 g every four hours)

           (2) **Carbapenem such as imipenem** (Primaxin, 500 mg every six hours) or meropenem (1 g every eight hours).

    5. **Dietary recommendations.** Outpatients should be instructed to consume clear liquids only. Clinical improvement should be evident after two to three days, after which the diet can be advanced slowly. Patients requiring hospitalization should receive clear liquids or NPO with intravenous hydration. Patients should consume a high fiber diet once the acute phase has resolved.

6. **Abscesses** amenable to percutaneous drainage should be treated. Laparotomy is necessary if abscesses cannot be drained or if drainage does not result in improvement. Surgery should proceed without delay if a patient's condition deteriorates (increased pain, more localized peritonitis or diffuse tenderness, increased white count).

7. **Two to six weeks after recovery**, patients should undergo an evaluation of the colon to exclude other diagnostic considerations (colon cancer) and to evaluate the extent of the diverticulosis. This is usually accomplished with a colonoscopy, although a flexible sigmoidoscopy plus barium enema is a reasonable alternative. Patients should be advised to consume a diet high in fiber.

8. **Prognosis.** Following successful conservative therapy for a first attack of diverticulitis, 30 to 40 percent of patients will remain asymptomatic, 30 to 40 percent will have episodic abdominal cramps without frank diverticulitis, and one-third will proceed to a second attack of diverticulitis.

9. After a second attack, elective surgery is not necessary for all patients who respond to medical therapy. Patients in whom elective surgery has been recommended following a single attack of diverticulitis include young patients (less than 40 or 50 years of age) and those who are immunosuppressed.

B. **Complicated diverticulitis**
1. **Peritonitis.** Diffuse peritonitis mandates resuscitation, broad-spectrum antibiotics, and emergency exploration.
   a. Ampicillin (2 g IV every six hours), gentamicin (1.5 to 2 mg/kg IV every 8 hours), and metronidazole (500 mg IV every 8 hours)
   b. Imipenem/cilastin (500 mg IV every six hours)
   c. Piperacillin-tazobactam (3.375 g IV every six hours)
2. **Obstruction.** Resection with primary anastomosis is usually possible; a colostomy is required if the bowel preparation is inadequate or on-table colonic lavage can be considered to permit primary anastomosis.
3. **Perforation.** Free intraperitoneal rupture of diverticulitis is unusual; however, such patients have high mortality rates of 20 to 30 percent. Treatment usually involves a two-stage procedure.
4. **Abscesses** occur in 16 percent of patients with acute diverticulitis without peritonitis and in 31 to 56 percent of those requiring surgery for diverticulitis. Percutaneous drainage now permits elective single stage surgery in 60 to 80 percent of patients; furthermore, in selected patients with contraindications to surgery, catheter drainage may be sufficient to relieve symptoms.

C. **Surgery.** Up to 30 percent of patients with uncomplicated diverticulitis require surgical intervention during the initial attack. Surgery is advised after a first attack of complicated diverticulitis or after two or more episodes of uncomplicated diverticulitis.

Indications for Surgery in Acute Diverticulitis

Absolute
Complications of diverticulitis: peritonitis, abscess (failed percutaneous drainage), fistula, obstruction
Clinical deterioration or failure to improve with medical therapy
Recurrent episodes
Intractable symptoms
Inability to exclude carcinoma

Relative Indications
  Symptomatic stricture
  Immunosuppression
  Right-sided diverticulitis
  Young patient

---

1. **Preoperative preparation.** A second- or third generation cephalosporin is administered or more broad-spectrum antibiotics, depending upon the degree of contamination. Regimens include cefazolin (Ancef [1 g IV every eight hours]) plus metronidazole (Flagyl [500 mg IV every 8 hours]); ampicillin-sulbactam (Unasyn [1.5 g IV every six hours]); or ticarcillin-clavulanate (Timentin 3.1 g IV every six hours]). Bowel preparation is often possible in nonemergent situations.
2. **Emergency sigmoid colectomy** with proximal colostomy is indicated for attacks of diverticulitis associated with sepsis, peritonitis, obstruction, or perforation.
3. **Elective sigmoid resection** is indicated for second or subsequent attacks of diverticulitis, or for attacks with complications managed nonoperatively (eg, percutaneous CT-guided drainage of an abscess), or carcinoma.
4. **Operative procedures**
   a. **Single-stage procedure.** This procedure is usually performed as an elective procedure after resolution of the acute attack of diverticulitis. The segment containing inflamed diverticulum (usually sigmoid colon) is resected with primary anastomosis. A bowel prep is required.
   b. **Two-stage procedure.** This procedure is indicated for acute diverticulitis with obstruction or perforation with an unprepared bowel. The first stage consists of resection of the involved segment of colon with end colostomy and either a mucous fistula or a Hartmann rectal pouch. The second stage consists of a colostomy take-down and reanastomosis after 2-3 months.

References: See page 294.

Acute Cystitis

Cystitis is an infection of the bladder. Acute cystitis in the healthy nonpregnant adult woman is considered to be uncomplicated. A complicated infection is associated with a condition that increases the risk of failing therapy. About 7.8% of girls and 1.6% of boys have had a symptomatic UTI. Approximately 50 to 60% of adult women have had a UTI at some time during their life. Young sexually active women have 0.5 episodes of acute cystitis per year.

I. Microbiology Clinical features
   A. Escherichia coli is the causative pathogen in 80 to 85% of episodes of acute uncomplicated cystitis. Staphylococcus saprophyticus is responsible for most other episodes, while Proteus mirabilis, Klebsiella species, enterococci or other uropathogens are isolated from a small proportion of patients.
   B. Acute uncomplicated cystitis is characterized by dysuria, usually in combination with frequency, urgency, suprapubic pain, and/or hematuria. Fever (>38°C), flank pain, costovertebral angle tenderness, and nausea or vomiting suggest pyelonephritis
   C. Vaginitis should be considered if there is vaginal discharge or odor, pruritus, dyspareunia, external dysuria, and the absence of frequency or urgency.

II. Diagnosis

A. Physical examination should include temperature, abdominal examination, and assessment for costovertebral angle tenderness. A pelvic examination is indicated if symptoms of urethritis or vaginitis are present.

B. Urinalysis. Pyuria is usually present with acute cystitis; its absence strongly suggests a noninfectious cause for the symptoms. An unspun voided midstream urine specimen should be examined with a hemocytometer; 10 or more leukocytes per mm^3 is considered abnormal. White blood cell casts in the urine are diagnostic of upper tract infection. Hematuria is common with UTI but not in urethritis or vaginitis. Microscopic evaluation of the urine for bacteriuria is generally not recommended for acute uncomplicated cystitis because pathogens in low quantities $\leq 10^4$ CFU/mL) are difficult to find on the wet mount or Gram stain.

C. Indications for voided midstream urine cultures
   1. Suspected complicated infection.
   2. The symptoms are not characteristic of UTI.
   3. The patient has persistent symptoms of UTI following treatment.
   4. UTI symptoms recur less than one month after treatment of a previous UTI.

D. Acute urethral syndrome. A CFU count $\geq 10^2$/mL should be considered positive on a midstream urine specimen in women with acute symptoms and pyuria. Some women with acute dysuria have neither bacteriuria nor pyuria. The symptoms usually resolve after antimicrobial therapy.

E. Urine dipsticks
   1. Dipsticks detect the presence of leukocyte esterase and nitrite; the former detect pyuria and the latter Enterobacteriaceae which convert urinary nitrate to nitrite. The leukocyte esterase test is a practical screening test with a sensitivity of 75 to 96% and specificity of 94 to 98%. A microscopic evaluation for pyuria or a culture is indicated with a negative leukocyte esterase test with urinary symptoms.
   2. The nitrite test is fairly sensitive and specific for detecting $\geq 10^5$ Enterobacteriaceae CFU per mL of urine. However, it lacks adequate sensitivity for detection of "low count" UTIs, or, in some cases, infections caused by common uropathogenic species.

III. Treatment

A. E. coli Resistance
   1. One-third or more of isolates demonstrate resistance to ampicillin and sulfonamides; these agents should not be used for empiric therapy. An increasing proportion of uropathogens demonstrate resistance to trimethoprim and/or TMP-SMX.
   2. The prevalence of resistance to nitrofurantoin among E. coli is less than 5%, although non-E. coli uropathogens are often resistant.
   3. Resistance to the fluoroquinolones remains well below 5%.

B. S. saprophyticus resistance. Three% are resistant to TMP-SMX, 1% to cephalothin, 0% to nitrofurantoin, and 0.4% to ciprofloxacin.

C. Recommendation
   1. Because of increasing fluoroquinolone resistance, TMP-SMX should be the first-line treatment for acute cystitis if the woman:
      a. Has no history of allergy to the drug.
      b. Has not been on antibiotics, especially TMP-SMX, in the past three months.
      c. Has not been hospitalized recently.
      d. If the prevalence of E. coli resistance to TMP-SMX in the area is not known to be more than 20% among women with acute uncomplicated cystitis.
   2. **A fluoroquinolone** is an appropriate choice for women who have an allergy to TMP-SMX or risk factors for TMP-SMX resistance and who have moderate to severe symptoms.

Oral Antibiotics for Acute Uncomplicated Cystitis		
Drug, dose	Dose and interval	Duration
Levofloxacin (Levaquin)	250 mg q24h	3 days
Ciprofloxacin (Cipro)	100 to 250 mg q12h **OR** 500 mg q24h	3 days 3 days
Gatifloxacin (Tequin)	400 mg single dose **OR** 200 mg q24h	3 days
Trimethoprim-sulfamethoxazole (Bactrim)	160/800 mg q12h	3 days
Trimethoprim	100 mg q12h	3 days
Cefpodoxime proxetil (Vantin)	100 mg q12h	3-7days
Nitrofurantoin macrocrystals (Macrobid)	50 mg q6h	7 days
Nitrofurantoin monohydrate macrocrystals (Macrobid)	100 mg q12h	7 days
Amoxicillin-clavulanate (Augmentin)	500 mg q12h	7 days

3. **Nitrofurantoin (Macrodantin** [for seven days]) should be used for women with mild-to-moderate symptoms who have allergy to TMP-SMX or risk factors for TMP-SMX resistance.
4. Urinary analgesia (phenazopyridine [Pyrimidine] 200 mg orally TID) is offered to those with severe dysuria (10%). Phenazopyridine is usually given for only one to two days.
5. Routine post-treatment cultures in non-pregnant women who have become asymptomatic after an episode of cystitis are not indicated. In patients whose symptoms do not resolve, urine culture and antimicrobial susceptibility testing should be performed. Empiric therapy should include a fluoroquinolone unless such an agent was used initially.

IV. **Acute complicated cystitis**
  A. Urinary tract infection may lead to serious complications in the person who is pregnant, very young or old, diabetic, immunocompromised, or who has an abnormal genitourinary tract.
  B. **Clinical presentation.** Acute complicated cystitis generally presents with dysuria, frequency, urgency, suprapubic pain, and/or hematuria. Fever (>38ºC), flank pain, costovertebral angle tenderness, and nausea or vomiting suggest the infection has extended beyond the bladder.
  C. **Bacteriology.** The spectrum of uropathogens causing complicated cystitis is much broader than that causing uncomplicated cystitis. Infection with Proteus, Klebsiella, Pseudomonas, Serratia, and Providencia species, and enterococci, staphylococci and fungi is more common in complicated

cystitis. These uropathogens, including E. coli, are much more likely to be resistant to common antimicrobials.

D. Diagnosis. Pyuria is present in almost all patients with complicated cystitis. Urine cultures with susceptibility testing should be obtained in complicated cystitis. A Gram stain may be helpful since the presence of Gram positive cocci, suggestive of enterococci, may influence the choice of empiric antibiotics.

E. Treatment

1. Complicated cystitis should be treated with an oral fluoroquinolone such as ciprofloxacin, levofloxacin, or gatifloxacin. The fluoroquinolones are well tolerated, provide a broad spectrum of activity covering most expected pathogens (including P. aeruginosa), and achieve high levels in the urine and urinary tract tissue. The recommended dose for ciprofloxacin (Cipro) is 500 mg PO twice daily, for levofloxacin (Levaquin) is 500 mg PO once daily, and for gatifloxacin (Tequin) is 400 mg PO once daily, each for 7 to 14 days.

2. Amoxicillin, nitrofurantoin and sulfa drugs are poor choices for empiric therapy in complicated cystitis because of the high prevalence of resistance.

3. Parenteral therapy is occasionally indicated for the treatment of complicated cystitis caused by multiply-resistant uropathogens, or for those patients who are allergic or intolerant to fluoroquinolones. Parenteral levofloxacin (500 mg) or gatifloxacin (400 mg), ceftriaxone (1 g), or an aminoglycoside (3 to 5 mg/kg of gentamicin or tobramycin) can be administered once daily. Patients initially given parenteral therapy can be switched to oral agents, usually a fluoroquinolone, after clinical improvement.

4. Gram positive cocci, suggestive of enterococci, may require the addition of ampicillin (1 g every six hours) or amoxicillin (500 mg PO every eight hours) to a treatment regimen.

5. If the patient does not show improvement within 24 to 48 hours, a repeat urine culture and ultrasound or computerized tomography should be considered to rule out urinary tract pathology.

6. The recommended duration of treatment for acute complicated cystitis is 7 to 14 days. A follow-up urine culture is not indicated in the asymptomatic patient.

V. Cystitis in young men. A small number of 15- to 50-year-old men suffer acute uncomplicated UTIs. Risk factors include homosexuality, intercourse with an infected female partner, and lack of circumcision.

A. Dysuria, frequency, urgency, suprapubic pain, or hematuria are typical of cystitis in men. The absence of pyuria suggests a non-infectious diagnosis. A midstream urine culture is recommended.

B. Other causes of infection. Urethritis must be considered in sexually active men; examination for penile ulcerations and urethral discharge, evaluation of a urethral swab specimen Gram stain, and diagnostic tests for N. gonorrheae and C. trachomatis are warranted. A urethral Gram stain demonstrating leukocytes and predominant Gram negative rods suggests E. coli urethritis.

C. Chronic prostatitis should also be considered, particularly in men who have had recurrent UTIs.

D. Treatment of cystitis. The etiologic agents causing uncomplicated urinary tract infections in men are similar to those in women. Thus, the TMP-SMX (Bactrim) is appropriate for empiric use in men, although 7-day regimens are recommended. Nitrofurantoin and beta-lactams should not be used in men with cystitis since they do not achieve reliable tissue concentrations and would be ineffective for occult prostatitis. Fluoroquinolones provide the best antimicrobial spectrum and prostatic penetration.

References: See page 294.

Acute Pyelonephritis

Urinary tract infections (UTIs) are common, especially in young children and sexually active women. UTI is defined either as a lower tract (acute cystitis) or upper tract (acute pyelonephritis) infection.

I. Clinical features

A. Acute uncomplicated pyelonephritis is suggested by flank pain, nausea/vomiting, fever (>38°C) and/or costovertebral angle tenderness. Frequency, dysuria, and suprapubic pain are found in the majority of patients whether infection is localized to the upper or lower tract.

B. Fever ≥ 37.8°C is strongly correlated with acute pyelonephritis. The examination should focus on temperature, abdomen, and costovertebral angle tenderness.

C. **Pelvic examination** may be indicated since pelvic inflammatory disease is a condition often mistaken for acute uncomplicated pyelonephritis. Pelvic examination does not need to be performed, however, in a woman with unilateral CVA pain and tenderness, fever, pyuria, and no vaginal symptoms.

Risk Factors for Occult Renal Infection or a Complicated Urinary Tract Infection	
Male sex Elderly Presentation in emergency department Hospital-acquired infection Pregnancy Indwelling urinary catheter Recent urinary tract instrumentation Childhood urinary tract infection	Functional or anatomic abnormality of the urinary tract Recent antimicrobial use Symptoms for more than seven days at presentation Diabetes mellitus Immunosuppression

II. Laboratory features

A. Pyuria is present in virtually all women with acute pyelonephritis; its absence strongly suggests an alternative diagnosis. Hematuria is common with urinary tract infection but not in urethritis or vaginitis. Most patients with acute pyelonephritis have leukocytosis and an elevated erythrocyte sedimentation rate and serum C-reactive protein.

B. Some patients with pyelonephritis may have colony counts of 10^3 to 10^4 CFU per mL. Blood cultures are positive in 10 to 20% of women with acute uncomplicated pyelonephritis.

C. A urinalysis should be performed to look for pyuria. White cell casts indicate a renal origin for the pyuria. Gram stain, usually performed on spun urine, may distinguish Gram negative from Gram positive infections. A pregnancy test should be performed if there is missed menses or lack of contraception.

D. Urine culture and antimicrobial susceptibility testing should be performed routinely in acute pyelonephritis.

E. Rapid methods for detection of bacteriuria, such as the nitrite test, should not be relied upon in the evaluation of patients with suspected pyelonephritis because tests lack adequate sensitivity for detection of "low count" urinary tract infection and common uropathogenic species. The nitrite test has a sensitivity of 35 to 80% and does not detect organisms unable to reduce nitrate to nitrite, such as enterococci and staphylococci.

F. Blood cultures are limited to those patients who warrant hospitalization.

III. **Treatment.** Microbiology of acute uncomplicated upper and lower urinary tract infection is rather limited with Escherichia coli accounting for 70 to 95% of infections and Staphylococcus saprophyticus 5 to 20%.

A. **Indications for admission to the hospital include:**
1. Inability to maintain oral hydration or take medications.
2. Patient noncompliance.
3. Uncertainty about the diagnosis.
4. Severe illness with high fevers, pain, and marked debility.
5. Outpatient therapy should generally be reserved for nonpregnant women with mild-to-moderate uncomplicated pyelonephritis who are compliant.

B. **Empiric antibiotic therapy**
1. Ampicillin and sulfonamides should not be used for empiric therapy because of the high rate of resistance. An increasing proportion of uropathogens demonstrate resistance to trimethoprim-sulfamethoxazole. In comparison, resistance to the fluoroquinolones and aminoglycosides is very low in uncomplicated UTIs.
2. **Oral agents.** In patients with acute uncomplicated pyelonephritis, an oral fluoroquinolone, such as ciprofloxacin (500 mg PO BID), levofloxacin (Levaquin [250 to 500 mg PO QD]), or gatifloxacin (Tequin [400 mg PO QD]), is recommended for outpatients as initial empiric treatment of infection caused by Gram negative bacilli. The newer fluoroquinolones, sparfloxacin, trovafloxacin and moxifloxacin, should be avoided because they may not achieve adequate concentrations in urine.
   a. Trimethoprim, trimethoprim-sulfamethoxazole or other agents can be used if the infecting strain is known to be susceptible. If enterococcus is suspected by the presence of small Gram positive cocci on Gram stain, amoxicillin (500 mg PO TID) should be added to the treatment regimen until the causative organism is identified.
   b. Cefixime (Suprax) and cefpodoxime proxetil (Vantin) also appear to be effective for the treatment of acute uncomplicated pyelonephritis. Cefixime is less effective against S. saprophyticus. Nitrofurantoin should not be used for the treatment of pyelonephritis since it does not achieve reliable tissue levels.

Parenteral Regimens for Empiric Treatment of Acute Uncomplicated Pyelonephritis	
Antibiotic, dose	**Interval**
Ceftriaxone (Rocephin), 1 g	q24h
Ciprofloxacin (Cipro), 200-400 mg	q12h
Levofloxacin (Levaquin), 250-500 mg	q24h
Ofloxacin (Floxin), 200-400 mg	q12 h
Gatifloxacin (Tequin), 400 mg	q24h
Gentamicin, 3-5 mg/kg (+ampicillin)	q24h
Gentamicin, 1 mg per kg (+ampicillin)	q8h
Ampicillin, 1-2 g (plus gentamicin)*	q6h

Antibiotic, dose	Interval
Aztreonam (Azactam), 1 g	q8-12h

˙Recommended regimen if enterococcus suspected.

3. **Parenteral therapy.** For hospitalized patients, ceftriaxone (Rocephin [1 gram IV QD]) is recommended if enterococcus is not suspected. Aminoglycosides (3 to 5 mg/kg) given once daily provide a therapeutic advantage compared with beta lactams because of their marked and sustained concentration in renal tissue.
   a. Ciprofloxacin, ofloxacin, levofloxacin and gatifloxacin are also effective for the parenteral treatment of uncomplicated pyelonephritis but should be used orally if the patient is able to tolerate oral medications since the costs are lower and serum levels are equivalent.
   b. If enterococcus is suspected based upon the Gram stain, ampicillin (1 to 2 g IV Q6h) plus gentamicin (1.0 mg/kg IV Q8h) or piperacillin-tazobactam (3.375 g IV Q8h) are reasonable broad spectrum empiric choices. Once-daily dosing of aminoglycosides is not recommended for serious probable enterococcal infection since this regimen may not provide adequate synergy against the organism.
C. **Duration.** Patients with acute uncomplicated pyelonephritis can often be switched to oral therapy at 24 to 48 hours. Patients should be evaluated for complicated pyelonephritis if they fail to defervesce or if bacteremia persists. A 14-day regimen is recommended. In sicker patients, a longer duration of treatment may be required (14 to 21 days).
D. **Posttreatment follow-up cultures** in an asymptomatic patient are not indicated. In women whose pyelonephritis symptoms resolve but recur within two weeks, a repeat urine culture and antimicrobial susceptibility testing should be performed. If the initially infecting species is isolated again with the same susceptibility profile, a renal ultrasound or computed tomographic (CT) scan should be performed. Retreatment with a two-week regimen using another agent should be considered.
E. **Urologic evaluation**
   1. Routine urologic investigation of young healthy women with acute uncomplicated pyelonephritis is generally not recommended. Ultrasound or CT scan should be considered if the patient remains febrile or has not shown clinical improvement after 72 hours of treatment. CT scan or renal ultrasound should be performed after two recurrences of pyelonephritis.

IV. **Acute complicated pyelonephritis**
A. **Clinical features.** In addition to flank pain, dysuria and fever, complicated urinary tract infections may also be associated with malaise, fatigue, nausea, or abdominal pain.
B. A urine Gram stain and culture should always be performed in patients with suspected complicated UTI. A colony count threshold of >10^3 CFU per mL should be used to diagnose symptomatic complicated infection except when urine cultures are obtained through a newly-inserted catheter in which case a level of >$10^{(2)}$ CFU per mL is evidence of infection.
C. **Microbiology.** E. coli is still the predominant uropathogen, but other uropathogens, including Citrobacter sp, Enterobacter sp, Pseudomonas aeruginosa, enterococci, Staphylococcus aureus, and fungi account for a higher proportion of cases compared with uncomplicated urinary tract infections.
D. **Treatment.** Patients with complicated pyelonephritis, including pregnant women, should be managed as inpatients. Underlying anatomic (eg, stones, obstruction), functional (eg, neurogenic bladder), or metabolic (eg, poorly controlled diabetes) defects should be corrected.

1. In contrast to uncomplicated UTI, S. aureus is relatively more likely to be found. For those patients with mild to moderate illness who can be treated with oral medication, a fluoroquinolone is the best choice for empiric therapy. Fluoroquinolones are comparable or superior to other broad spectrum regimens, including parenteral therapy. Sparfloxacin, trovafloxacin and moxifloxacin are not effective.
2. Antimicrobial regimen can be modified when the infecting strain susceptibilities are known. Patients on parenteral regimens can be switched to oral treatment, generally a fluoroquinolone, after clinical improvement. Patients undergoing effective treatment with an antimicrobial to which the infecting pathogen is susceptible should have definite improvement within 24 to 48 hours and, if not, a repeat urine culture and imaging studies should be performed.
3. At least 10 to 14 days of therapy is recommended. Urine culture should be repeated one to two weeks after the completion of therapy. Suppressive antibiotics may be considered with complicated pyelonephritis and a positive follow-up urine culture.

Parenteral Regimens for Empiric Treatment of Acute Complicated Pyelonephritis

Antibiotic, dose	Interval
Cefepime (Maxipime) , 1 g	q12 hours
Ciprofloxacin (Cipro), 400 mg	q12 hours
Levofloxacin (Levaquin), 500 mg	q24 hours
Ofloxacin (Floxin), 400 mg	q12 hours
Gatifloxacin (Tequin), 400 mg	q24 hours
Gentamicin, 3-5 mg/kg (+ ampicillin)*	q24 hours
Gentamicin, 1 mg per kg (+ ampicillin)*	q8 hours
Ampicillin, 1-2 g (+ gentamicin)*	q6 hours
Ticarcillin-clavulante (Timentin), 3.2 g	q8 hours
Piperacilin-tazobactam (Zosyn), 3.375 g*	q6-8 hours
Imipenem-cilastatin, 250-500 mg	q6-8 hours

*Recommended regimen if enterococcus suspected

References: See page 294.

Genital Herpes Simplex Virus Infection

The seroprevalence of herpes simplex virus type-2 (HSV-2) is 17 percent. HSV-2 remains the causative agent for most genital herpes infections. Recurrences are common following primary genital herpes. About 89 percent have one recurrence. And 38 percent of patients have six recurrences and 20 percent have more than ten.

I. **Types of infection**
   A. **Primary infection** refers to infection in a patient without preexisting antibodies to HSV-1 or HSV-2.
   B. **Nonprimary first episode infection** refers to the acquisition of genital HSV-1 in a patient with preexisting antibodies to HSV-2 or the acquisition of genital HSV-2 in a patient with preexisting antibodies to HSV-1.
   C. **Recurrent infection** refers to reactivation of genital HSV in which the HSV type recovered in the lesion is the same type as antibodies in the serum
   D. Each of these types can be either symptomatic or asymptomatic (also called subclinical).

II. Clinical features

A. **Acute primary and recurrent infection.** The initial presentation can be severe with painful genital ulcers, dysuria, fever, tender local inguinal lymphadenopathy, and headache. In other patients, however, the infection is mild, subclinical, or entirely asymptomatic.

B. Recurrent infection is typically less severe than primary or nonprimary first episode infection.

C. **Primary infection.** The average incubation period after exposure is four days (range two to twelve days). Patients with primary infections usually have multiple, bilateral, ulcerating, pustular lesions which resolve after a mean of 19 days.

D. **Other symptoms and signs in these first episode infections:**
  1. Systemic symptoms, including fever, headache, malaise, and myalgias — 67 percent
  2. Local pain and itching — 98 percent
  3. Dysuria — 63 percent
  4. Tender lymphadenopathy — 80 percent

E. **Recurrent infection** is more common with HSV-2 than HSV-1 (60 versus 14 percent with HSV-1). The frequency of recurrences may correlate with the severity of the initial primary infection.

F. Subclinical infection (asymptomatic viral shedding). After resolution of the primary genital HSV infection, intermittent viral shedding in the absence of genital lesions has been documented in both men and women

G. **Diagnosis.** Among patients with genital herpes who present with a genital ulcer, the primary differential diagnosis includes syphilis chancroid, and drug eruptions, and Behcet's disease.
  1. The clinical diagnosis of genital herpes should be confirmed by laboratory testing.
  2. Viral culture. If active genital lesions are present, the vesicle should be unroofed for sampling of vesicular fluid for culture. However, the overall sensitivity of viral culture of genital lesions is only 50 percent.
  3. Polymerase chain reaction. While viral culture is the standard diagnostic method for isolating HSV, real-time HSV PCR assays have emerged as a more sensitive method to confirm HSV infection.
  4. Direct fluorescent antibody. Many diagnostic laboratories provide a rapid type-specific direct fluorescent antibody (DFA) test to detect HSV in clinical specimens. This test is specific, reproducible, and less expensive than current real-time HSV PCR assays.

III. Treatment

A. **Acyclovir, famciclovir, and valacyclovir,** which is a prodrug that is converted acyclovir, appear to have equivalent efficacy for the treatment of genital herpes and for the suppression of recurrent infection. Famciclovir and valacyclovir have greater oral availability than acyclovir.

B. Pain control with topical agents or opioid medications should be administered.

C. Although there is no difference in efficacy, acyclovir is substantially less expensive than famcicovir and valacyclovir.

D. **Acyclovir (Zovirax)** dose is 400 mg PO three times per day or 200 mg PO five times per day for 7 to 10 days There is no clinical benefit from higher doses.

E. Patients with primary genital herpes infections accompanied by more severe clinical manifestations, such as aseptic meningitis, may be treated with intravenous **acyclovir** (5 to 10 mg/kg every eight hours for five to seven days).
  1. **Famciclovir (Famvir)** dose is 250 mg PO three times daily for seven to ten days.
  2. **Valacyclovir (Valtrex)** dose is 1000 mg PO twice daily for seven to ten days.

Dosage Regimens for Primary Genital Herpes Infection	
Drug	Dosage
Acyclovir (Zovirax)	400 mg three times daily for 7-10 days
Famciclovir (Famvir)	250 mg three times daily for 7-10 days
Valacyclovir (Valtrex)	1 g twice daily for 7-10 days

F. **Recurrent episodes.** When compared to primary infection, recurrent genital HSV is typically less severe, with fewer lesions that are often in a unilateral, rather than bilateral distribution. In addition, treatment of the primary infection does not appear to reduce the frequency of subsequent recurrences.

G. **Recommendations.** Antiviral therapy of recurrent episodes is most likely to be effective if started within the first 24 hours.
   1. Although there is no difference in efficacy, acyclovir is substantially less expensive.
   2. The recommended dose of acyclovir is 800 mg PO three times daily for two days or 400 mg PO three times daily for three to five days.
   3. The recommended dose of famciclovir is 125 mg PO two times daily for three to five days.
   4. The recommended dose of valacyclovir is 500 mg PO twice daily for three days.

Dosages of Antiviral Agents for Treatment of Episodic Genital Herpes	
Drug	Dosage
Acyclovir (Zovirax)	400 mg three times daily daily for 3-5 days 800 mg twice daily for 2 days
Famciclovir (Famvir)	125 mg twice daily for 3-5 days
Valacyclovir (Valtrex)	500 mg twice daily for 3 days

H. **Suppression of recurrence and asymptomatic shedding.** Suppressive therapy diminishes the frequency of viral shedding, reduces the rates of reactivation, and decreases transmission to uninfected partners.
   1. Suppressive therapy can diminish viral shedding and the rate of clinical recurrence.
   2. The recommended dose regimens for the prevention of recurrent infection are as follows. Although there is no difference in efficacy, acyclovir is substantially less expensive.
      a. Acyclovir. 400 mg twice daily.
      b. Famciclovir. 250 mg PO two times daily.
      c. Valacyclovir. 500 mg once daily; a higher dose of 500 mg twice daily or 1000 mg once daily is recommended in patients with ≥ 10 recurrences per year.

Dosages and Characteristics of Chronic Suppressive Treatment Regimens for Recurrent Genital Herpes Infection			
Drug	Dosage	Decrease in recurrence rate (percentage)	Use in patients with ≥6 recurrences per year
Acyclovir (Zovirax)	400 mg twice daily	78 to 79	Yes
Famciclovir (Famvir)	250 mg twice daily	79	Yes
Valacyclovir (Valtrex)	1 g once daily	78 to 79	Yes
	250 mg twice daily	78 to 79	Yes
	500 mg once daily	71	No

   I. **STD screening.** Patients with genital herpes should be screened for
      other sexually transmitted diseases.
   J. **Prevention.** Behavioral changes, including condom use, may prevent
      the spread of genital HSV.
IV. **Counseling**
   A. Patients should be counseled that the acquisition of HSV can be
      asymptomatic and only serologic testing can determine if their infection
      was recently acquired. They should be educated about the probability of
      recurrence (60%).
   B. All persons with genital HSV infection should be encouraged to inform
      their current and future sex partners that they have genital herpes.
      Serologic testing should be considered for those who are asymptomatic
      to determine the risk of HSV acquisition.
   C. Couples who are serologically discordant should be advised to use
      condoms to decrease the risk of transmission and to abstain from
      intercourse when active lesions or prodromal symptoms are present.
      Patients may also be counseled that suppressive therapy may decrease
      the risk of transmission to the sexual partner.
References: See page 294.

Herpes Zoster and Postherpetic Neuralgia

Following primary infection with varicella-zoster virus (VZV), which causes
chickenpox, latent infection is established in the sensory dorsal root ganglia.
Reactivation of endogenous latent VZV infection within the sensory ganglia
results in herpes zoster or "shingles", characterized by a painful, unilateral
vesicular eruption in a restricted dermatomal distribution.

I. **Epidemiology**
   A. Cumulative lifetime incidence is 10 to 20 percent of the population. Older
      age groups have the highest incidence of zoster, because of the decline in
      VZV-specific cell mediated immunity. Approximately 4 percent of individu-
      als will experience a second episode of herpes zoster.
   B. Herpes zoster cases has the highest incidence (5 to 10 cases per 1,000
      persons) after the sixth decade.
   C. The incidence of shingles is significantly lower in black subjects versus
      white (5 versus 16 percent).
   D. HIV-infected patients. Herpes zoster preferentially occurs in
      immunosuppressed patients, including transplant recipients and
      HIV-infected patients. The development of herpes zoster suggests the

need for assessment of HIV-1 seropositivity in populations at risk for HIV-1 infection.

II. Natural history and infectivity

    A. Approximately 75 percent of patients patients have prodromal pain in the dermatome where the rash subsequently appears. The rash appears as grouped vesicles or bullae which evolve into pustular or occasionally hemorrhagic lesions within three four days. In immunocompetent hosts, the lesions crust by day 7 to 10 and are no longer infectious; crusting of the rash occurs within three to four weeks. Recurrence of clinical zoster in the immunocompetent host is rare.

    B. Pain is the most common symptom of zoster and can precede the rash by days to weeks; prodromal pain may be constant or intermittent. The pain is a deep "burning", "throbbing" or "stabbing" sensation.

    C. Zoster is generally limited to one dermatome in normal hosts, but can occasionally affect two or three neighboring dermatomes.

    D. The thoracic and lumbar dermatomes are the most commonly involved sites of herpes zoster. Zoster keratitis or zoster ophthalmicus can result from involvement of the ophthalmic branch of the trigeminal cranial nerve. These can be sight-threatening infections.

    E. Fewer than 20 percent of patients have significant systemic symptoms, such as headache, fever, malaise, or fatigue.

III. Complications in immunocompetent patients.

    A. Complications of herpes zoster include ocular, neurologic, bacterial superinfection of the skin and postherpetic neuralgia. Herpes zoster may also extend centrally which can result in meningeal inflammation and clinical meningitis. Occasionally VZV reactivation affects motor neurons in the spinal cord and brain stem resulting in motor neuropathies.

    B. Postherpetic neuralgia. Approximately 10 to 15 percent of all patients with herpes zoster will develop postherpetic neuralgia (PHN); individuals older than 60 years account for 50 percent of these cases. PHN has been generally defined as the persistence of sensory symptoms (pain, numbness, dysesthesias, allodynia, which is pain precipitated by movement) in the affected dermatome for >30 days after the onset of zoster.

        1. Prodromal sensory symptoms were associated with a twofold higher prevalence of PHN.

        2. Immunosuppressed individuals (HIV, transplant, connective tissue disease) had higher PHN prevalence.

        3. Treatment of herpes zoster with steroids does not reduce the prevalence of PHN.

        4. Acyclovir therapy does not reduce the prevalence of PHN.

        5. The current standard therapeutic approach has employed tricyclic antidepressants (amitriptyline, desipramine) alone or in combination with carbamazepine or opioids. Tricyclic antidepressants may be contraindicated in elderly patients with cardiovascular disease. Intrathecal corticosteroids were effective in one study of patients with intractable PHN.

        6. Gabapentin (Neurontin), a structural analog of gamma-aminobutyric acid (GABA) significantly reduces in daily pain score. Gabapentin is moderately effective for PHN approach to the management of PHN.

IV. Treatment and prevention of herpes zoster

    A. Uncomplicated herpes zoster

        1. Antiviral therapy should be initiated within 72 hours in patients older than 50 years of age. Treatment 72 hours after the onset of lesions should be considered if new lesions are still appearing at that time.

        2. The benefit of ACV therapy was less marked in patients under the age of 50 years. Therapy can be considered on an individual basis in younger patients based upon predictors of PHN such as the severity of the acute pain and rash and history of prodromal pain.

        3. Valacyclovir (1000 mg three times per day for seven days) is recommmended because compared to ACV, valacyclovir was associated with more rapid resolution of acute neuritis and a shorter duration of PHN. However, if cost is an issue, then ACV (800 mg every four hours [five times/day] for seven to ten days) may be preferred. If famciclovir is used, the dosage is 500 or 750 mg three times daily.

Treatment Options for Herpes Zoster	
Medication	**Dosage**
Acyclovir (Zovirax)	800 mg orally five times daily for 7 to 10 days 10 mg per kg IV every 8 hours for 7 to 10 days
Famciclovir (Famvir)	500 mg orally three times daily for 7 days
Valacyclovir (Valtrex)	1,000 mg orally three times daily for 7 days
Prednisone (Deltasone)	30 mg orally twice daily on days 1 through 7; then 15 mg twice daily on days 8 through 14; then 7.5 mg twice daily on days 15 through 21 2 (2 to 4) for days 1 through 7 2 (1 to 3) for days 8 through 14 1 (1 to 2) for days 15 to 21

4. **Prednisone** combined with antiviral therapy should be considered only in patients with severe symptoms at initial presentation who do not have a specific contraindication to steroid use. Dosage is 40 mg of prednisone daily with a taper over seven to ten days with the last dose coinciding with the end of antiviral therapy.
5. **Analgesia for herpetic neuralgia.** Nonsteroidal antiinflammatory drugs are usually not effective. Opioid therapy, such as oxycodone/acetaminophen, is preferred.

V. Treatment of postherpetic neuralgia
  A. Although postherpetic neuralgia is generally a self-limited condition, it can last indefinitely.

Treatment Options for Postherpetic Neuralgia	
Medication	**Dosage**
Topical agents	
Capsaicin cream (Zostrix)	Apply to affected area three to five times daily.
Lidocaine (Xylocaine) patch	Apply to affected area every 4 to 12 hours as needed.
Tricyclic antidepressants	
Amitriptyline (Elavil)	0 to 25 mg orally at bedtime; increase dosage by 25 mg every 2 to 4 weeks until response is adequate, or to maximum dosage of 150 mg per day.
Nortriptyline (Pamelor)	0 to 25 mg orally at bedtime; increase dosage by 25 mg every 2 to 4 weeks until response is adequate, or to maximum dosage of 125 mg per day.
Imipramine (Tofranil)	25 mg orally at bedtime; increase dosage by 25 mg every 2 to 4 weeks until response is adequate, or to maximum dosage of 150 mg per day.

Medication	Dosage
Desipramine (Norpramin)	25 mg orally at bedtime; increase dosage by 25 mg every 2 to 4 weeks until response is adequate, or to maximum dosage of 150 mg per day.
Anticonvulsants	
Phenytoin (Dilantin)	100 to 300 mg orally at bedtime; increase dosage until response is adequate or blood drug level is 10 to 20 µg per mL (40 to 80 µmol per L).
Carbamazepine (Tegretol)	100 mg orally at bedtime; increase dosage by 100 mg every 3 days until dosage is 200 mg three times daily, response is adequate or blood drug level is 6 to12 µg per mL (25.4 to 50.8 µmol per L).
Gabapentin (Neurontin)	100 to 300 mg orally at bedtime; increase dosage by 100 to 300 mg every 3 days until dosage is 300 to 900 mg three times daily or response is adequate.

B. Analgesics
   1. Capsaicin is more efficacious than placebo but must be applied to the affected area three to five times daily. Pain will likely increase during the first few days to a week after capsaicin therapy is initiated.
   2. Lidocaine patches reduce pain intensity, with minimal systemic absorption. The effect lasts only four to 12 hours with each application.
   3. Acetaminophen and nonsteroidal anti-inflammatory drugs are useful for potentiating the pain-relieving effects of narcotics.
C. Tricyclic Antidepressants
   1. Tricyclic antidepressants can be effective adjuncts in reducing pain. Tricyclic antidepressants commonly used in the treatment of postherpetic neuralgia include amitriptyline (Elavil), nortriptyline (Pamelor), imipramine (Tofranil) and desipramine (Norpramin).
   2. The tricyclic antidepressants may cause sedation, dry mouth, postural hypotension, blurred vision and urinary retention. Nortriptyline is better tolerated.
D. Gabapentin is effective in treating the pain of postherpetic neuralgia. The dosages required for analgesia are often lower than those used in the treatment of epilepsy.
E. Transcutaneous electric nerve stimulation (TENS), biofeedback and nerve blocks are also sometimes used.
References: See page 294.

Herpes Simplex Virus Type 1 Infection

Herpes simplex virus type 1 (HSV-1) is the etiologic agent of vesicular lesions of the oral mucosa commonly referred to as "cold sores." HSV-1 can also cause clinical disease in the genitalia, liver, lung, eye, and central nervous system.

I. Primary infection
   A. Inoculation of HSV-1 at mucosal surfaces or skin sites permits entry of the virus into the epidermis, the dermis, and eventually to sensory and autonomic nerve endings. Disease is characterized by sudden appearance of multiple vesicular lesions on an inflammatory, erythematous base. Primary infection may also be associated with systemic symptoms, such as fever and malaise. The severity of symptoms and the number of lesions is considerably less with reactivation.

    B. The lesions can be painful and last for 10 to 14 days. Vesicles are usually grouped in a single anatomic site.

    C. Although the symptoms can be severe, most primary HSV-1 infections are asymptomatic. Only 20 to 25 percent of patients with HSV-1 antibodies and 10 to 20 percent of those with HSV-2 antibodies have a history of oral-labial or genital infections.

II. Recurrent infection

    A. Once HSV infection has occurred, the virus lives in a latent state in nerve cell bodies in ganglion neurons and can reactivate.

    B. In contrast to primary HSV-1, recurrent HSV-1 is rarely associated with systemic signs or symptoms except for local lymphadenopathy. Prodromal symptoms may herald the onset of a reactivation episode, such as pain, burning, tingling, and pruritus. These symptoms may last from 6 to 53 hours prior to the appearance of the first vesicles.

    C. Subclinical shedding is common in both immunocompetent and immunocompromised patients.

    D. **Immunocompetent hosts.** Recurrent episodes are usually of shorter duration than the primary episode. The median time from onset of prodromal symptoms to healing of the lesion is five days.

    E. **Precipitating factors** for HSV-1 recurrence include exposure to sunlight, fever, menstruation, emotional stress, and trauma to the area of primary infection.

    F. **Recurrences** occur as frequently as once per month (24 percent) or as infrequently as twice per year (19 percent).

    G. **Immunocompromised hosts.** The initial containment of HSV infection requires intact cellular immunity. Thus, immunocompromised hosts are at risk for increased frequency and severity of recurrent HSV infections. They are also at risk for dissemination of infection, which may include the lungs or gastrointestinal tract.

    H. **HIV infection.** Patients with advanced HIV infection (CD4 count <200 cells/μL) are at increased risk for recurrent and extensive HSV infections. HSV infections can occur anywhere on the skin, often presenting as extensive oral or perianal ulcers. HIV-infected patients can also develop esophagitis, colitis, chorioretinitis, acute retinal necrosis, tracheobronchitis, and pneumonia.

III. Oral infections

    A. **Gingivostomatitis and pharyngitis** are the most frequent clinical manifestations of first-episode HSV-1 infection. Herpes labialis is the most frequent sign of reactivation disease.

    B. **Children.** Primary HSV-1 oral infection usually presents as gingivostomatitis in children. After a brief incubation period (median 6 to 8 days, range 1 to 26 days), fever, pharyngitis and painful vesicular lesions develop suddenly. Lesions can occur anywhere on the pharyngeal and oral mucosa and progress over several days, eventually involving the soft palate, buccal mucosa, tongue, and the floor of the mouth. Gingivitis and extensions to lips and cheeks can be seen.

    C. Common systemic symptoms and signs include fever, malaise, myalgias, irritability, and cervical lymphadenopathy. Transmission can occur through close contact with oral lesions.

    D. Adults. Primary oral HSV-1 infection in adults can present as severe pharyngitis, fever, malaise, myalgia and cervical lymphadenopathy. Severe mouth pain and fever usually persist for two to eight days, during which time vesicles crust over and heal; cervical lymphadenopathy may persist for weeks.

    E. Recurrences involving the oral cavity and lips are common. Lesions progress from vesicle to crust in about eight days, with significant diminution of pain after the first 24 hours.

    F. Differential diagnosis. Recurrent aphthous ulcers, which are most often confused with HSV infection, are never preceded by vesicles and occur exclusively on mucosal surfaces such as the inner surfaces of lips, buccal mucosa, ventral tongue, and mucobuccal fold in the anterior part of the oral cavity. In contrast, recurrent oral HSV-1 lesions ("cold sores") occur at the border of the vermillion (ie, the colored portion of the lips).

  G. Other diseases that present with oral lesions and/or severe pharyngitis include aphthous stomatitis, syphilis, bacterial pharyngitis, enteroviruses (eg, herpangina), Epstein-Barr virus, and Stevens-Johnson syndrome.

IV. Skin infections

  A. HSV-1 can cause primary infection anywhere on the skin, especially if there is disruption of skin integrity. Primary infections begin with a typical prodrome of pruritus and pain, followed by the development of vesicular lesions. Associated symptoms include neuralgia and lymphadenopathy.

  B. There are also a variety of syndromes associated with HSV-1 infection of the skin: HSV infection of the finger, known as herpetic whitlow, can occur as a complication of primary oral or genital herpes by inoculation of the virus through a break in the skin barrier.

V. Genital HSV-1 infections. The majority of genital HSV infections are due to HSV-2. Genital HSV-1 infection is transmitted through oral-genital contact.

VI. Ocular infections. Primary ocular HSV infections occur in less than 5 percent of patients, but can cause significant morbidity due to keratitis and acute retinal necrosis.

  A. **Keratitis.** Recurrent HSV-1 keratitis continues to be a leading cause of corneal blindness. HSV keratitis has an acute onset with symptoms of pain, visual blurring, and discharge. Physical examination is notable for chemosis, conjunctivitis, and characteristic dendritic lesions of the cornea.

  B. Use of topical steroid drops can exacerbate the infection and lead to blindness.

  C. **Recurrent infection.** The acute disease is usually self-limited. Recurrences are common. Recurrent superficial keratitis heals without affecting vision. In comparison, recurrent attacks involving stromal tissue may lead to blindness.

  D. Acute retinal necrosis (ARN) is a rare, potentially blinding retinal disease resulting from ocular infection with HSV or varicella-zoster virus (VZV).

VII. Neurologic syndromes. HSV-1 causes sporadic cases of encephalitis, characterized by the rapid onset of fever, headache, seizures, focal neurologic signs, and impaired consciousness. Other neurologic syndromes include aseptic meningitis, autonomic dysfunction, transverse myelitis, benign recurrent lymphocytic meningitis, and Bell's palsy.

VIII. Diagnosis

  A. **Viral culture.** The diagnosis of HSV infection is generally based upon tissue culture identification. Recovery of virus from secretions is possible in only 7 to 25 percent of patients with active lesions.

  B. **Polymerase chain reaction.** While viral culture has remained the standard diagnostic method for isolating HSV, real-time HSV PCR assays have emerged as a more sensitive method to confirm HSV infection in clinical specimens obtained from genital ulcers, mucocutaneous sites, and cerebrospinal fluid.

IX. Treatment and prevention of herpes simplex virus type 1 infection

  A. Children with gingivostomatitis often require either topical or oral analgesics and, in severe cases, intravenous rehydration. Short-term relief can be achieved with viscous lidocaine. Zilactin, a nonprescription topical medication may be used to protect lesions. Ziladent, a similar agent with benzocaine can provide pain relief for up to six hours. In more severe cases, oral opiate elixirs may be required.

  B. Acyclovir may be beneficial if begun early during primary (or recurrent) infections (400 mg PO three times per day or 200 mg PO five times per day or 15 mg/kg up to a dose of 200 mg PO, with each dose taken five times daily for seven days).

  C. Topical acyclovir 5 percent is minimally effective in the treatment of primary oral lesions since it has poor penetration.

D. Recurrent herpes labialis is usually not treated with antivirals unless a prodromal stage before the appearance of lesions can be identified. In these cases oral acyclovir or penciclovir cream can be prescribed for four days duration.

Dosage Regimens for Primary Genital Herpes Infection	
Drug	**Dosage**
Acyclovir (Zovirax)	200-400 mg three times daily for 10 days
Famciclovir (Famvir)	250 mg three times daily for 10 days
Valacyclovir (Valtrex)	1 g twice daily for 10 days

E. Suppressive therapy to prevent recurrences
  1. Chronic suppression has proven helpful in preventing HSV recurrences, decreasing in occurrence of new lesions by 50 to 78 percent in immunocompetent patients on prophylactic regimens of oral acyclovir. The number of recurrences per four months is lower with acyclovir (0.85 versus 1.80 with placebo). A daily suppressive regimen (Zovirax, 200 mg three to five times daily) has been shown to be safe and effective when used continuously for up to one year.
  2. Valacyclovir (Valtrex, 500 mg once daily) helps prevent recurrences (60 versus 38 percent), and the time to first recurrence is significantly longer (13 versus 9.6 weeks).
  3. Short-term antiviral prophylaxis can also be considered in UV light-induced HSV recurrences.

References: See page 294.

Early Syphilis

Syphilis is a chronic infection caused by the bacterium Treponema pallidum (Tp). Early syphilis is defined as the stages of syphilis that typically occur within the first year after infection. Early latent syphilis is defined as asymptomatic infection, with positive serology and a negative physical examination, when the date of infection can be established as having occurred within one year's time. Early syphilis is a reportable infection.

I. Clinical manifestations
  A. Early syphilis begins when an uninfected person acquires Tp, usually via direct contact with an infectious lesion during sex. The spirochete gains access at sites of minor trauma. Transmission occurs in one-third of patients exposed to early syphilis.
  B. Primary syphilis. After an average incubation period of two to three weeks, a painless papule appears at the site of inoculation. This soon ulcerates to produce the classic chancre of primary syphilis, a one to two centimeter ulcer with a raised, indurated margin. The ulcer has a non-exudative base and is associated with regional lymphadenopathy. Most lesions are seen on the genitalia. Chancres heal spontaneously within three to six weeks.
  C. Secondary syphilis. Weeks to a few months later, 25% of individuals with untreated infection will develop a systemic illness that represents secondary syphilis. Secondary syphilis can produce a wide variety of symptoms.
    1. **Rash** is the most characteristic finding of secondary syphilis. The rash is classically a symmetric papular eruption involving the entire trunk and extremities including the palms and soles. Individual lesions are discrete red or reddish-brown and measure 0.5 to 2 cm. They are often

scaly but may be smooth and rarely pustular. The involvement of the palms and soles is an important clue to the diagnosis of secondary syphilis.

2. Large, raised, gray to white lesions, involving warm, moist areas such as mucous membranes in the mouth or perineum, may develop in some patients during secondary syphilis. These are referred to as condyloma lata.

3. **Systemic symptoms** include fever, headache, malaise, anorexia, sore throat, myalgias, and weight loss.

4. **Diffuse lymphadenopathy.** Most patients with secondary syphilis have lymph node enlargement with palpable nodes present in the inguinal, axillary, posterior cervical, femoral, and/or epitrochlear regions. These nodes are generally minimally tender, firm, and rubbery in consistency.

5. **Alopecia.** "Moth-eaten" alopecia is occasionally seen among patients presenting with secondary syphilis. This condition is usually reversible with treatment.

6. **Neurologic abnormalities.** Central nervous system (CNS) syphilis may occur within the first few weeks after initial infection or up to 25 years later.

   a. The acute manifestations of secondary syphilis (including the neurologic abnormalities) typically resolve spontaneously, even in the absence of therapy.

   b. Indications for lumbar puncture are symptoms of meningitis or focal neurologic findings.

   c. **Early syphilis in HIV-infected patients.** There is a strong association between syphilis and the human immunodeficiency virus (HIV) infection.

   d. **Latent syphilis** refers to the period during which patients infected with Tp have no symptoms but have infection demonstrable by serologic testing. Early latent syphilis is defined as infection of one year's duration or less. All other cases are referred to as late latent syphilis or latent syphilis of unknown duration. A longer duration of therapy is recommended for patients with late latent syphilis.

II. **Diagnosis.** The chancre of primary syphilis is best diagnosed by darkfield microscopy, while secondary syphilis is reliably diagnosed by serologic testing.

A. **Serologic testing for syphilis**

1. **Darkfield microscopy.** The most rapid method for diagnosing primary and secondary syphilis is direct visualization of the spirochete from moist lesions by darkfield microscopy.

2. **Serologic tests.** Most patients suspected of having syphilis must be diagnosed by serologic testing. There are two types of serologic tests for syphilis: nontreponemal tests such as the Venereal Disease Research Laboratory (VDRL) test and the Rapid Plasma Reagin (RPR) test, and treponemal tests such as the fluorescent treponemal antibody absorption (FTA-ABS) test, the microhemagglutination test for antibodies to Treponema pallidum (MHA-TP), and the Treponema pallidum particle agglutination assay (TPPA).

   a. **Nontreponemal tests** are based upon the reactivity of serum from patients with syphilis to a cardiolipin-cholesterol-lecithin antigen. These tests measure IgG and IgM antibodies and are used as the screening test for syphilis. Positive tests are usually reported as a titer of antibody, and they can be used to follow the response to treatment in many patients.

   b. **Treponemal tests** are used as confirmatory tests when the nontreponemal tests are reactive. These tests all use T. pallidum antigens and are based upon the detection of antibodies directed against treponemal cellular components.

3. **Algorithm for screening and testing.** Serologic testing to diagnose syphilis is performed in two settings: screening of patients at increased risk and evaluation of patients with suspected disease.

a. Screening is recommended for all pregnant women and people at higher risk of acquiring syphilis (MSM who engage in high risk behaviors, commercial sex workers, persons who exchange sex for drugs, and those in adult correctional facilities).
b. Screening begins with a nontreponemal test such as the VDRL; a reactive specimen is then confirmed with a treponemal test such as the FTA-ABS.
c. The most common cause of a false negative syphilis serologic test is performance prior to the development of antibodies. Twenty to 30 percent of patients presenting with a chancre will not yet have developed a reactive serologic test for syphilis.

4. **Monitoring the response to therapy.** The following reductions in reagin antibody titers are noted after recommended antibiotic therapy:
   a. Among patients with primary and secondary syphilis, a fourfold decline by six months and an eightfold decline by 12 months.
   b. Compared to those with primary and secondary syphilis, the rate of decline is slower among patients with early latent syphilis — fourfold decline by 12 months.

Causes of False-positive Tests for Syphilis

Nontreponemal tests (VDRL, RPR) - acute	Nontreponemal tests (VDRL, RPR) - chronic	Treponemal tests (FTA-ABS, MHA-TP)
Pneumococcal pneumonia	Chronic liver disease	Lyme borreliosis
Scarlet fever	Malignancy (advanced)	Leprosy
Leprosy	Injection drug use	Malaria
Lymphogranuloma venereum	Myeloma	Infectious mononucleosis
Relapsing fever	Advanced age	Relapsing fever
infective endocarditis	Connective tissue disease	Leptospirosis
Malaria	Multiple transfusions	Systemic lupus erythematosus
Rickettsial infections		
Psittacosis		
Leptospirosis		
Chancroid		
Tuberculosis		
Mycoplasma infections		
Trypanosomiasis		
Varicella infections		
HIV		
Measles		
Infectious mononucleosis		
Mumps		
Viral hepatitis		
Pregnancy		

Indications for cerebrospinal fluid examination in patients with reactive syphilis serologic tests

Signs of neurosyphilis
    Weakness, pain, paresthesias, sensory changes in the legs
    Hyperactive deep tendon reflexes (later, absent DTRs)
    Loss of vibratory and position sense in the legs
    Broad-based, stamping gait
    Fecal or urinary incontinence
    Confusion, psychotic behavior, dementia

Signs of ophthalmic syphilis
    Chorioretinitis
    Acute optic neuritis
    Optic atrophy
    Pupillary abnormalities (small, fixed pupils that do not react to light)

Evidence of active tertiary syphilis
    Cardiovascular syphilis (aortic aneurysm, aortic regurgitation)
    Late benign syphilis (gummatous syphilis): most frequently involving bones, skin

Treatment failure
    In primary and secondary syphilis:
        Failure of non-treponemal test titer to decline fourfold after six months
        Failure of non-treponemal test titer to decline eightfold after twelve months
    In early latent syphilis
        Failure of non-treponemal test titer to decline fourfold after twelve months

HIV-infected patients with late latent syphilis or latent syphilis of unknown duration

III. Treatment of early syphilis

A. A single dose of benzathine penicillin G (2.4 million units IM) is standard therapy for all forms of early syphilis.

B. The single dose of benzathine penicillin as therapy is only appropriate when it is possible to document that there was a non-reactive syphilis serologic within the past year or if there is good documentation of the chancre of primary syphilis serology within the past year. Otherwise it should be referred to as latent syphilis of unknown duration for which three doses of benzathine penicillin at weekly intervals are recommended.

C. Some patients do not respond, based upon failure of serum VDRL titers to decrease at least fourfold over 6 to 12 months of follow-up. Some of these cases may be due to reinfection. Such treatment failures are managed by giving another course of benzathine penicillin, and all sexual contacts.

D. Patients with early syphilis who are allergic to penicillin may be treated with 14 days of either doxycycline (100 mg PO BID) or tetracycline (500 mg PO QID).

E. Azithromycin has also been considered an option for penicillin-allergic patients. Azithromycin should be avoided in regions where azithromycin resistance is relatively common and in patients with frequent macrolide use (eg, MAC prophylaxis in HIV-infected patients).

F. There is no alternative to penicillin for the treatment of syphilis during pregnancy; penicillin allergic pregnant patients should be desensitized to penicillin.

Stages of Syphilitic Infection			
Stage	Clinical manifestations	Diagnosis (sensitivity)	Treatment
Primary	Chancre	Dark-field micros-	Penicillin G benzathine, 2.4

Stage	Clinical manifestations	Diagnosis (sensitivity)	Treatment
syphilis		copy of skin lesion (80%) Nontreponemal tests (78% to 86%) Treponemal-specific tests (76% to 84%)	million units IM (single dose) Alternatives in nonpregnant patients with penicillin allergy: doxycycline (Vibramycin), 100 mg orally twice daily for 2 weeks; tetracycline, 500 mg orally four times daily for 2 weeks; ceftriaxone (Rocephin), 1 g once daily IM or IV for 8 to 10 days; or azithromycin (Zithromax), 2 g orally (single dose)
Secondary syphilis	Skin and mucous membranes: diffuse rash, condyloma latum, other lesions Renal system: glomerulonephritis, nephrotic syndrome Liver: hepatitis Central nervous system: headache, meningismus, cranial neuropathy, iritis and uveitis Constitutional symptoms: fever, malaise, generalized lymphadenopathy, arthralgias, weight loss, others	Dark-field microscopy of skin lesion (80%) Nontreponemal tests (100%) Treponemal-specific tests (100%)	Same treatments as for primary syphilis
Latent syphilis	None	Nontreponemal tests (95% to 100%) Treponemal-specific tests (97% to 100%)	Early latent syphilis: same treatments as for primary and secondary syphilis Late latent syphilis: penicillin G benzathine, 2.4 million units IM once weekly for 3 weeks Alternatives in nonpregnant patients with penicillin allergy: doxycycline, 100 mg orally twice daily for 4 weeks; or tetracycline, 500 mg orally four times daily for 4 weeks
Tertiary (late) syphilis	Gummatous disease, cardiovascular disease	Nontreponemal tests (71% to 73%) Treponemal-specific tests (94% to	Same treatment as for late latent syphilis

Stage	Clinical manifestations	Diagnosis (sensitivity)	Treatment
		96%)	
Neuro-syphilis	Seizures, ataxia, aphasia, paresis, hyperreflexia, personality changes, cognitive disturbance, visual changes, hearing loss, neuropathy, loss of bowel or bladder function, others	Cerebrospinal fluid examination	Aqueous crystalline penicillin G, 3 to 4 million units IV every 4 hours for 10 to 14 days; or penicillin G procaine, 2.4 million units IM once daily, plus probenecid, 500 mg orally four times daily, with both drugs given for 10 to 14 days

References: See page 294.

Pulmonary Tuberculosis

Mycobacterium tuberculosis infection most commonly affects the lungs. Pulmonary manifestations of tuberculosis (TB) include primary, reactivation, endobronchial, and lower lung field infection.

I. **Primary tuberculosis**
   A. **Fever** is the most common symptom, occurring in 70 percent of patients. Fever is low grade but could be as high as 39ºC and usually last for14 to 21 days. Fever usually resolves in 10 weeks.
   B. Symptoms in addition to fever are present only in 25 percent of patients, and include chest pain and pleuritic chest pain.
   C. The physical examination is usually normal; pulmonary signs include pain to palpation and signs of an effusion.
   D. **Radiographic abnormalities.** The most common abnormality on chest radiography is hilar adenopathy, occurring in 65 percent. Hilar changes can be seen as early as one week after skin test conversion and within two months in all cases. These radiographic findings resolve slowly, often over a period of more than one year.
   E. One-third of converters developed pleural effusions. Pulmonary infiltrates occur in 27 percent. Perihilar and right sided infiltrates are the most common, with ipsilateral hilar enlargement. Lower and upper lobe infiltrates are observed in 33 and 13 percent of adults, respectively. Most infiltrates resolved over months to years.

II. **Reactivation tuberculosis**
   A. Reactivation TB represents 90 percent of adult cases, and results from reactivation of a previously dormant focus seeded at the time of the primary infection. The apical posterior segments of the lung are frequently involved.
   B. Symptoms typically began insidiously and are present for weeks or months before diagnosis. One-half to two-thirds of patients develop cough, weight loss and fatigue. Fever and night sweats or night sweats alone are present in one-half. Chest pain and dyspnea each are reported in one-third of patients, and hemoptysis in one-quarter.
   C. The cough of TB may be mild initially and may be non-productive or productive of only scant sputum. Initially, it may be present only in the morning. As the disease progresses, cough becomes more continuous and productive of yellow or yellow-green sputum. Frank hemoptysis is present later.

D. Dyspnea can occur when patients have extensive parenchymal involvement, pleural effusions, or a pneumothorax. Pleuritic chest pain is not common.

E. **Physical findings of pulmonary TB** are usually absent in mild or moderate disease.

    1. Dullness with decreased fremitus may indicate pleural thickening or effusion. Rales may be heard only after a short cough (post-tussive rales).

    2. When large areas of the lung are involved, signs of consolidation, such as whispered pectoriloquy or tubular breath sounds, may be heard. Extrapulmonary signs include clubbing and findings at other sites of involvement.

F. **Laboratory findings** are usually normal in pulmonary TB. Late in the disease, hematologic changes may include normocytic anemia, leukocytosis, or, more rarely, monocytosis. Hyponatremia may be associated with the syndrome of inappropriate antidiuretic hormone secretion (SIADH) or rarely with adrenal insufficiency.

G. **Radiographic abnormalities**

    1. **Reactivation TB** typically involves the apical-posterior segments of the upper lobes (80 to 90 percent), followed in frequency by the superior segment of the lower lobes and the anterior segment of the upper lobes; 19 to 40 percent also have cavities, with visible air-fluid levels.

    2. **Computed tomographic (CT) scanning** is more sensitive than plain chest radiography for diagnosis. CT scan may show a cavity or centrilobular lesions, nodules and branching linear densities.

III. **Targeted tuberculin testing and treatment of latent tuberculosis infection**

A. **Targeted tuberculin testing** for latent tuberculosis infection (LTBI) identifies persons at high risk for developing TB who would benefit by treatment of LTBI, if detected. Persons with increased risk for developing TB include those who have had recent infection with Mycobacterium tuberculosis and those who have clinical conditions that are associated with an increased risk for progression of LTBI to active TB. Targeted tuberculin testing programs should be conducted only among groups at high risk.

B. For persons who are at highest risk for developing active TB (ie, HIV infection, immunosuppressive therapy, recent close contact with persons with infectious TB, or who have abnormal chest radiographs consistent with prior TB), >5 mm of induration is considered positive.

IV. **Clinical and laboratory monitoring**

A. Baseline laboratory testing is not routinely indicated for all patients at the start of treatment for LTBI. Patients whose initial evaluation suggests a liver disorder should have baseline hepatic measurements of serum aspartate aminotransferase (AST) or alanine aminotransferase(ALT) and bilirubin.

Groups at High Risk for Tuberculosis

Persons with recent Mycobacterium tuberculosis infection (within the past 2 years) or
a history of inadequately treated tuberculosis

Close contacts of persons known or suspected to have tuberculosis

Persons infected with the human immunodeficiency virus

Persons who inject illicit drugs or use other locally identified high-risk substances (eg
crack cocaine)

Residents and employees of high-risk congregate settings (eg correctional institutions, nursing homes, mental institutions or shelters for the homeless)

Health-care workers who serve high-risk clients

Foreign-born persons including children who have recently arrived (within 5 years)
from countries that have a high incidence or prevalence of tuberculosis (Africa
Asia and Latin America)

Some medically underserved low-income populations

High-risk racial or ethnic minority populations as defined locally

Elderly persons

Children less than 4 years of age or infants children and adolescents who have been
exposed to adults in high-risk categories

Persons with medical conditions known to increase the risk of tuberculosis:

    Chest radiograph findings suggestive of previous tuberculosis in a person who
received inadequate treatment or no treatment

    Diabetes mellitus

    Silicosis

    Organ transplantation

    Prolonged corticosteroid therapy (eg prednisone in a 15 mg or more per day for
1 month

    Other immunosuppressive therapy

    Cancer of the head and neck

    Hematologic and reticuloendothelial diseases (eg leukemia and lymphoma)

    End-stage renal disease

    Intestinal bypass or gastrectomy

    Chronic malabsorption syndromes

    Weight that is 10 percent or more below ideal body weight

Interpretation of the Purified Protein Derivative Tuberculin Skin Test

I. An induration of 5 mm or more is classified as positive in persons with any of the
following:
   - A. Human immunodeficiency virus infection
   - B. Recent close contact with persons who have active tuberculosis
   - C. Chest radiographs showing fibrosis (consistent with healed tuberculosis)

II. An induration of 10 mm or more is classified as positive in all persons who do not
meet any of the criteria in section I but have other risk factors for tuberculosis

III. An induration of 15 mm or more is positive in persons who do not meet any of the
criteria from sections I or II.

IV. Recent tuberculin skin test conversion is defined as an increase in induration of
10 mm or more within a two-year period, regardless of age.

V. In health-care workers, the recommendations in sections I, II and III generally
should be followed. In facilities where tuberculosis patients frequently receive
care, the optimal cut-off point for health-care workers with no other risk factors
may be an induration of 10 mm or greater.

    B. Baseline testing is also indicated for patients with HIV infection, pregnant
women, and women in the immediate postpartum period (ie, within three
months of delivery), persons with a history of chronic liver disease (eg,
hepatitis B or C, alcoholic hepatitis, or cirrhosis), alcoholics, and persons
at risk for chronic liver disease. Baseline testing is not routinely indicated
in older persons. Hepatitis and end-stage liver disease are relative
contraindications to the use of isoniazid or pyrazinamide for treatment of
LTBI.

    C. Routine laboratory monitoring during treatment of LTBI is indicated for
persons whose baseline liver function tests are abnormal and other

persons at risk for hepatic disease. Isoniazid should be withheld if transaminase levels exceed three times the upper limit of normal if associated with symptoms and five times the upper limit of normal if the patient is asymptomatic.

D. Chest radiograph is indicated for all persons being considered for treatment of LTBI to exclude active pulmonary TB.

E. If chest radiographs are normal and no symptoms consistent with active TB are present, tuberculin-positive persons may be candidates for treatment of LTBI. If radiographic or clinical findings are consistent with pulmonary or extrapulmonary TB, further studies (eg, medical evaluation, bacteriologic examinations, and a comparison of the current and old chest radiographs) should be done to determine if treatment for active TB is indicated.

F. Sputum examination is not indicated for most persons being considered for treatment of LTBI. However, persons with chest radiographic findings suggestive of prior, healed TB infections should have three consecutive sputum samples, obtained on different days, submitted for AFB smear and culture. HIV-infected persons with respiratory symptoms who are being considered for treatment of LTBI should also have sputum specimens submitted for mycobacterial examination, even if the chest radiograph is normal. If the results of sputum smears and cultures are negative, the person is a candidate for treatment of LTBI.

V. Treatment of tuberculosis

Drug regimens for culture-positive tuberculosis caused by drug-susceptible organisms					
Regi-men	Drugs	Interval and doses, mini-mal duration	Regi-men	Drugs	Interval and doses, minimal duration
1	INH RIF PZA EMB	Seven days per week for 56 doses (8 wk) or 5 d/wk for 40 doses (8 wk)	1a	INH/RIF	Seven days per week for 126 doses (18 wk) or 5 d/wk for 90 doses (18 wk)
			1b	INH/RIF	Twice weekly for 36 doses (18 wk)
			1c	INH/RPT	Once weekly for 18 doses (18 wk)
2	INH RIF PZA EMB	Seven days per week for 14 doses (2 wk), then twice weekly for 12 doses (6 wk) or 5 d/wk for 10 doses (2 wk), then twice weekly for 12 doses (6 wk)	2a	INH/RIF	Twice weekly for 36 doses (18 wk)
			2b	INH/RPT	Once weekly for 18 doses (18 wk)
3	INH RIF PZA EMB	Three times weekly for 24 doses (8 wk)	3a	INH/RIF	Three times weekly for 54 doses (18 wk)

Regimen	Drugs	Interval and doses, minimal duration	Regimen	Drugs	Interval and doses, minimal duration
4	INH RIF EMB	Seven days per week for 56 doses (8 wk) or 5 d/wk for 40 doses (8 wk)	4a	INH/RIF	Seven days per week for 217 doses (31 wk) or 5 d/wk for 155 doses (31 wk)
			4b	INH/RIF	Twice weekly for 62 doses (31 wk)

Treatment of latent tuberculosis infection

Drugs	Duration (mo)	Interval	HIV-	HIV+
Isoniazid	9	Daily	preferred	preferred
		Twice weekly	acceptable alternative	acceptable alternative
Isoniazid	6	Daily	acceptable alternative	offer when others cannot be given
		Twice weekly	acceptable alternative	offer when others cannot be given
Rifampin-pyrazinamide	2	Daily	acceptable alternative	preferred
	2-3	Twice weekly	offer when others cannot be given	offer when others cannot be given
Rifampin	4	Daily	acceptable alternative	acceptable alternative

Treatment of Active Tuberculosis: First-Line Medications

Drug	Daily dosing	Twice-weekly dosing	Thrice-weekly dosing	Adverse reactions
Isoniazid (INH)	Children: 10 mg per kg PO or IM Adults: 300 mg PO or IM Max: 300 mg Children: 20-40 mg/kg PO/IM	Adults: 15 mg per kg PO or IM Maximum: 300 mg Children: 20 to 40 mg per kg PO or IM	Adults: 15 mg per kg PO or IM Maximum: 300 mg	Elevation of hepatic enzyme levels, hepatitis, neuropathy, central nervous system effects

Drug	Daily dosing	Twice-weekly dosing	Thrice-week-ly dosing	Adverse re-actions
Rifampin (Rifadin)	Children: 10 to 20 mg per kg PO or IV Adults: 10 mg per kg PO or IV Maximum: 600 mg Children: 10 to 20 mg per kg PO or IV	Adults: 10 mg per kg PO or IV Maximum: 600 mg Children: 10 to 20 mg per kg PO or IV	Adults: 10 mg per kg PO or IV Maximum: 600 mg	Orange discoloration of secretions and urine, gastrointestinal tract upset, hepatitis, bleeding problems, flu-like symptoms, drug interactions, rash
Pyrazinamide	Children: 20 to 30 mg per kg PO Adults: 25 mg per kg PO	Maximum: 2 g Children: 50 to 70 mg per kg PO Adults: 50 to 70 mg per kg PO	Maximum: 4 g Children: 50 to 70 mg per kg PO Adults: 50 to 70 mg per kg PO Maximum: 3 g	Gastrointestinal tract upset, hepatitis, hyperuricemia, arthralgias
Ethambutol (Myambutol)	Children and adults: 15 to 25 mg per kg PO	Children and adults: 50 mg per kg PO	Children and adults: 25 to 30 mg per kg PO	Optic neuritis

VI. Monitoring
    A. Baseline and follow-up studies. Patients receiving combination antituberculous therapy with first-line drugs should undergo baseline measurement of hepatic enzymes (AST, bilirubin, alkaline phosphatase), platelet count, serum creatinine, and hepatitis B serology prior to the initiation of therapy. Testing of visual acuity and red-green color discrimination should be obtained when treatment includes EMB.

    B. Repeated monthly measurements should be obtained in the following settings:
        1. The baseline results are abnormal
        2. A drug reaction is suspected
        3. HIV infection
        4. Liver disease (eg, hepatitis B or C, alcohol abuse)
        5. Women who are pregnant or in the first three months postpartum
        6. Patients receiving combination therapy with pyrazinamide

    C. Response to treatment. The overall treatment success rate for tuberculosis worldwide is 82 percent.

    D. AFB smears. Patients being treated for pulmonary tuberculosis should submit a sputum specimen for microscopic examination and culture at a minimum of monthly intervals until two consecutive specimens are negative on culture.

References: See page 294.

Tetanus Prophylaxis

History of Two Primary Immunizations:
  Low risk wound - Tetanus toxoid 0.5 mL IM.
  Tetanus prone - Tetanus toxoid 0.5 mL IM + Tetanus immunoglobulin (TIG)
    250-500 U IM.
Three Primary and 10 yrs since last Booster:
  Low risk wound - Tetanus toxoid, 0.5 mL IM.
  Tetanus prone - Tetanus toxoid, 0.5 mL IM.
Three Primary and 5-10 yrs since last Booster:
  Low risk wound - None
  Tetanus prone - Tetanus toxoid, 0.5 mL IM.
Three Primary and ≤5 yrs since last Booster:
  Low risk wound - None
  Tetanus prone - None

Conjunctivitis

Conjunctivitis is the most likely diagnosis in a patient with a red eye and discharge. Most infectious conjunctivitis is viral in adults and children.

I. Etiology and clinical manifestations
  A. Acute conjunctivitis can be classified as infectious or noninfectious and further divided into four main types:
    1. Infectious: Bacterial or viral
    2. Noninfectious: Allergic nonallergic

Differential Diagnosis of Red Eye	

Conjunctivitis
  Infectious
    Viral
    Bacterial (eg, staphylococcus, Chlamydia)
  Noninfectious
    Allergic conjunctivitis
    Dry eye
    Toxic or chemical reaction
    Contact lens use
    Foreign body
    Factitious conjunctivitis
	Keratitis
	    Infectious. Bacterial, viral, fungal
	    Noninfectious. Recurrent epithelial erosion, foreign body
	Uveitis
	Episcleritis/scleritis
	Acute glaucoma
	Eyelid abnormalities
	Orbital disorders
	    Preseptal and orbital cellulitis
	    Idiopathic orbital inflammation (pseudotumor)

  B. Bacterial conjunctivitis is commonly caused by Staphylococcus aureus, Streptococcus pneumoniae, Haemophilus influenzae, and Moraxella catarrhalis.
    1. Bacterial conjunctivitis is highly contagious; it is spread by direct contact with the patient and his secretions or with contaminated objects.
    2. Bacterial conjunctivitis usually causes unilateral redness and discharge. Similar to viral and allergic conjunctivitis, the affected eye often is "stuck shut" in the morning. The purulent discharge continues throughout the day. The discharge is thick and globular; it may be yellow, white, or green. The appearance differs from that of viral or allergic conjunctivitis, which presents with a mostly watery discharge during the day, with a scanty, stringy component that is mucus rather than pus.

C. Hyperacute bacterial conjunctivitis

1. N. gonorrhoeae can cause a hyperacute bacterial conjunctivitis that is severe and sight-threatening, requiring immediate ophthalmologic referral. Concurrent urethritis is typically present.

2. The eye infection is characterized by a profuse purulent discharge. Other symptoms include redness, irritation, and tenderness to palpation. There is typically marked chemosis, lid swelling, and tender preauricular adenopathy. Gram negative diplococci can be identified on Gram stain of the discharge. These patients require hospitalization for systemic and topical therapy.

D. Viral conjunctivitis is typically caused by adenovirus. The conjunctivitis may be followed by adenopathy, fever, pharyngitis, and upper respiratory tract infection. Viral conjunctivitis is highly contagious; it is spread by direct contact with the patient and his or her secretions or with contaminated objects and surfaces.

1. Viral conjunctivitis presents as injection, watery or mucoserous discharge, and a burning, sandy, or gritty feeling in one eye. Patients may have morning crusting followed by watery discharge with some scanty mucus throughout the day. The second eye usually becomes involved within 24 to 48 hours.

2. On examination there typically is only mucoid discharge on the lower lid in the corner of the eye. Usually there is profuse tearing rather than discharge. The tarsal conjunctiva may have a follicular or "bumpy" appearance. An enlarged and tender preauricular node may be present.

3. Viral conjunctivitis is a self-limited process. The symptoms frequently get worse for the first three to five days, with very gradual resolution over the following one to two weeks.

E. Allergic conjunctivitis is caused by airborne allergens, which cause local mast cell degranulation and the release of histamine.

1. It typically presents as bilateral redness, watery discharge, and itching. Itching is the cardinal symptom of allergy, distinguishing it from a viral etiology, which is more typically described as grittiness, burning, or irritation. Eye rubbing can worsen symptoms. Patients with allergic conjunctivitis often have a history of atopy, seasonal allergy, or specific allergy (eg, to cats).

2. Similar to viral conjunctivitis, allergic conjunctivitis causes diffuse injection with a follicular appearance to the tarsal conjunctiva and profuse watery or mucoserous discharge. There may be morning crusting. It is the complaint of itching and the history of allergy or hay fever and a recent exposure allows the distinction between allergic and viral conjunctivitis; the clinical findings are the same.

II. Diagnosis

A. Conjunctivitis is a diagnosis of exclusion. Conjunctivitis causes red eye and discharge; however, the vision is normal and there is no evidence of keratitis, iritis, or glaucoma.

B. Patients with all types of conjunctivitis complain of morning crusting and daytime redness and discharge. On examination, there should be no focal pathology in the lids such as hordeolum (stye), cancerous mound or ulceration, or blepharitis (diffuse eyelid margin thickening and hyperemia with lash crusts). The redness or injection should be diffuse. Foreign body, pterygium, or episcleritis should be considered if the conjunctival injection is localized rather than diffuse.

C. Cultures are not necessary for the initial diagnosis and therapy of conjunctivitis.

D. Red flags for more serious problems that should prompt evaluation by an ophthalmologist:
1. Reduction of visual acuity
2. Ciliary flush: A pattern of injection in which the redness is most pronounced in a ring at the limbus (the limbus is the transition zone between the cornea and the sclera).

3. Photophobia.
4. Severe foreign body sensation that prevents the patient from keeping the eye open.
5. Corneal opacity.
6. Fixed pupil.
7. Severe headache with nausea.

III. **Therapy.** Bacterial conjunctivitis is likely to be self-limited, although treatment shortens the clinical course and reduces person-to-person spread.

    A. **Bacterial conjunctivitis** is treated with erythromycin ophthalmic ointment (Ilotycin and generic), or sulfa ophthalmic drops (Sulf-10, Bleph-10, Sulamyd, or as a 10% generic solution). The dose is 1/2" (1.25 cm) of ointment deposited inside the lower lid or 1 to 2 drops instilled four times daily for five to seven days. The dose may be reduced from four times daily to twice daily, if there is improvement in symptoms after three days.

        1. Ointment is preferred over drops for children, drops are preferable for adults because ointments blur vision for 20 minutes after the dose is administered.

        2. Alternative therapies include bacitracin ointment, sulfacetamide ointment, polymyxin-bacitracin ointment (Polysporin), or fluoroquinolone drops (Ciloxan, Ocuflox, Quixin, Zymar, Vigamox). Aminoglycosides are poor choices since they are toxic to the corneal epithelium and can cause a reactive keratoconjunctivitis.

        3. The fluoroquinolones are effective and well tolerated; they are the treatment of choice for corneal ulcers and are extremely effective against pseudomonas. Conjunctivitis in a contact lens wearer should be treated with a fluoroquinolone because of the high incidence of pseudomonas infection.

        4. Contact lens wearers with a red eye should discontinue contact lens wear. Contact lens wear can resume when the eye is white and has no discharge for 24 hours after the completion of antibiotic therapy. The lens case should be discarded and the lenses subjected to overnight disinfection or replaced if disposable.

    B. **Viral conjunctivitis.** Some patients derive symptomatic relief from topical antihistamine/decongestants. These are available over the counter (Naphcon-A, OcuHist, generics). Warm or cool compresses may provide additional symptomatic relief.

    C. **Allergic conjunctivitis.** There are numerous therapies available for allergic conjunctivitis (see below).

References: See page 294.

Gastrointestinal Disorders

Gastroesophageal Reflux Disease

Gastroesophageal reflux disease is caused by the combination of excess reflux of gastric juice and impaired clearance of this refluxate from the esophagus. GERD is defined as symptoms or tissue damage caused by reflux of gastric contents with or without esophageal inflammation.

I. Clinical manifestations
   A. Typical symptoms of GERD are heartburn and regurgitation; atypical symptoms include odynophagia, dysphagia, chest pain, cough, and reactive airway disease. Up to half of the general population has monthly heartburn or regurgitation.
   B. Heartburn, the most common symptom of GERD, is a substernal burning sensation that rises from the upper abdomen into the chest and neck. Dysphagia, the sensation that swallowed material is lodged in the chest, may be caused by esophageal inflammation or impaired motility. Esophageal cancer also is an important differential diagnostic consideration when dysphagia is the presenting complaint.

Symptoms of GERD	
Heartburn (pyrosis)	Chronic cough
Regurgitation	Nocturnal cough
Dysphagia	Asthma
Water brash	Dyspepsia
Globus	Hiccups
Odynophagia	Chest pain
Hoarseness	Nausea

   C. Chest pain due to GERD can mimic angina. Extraesophageal manifestations of GERD include asthma, chronic cough, sinusitis, pneumonitis, laryngitis, hoarseness, hiccups, and dental disease. Complications of long-standing GERD include esophageal stricture and Barrett's esophagus.

Differential diagnostic considerations in GERD	
Esophageal neoplasm	Nonulcer dyspepsia
Infectious esophagitis	Coronary artery disease
Caustic esophagitis	Hepatobiliary disease
Pill esophagitis	Esophageal motility disorders
Gastritis	Cholelithiasis
Peptic ulcer disease	

II. Diagnosis
   A. Diagnosis of GERD is often based on clinical findings and confirmed by the response to therapy. Diagnostic evaluation should be pursued if symptoms are chronic or refractory to therapy or if esophageal or extra-esophageal complications are suspected.

Indications for esophageal endoscopy in patients with GERD

Dysphagia or odynophagia
Persistent or progressive symptoms despite therapy
Esophageal symptoms in an immunocompromised patient
Mass, stricture, or ulcer on upper gastrointestinal barium study
Gastrointestinal bleeding or iron deficiency anemia
At least 10 years of GERD symptoms (screen for Barrett's esophagus)

    B. Ambulatory esophageal pH monitoring is performed by placing a pH electrode just above the lower esophageal sphincter. This test has a sensitivity of 60-100%.

    C. Short PPI trials are useful for diagnosis of GERD and have a sensitivity of 70 to 90% and specificity of 55 to 85%.

III.   **Treatment options**

    A. Lifestyle modification. Strategies include elevation of the head of the bed 6 to 8 in; reduced consumption of fatty foods, chocolate, alcohol, colas, red wine, citrus juices, and tomato products; avoidance of the supine position after meals; not eating within 3 hours of bedtime; avoidance of tight-fitting clothing; weight loss if obese; and smoking cessation.

    B. Although H_2-blockers are less expensive than PPIs, PPIs provide superior acid suppression, healing rates and symptom relief. Therefore, PPIs may be more cost-effective than H_2-blockers, especially in patients with more severe acid-peptic disorders, because of their lower and less frequent dosing requirements and their comparatively shorter duration of required therapy.

    C. Histamine$_2$-blockers are used extensively. The four available agents, cimetidine (Tagamet), famotidine (Pepcid), nizatidine (Axid), and ranitidine (Zantac), are equivalent. Dosage must be reduced in patients with renal failure. In general, doses of H_2 blockers required to control GERD symptoms and heal esophagitis are two to three times higher than those needed for treatment of peptic ulcer disease. Rates of symptom control and healing are about 50%.

        1. Cimetidine (Tagamet), 800 mg twice daily; **ranitidine (Zantac)**, 150 mg four times daily; **famotidine (Pepcid)**, 40 mg twice daily; and **nizatidine (Axid)**, 150 mg twice daily.

    D. Proton pump inhibitors (PPIs) irreversibly bind and inhibit the proton pump.

        1. The five available PPIs, esomeprazole (Nexium), lansoprazole (Prevacid), omeprazole (Prilosec), pantoprazole (Protonix), and rabeprazole (AcipHex), have similar pharmacologic activities. PPIs should be taken 20 to 30 minutes before the first meal of the day. PPIs are more effective than are H2 blockers.

        2. In contrast to the other Proton Pump Inhibitors (PPIs), rabeprazole (AcipHex) forms a partially reversible bond with the proton pump. Therefore, it may have a more sustained acid-suppressing effect than the other PPIs. Rabeprazole and pantoprazole, seem to have fewer drug interactions. Pantoprazole is the least expensive.

Proton Pump Inhibitors	
Drug	**Dosage**
Esomeprazole - *Nexium*	20 mg or 40 mg, 20 to 30 minutes before the first meal of the day
Lansoprazole - *Prevacid*	30 mg, 20 to 30 minutes before the first meal of the day

Drug	Dosage
Omeprazole - *Prilosec*, generic	20 mg/day, 20 to 30 minutes before the first meal of the day
Pantoprazole - *Protonix*	40 mg PO, 20 minuted before the first meal of the day or IV once daily
Rabeprazole - *AcipHex*	20 mg/day, 20 to 30 minutes before the first meal of the day

E. Surgical treatment. The most common of the antireflux procedures used to treat GERD is the Nissen fundoplication, which is a laparoscopic procedure. A portion of the stomach is wrapped around the distal esophagus. Indications include patient preference for surgical treatment over prolonged medical therapy, incomplete control despite medical therapy, and refractory manifestations of reflux (eg, pneumonia, laryngitis, asthma).

IV. Management considerations

A. Patients with frequent or unrelenting symptoms or esophagitis, or both, should be treated from the outset with a PPI once or twice daily as appropriate.

B. Refractory GERD. Increasing the dosage of PPIs often can control GERD in patients receiving a single daily dose. Sometimes switching to a different PPI can improve symptoms. Antireflux surgical treatment is an alternative.

Alternative diagnoses in patients with refractory GERD

Esophageal hypersensitivity (visceral hyperalgesia) Achalasia Distal esophageal cancer Stricture NSAID-induced symptoms Infection (eg, Candida, herpes, cytomegalovirus esophagitis)	Caustic exposure Impaired gastric emptying Eosinophilic gastroenteritis Bile acid reflux Nonulcer dyspepsia Pill esophagitis

References: See page 294.

Helicobacter Pylori Infection and Peptic Ulcer Disease

The spiral-shaped, gram-negative bacterium *Helicobacter pylori* is found in gastric mucosa or adherent to the lining of the stomach. Acute infection is most commonly asymptomatic but may be associated with epigastric burning, abdominal distention or bloating, belching, nausea, flatulence, and halitosis. *H. pylori* infection can lead to ulceration of the gastric mucosa and duodenum and is associated with malignancies of the stomach. The prevalence of *H. pylori* infection is as high as 52 percent.

I. Pathophysiology

A. Helicobacter pylori (HP), a spiral-shaped, flagellated organism, is the most frequent cause of peptic ulcer disease (PUD). Nonsteroidal anti-inflammatory drugs (NSAIDs) and pathologically high acid-secreting states (Zollinger-Ellison syndrome) are less common causes. More than 90% of ulcers are associated with H. pylori. Eradication of the organism cures and prevents relapses of gastroduodenal ulcers.

    B. Complications of peptic ulcer disease include bleeding, duodenal or gastric perforation, and gastric outlet obstruction (due to inflammation or strictures).

II. Clinical evaluation

    A. Symptoms of PUD include recurrent upper abdominal pain and discomfort. The pain of duodenal ulceration is often relieved by food and antacids and worsened when the stomach is empty (eg, at nighttime). In gastric ulceration, the pain may be exacerbated by eating.

    B. Nausea and vomiting are common in PUD. Hematemesis ("coffee ground" emesis) or melena (black tarry stools) are indicative of bleeding.

    C. Physical examination. Tenderness to deep palpation is often present in the epigastrium, and the stool is often guaiac-positive.

Presentation of Uncomplicated Peptic Ulcer Disease

Epigastric pain (burning, vague abdominal discomfort, nausea)
    Often nocturnal
    Occurs with hunger or hours after meals
    Usually temporarily relieved by meals or antacids
    Persistence or recurrence over months to years
    History of self-medication and intermittent relief

    D. NSAID-related gastrointestinal complications. NSAID use and *H pylori* infection are independent risk factors for peptic ulcer disease. The risk is 5 to 20 times higher in persons who use NSAIDs than in the general population. Misoprostol (Cytotec) has been shown to prevent both NSAID ulcers and related complications. The minimum effective dosage is 200 micrograms twice daily; total daily doses of 600 micrograms or 800 micrograms are significantly more effective.

III. Indications for testing and treatment

    A. In the absence of alarm symptoms for cancer or complicated ulcer disease, the approach to testing in patients with dyspepsia can be divided into four clinical scenarios: (1) known peptic ulcer disease, currently or previously documented; (2) known nonulcer dyspepsia; (3) undifferentiated dyspepsia, and (4) gastroesophageal reflux disease (GERD).

    B. Peptic ulcer disease. Treatment of *H. pylori* infection in patients with ulcers almost always cures the disease and reduces the risk for perforation or bleeding.

    C. Nonulcer disease. There is no convincing evidence that empiric eradication of *H. pylori* in patients with nonulcer dyspepsia improves symptoms.

    D. Undifferentiated dyspepsia. A test-and-treat strategy is recommended in which patients with dyspepsia are tested for the presence of *H. pylori* with serology and treated with eradication therapy if the results are positive. Endoscopy is reserved for use in patients with alarm signs or those with persistent symptoms despite empiric therapy.

Alarm Signs for Risk of Gastric Cancer of Complicated Ulcer Disease

Older Than 45 years	Abdominal mass
Rectal bleeding or melena	Jaundice
Weight los of >10 percent of body weight	Family history of gastric cancer
Anemia	Previous history of peptic ulcer
Dysphagia	Anorexia/early satiety

Evaluation for Helicobacter pylori-Related Disease	
Clinical scenario	**Recommended test**
Dyspepsia in patient with alarm symptoms for cancer or complicated ulcer (eg, bleeding, perforation)	Promptly refer to a gastroenterologist for endoscopy.
Known PUD, uncomplicated	Serology antibody test; treat if result is positive.
Dyspepsia in patient with previous history of PUD not previously treated with eradication therapy	Serology antibody test; treat if result is positive.
Dyspepsia in patient with PUD previously treated for *H. pylori*	Stool antigen or urea breath test; if positive, treat with regimen different from the one previously used; retest to confirm eradication. Consider endoscopy.
Undifferentiated dyspepsia (without endoscopy)	Serology antibody test; treat if result is positive.
Documented nonulcer dyspepsia (after endoscopy)	Unnecessary
GERD	Unnecessary
Asymptomatic with history of documented PUD not previously treated with eradication therapy	Serology antibody test; treat if result is positive.
Asymptomatic	Screening unnecessary

   E. Gastroesophageal Reflux Disease. *H. pylori* infection does not increase
      the risk of GERD. Eradication therapy does not eliminate GERD symptoms (sensation of burning and regurgitation.
IV. Helicobacter pylori Tests
   A. Once testing and eradication are chosen, several diagnostic tests are
      available. Unless endoscopy is planned, a practical approach is to use
      serology to identify initial infection, and use the stool antigen test or urea
      breath test to determine cure, if indicated.

Noninvasive Testing Options for Detecting Helicobacter pylori				
Test	**What does it measure?**	**Sensitivity**	**Test of cure?**	**Comments**
Serology: laboratory-based ELISA	IgG	90 to 93	No	Accurate; convenient for initial infection; titers may remain positive after one year
Whole blood: office-based ELISA	IgG	50 to 85	No	Less accurate but fast, convenient

Test	What does it measure?	Sensitiv- ity	Test of cure?	Comments
Stool: HpSA	*H. pylori* anti- gens	95 to 98	Yes	Relatively conve- nient and available
Urea breath test	Urease activ- ity	95 to 100	Yes	Sensitivity reduced by acid suppression

- **B. Endoscopy and Biopsy.** Alarm symptoms for cancer or ulcer complica- tion warrant prompt endoscopic evaluation. A gastric antral biopsy specimens is considered the gold standard for detecting the presence of *H. pylori.* Cultures of biopsy specimens obtained during endoscopy can be tested for antimicrobial resistance in cases of treatment failure.
- **C. Serology/ELISA.** When endoscopy is not performed, the most commonly used diagnostic approach is the laboratory-based serologic antibody test. This enzyme-linked immunosorbent assay (ELISA) detects IgG antibod- ies to *H. pylori,* indicating current or past infection. A positive serologic test suggests active infection in patients who have not undergone eradi- cation therapy. The serologic test results may not revert to negative once the organism is eradicated; therefore, the test is not used to identify persistent infection.
- **D. Stool testing with enzyme-linked immunoassay** for *H. pylori* antigen in stool specimens is highly sensitive and specific, the stool antigen test reverts to negative from five days to a few months after eradication of the organism, with 90 percent specificity. This test is useful in confirming eradication, and, because it is office-based, is less costly and more convenient than the urea breath test. False-positive results may occur even four weeks following eradication therapy.
- **E. Urea Breath Test.** The urea breath test is a reliable test for cure and can detect the presence or absence of active *H. pylori* infection with greater accuracy than the serologic test. It is usually administered in the hospital outpatient setting because it requires time and special equipment.

V. Treatment Regimens for Helicobacter Pylori
A. Initial treatment
1. The regimen of choice is triple therapy with a proton pump inhibitor (eg, lansoprazole 30 mg twice daily, omeprazole (Prilosec) 20 mg twice daily, pantoprazole (Protonix) 40 mg twice daily, rabeprazole (AcipHex) 20 mg twice daily, or esomeprazole (Nexium) 40 mg once daily), amoxicillin (1 g twice daily), and clarithromycin (500 mg twice daily) for two weeks (10 days may be adequate). The combination of lansoprazole, amoxicillin and clarithromycin is available in a daily-dose package, Prevpac.
2. Metronidazole (Flagyl [500 mg twice daily]) can be substituted for amoxicillin but only in penicillin-allergic individuals since metronidazole resistance is common.
3. A proton pump inhibitor (PPI) may be combined with bismuth (525 mg four times daily) and two antibiotics (eg, metronidazole 500 mg four times daily and tetracycline 500 mg four times daily) for two weeks. One week of bismuth based treatment may be sufficient as long as it is given with a PPI.

Triple Therapy Regimens for *Helicobacter pylori* Infection		
Treatment (10 to 14 days of therapy recommended)	**Convenience factor**	**Tolerability**
1. Omeprazole (Prilosec), 20 mg two times daily *or* Lansoprazole (Prevacid), 30 mg two times daily *plus* Metronidazole (Flagyl), 500 mg two times daily *or* Amoxicillin, 1 g two times daily *plus* Clarithromycin (Biaxin), 500 mg two times daily **Prepackaged triple-therapy(Prevpac):** taken bid for 14 days; consists of 30 mg lansoprazole, 1 g amoxicillin, and 500 mg clarithromycin.	Twice-daily dosing	Fewer significant side effects, but more abnormal taste versus other regimens
2. Ranitidine bismuth citrate (Tritec), 400 mg twice daily *plus* Clarithromycin, 500 mg twice daily *or* Metronidazole, 500 mg twice daily *plus* Tetracycline, 500 mg twice daily *or* Amoxicillin, 1 g twice daily 92 (RMA)	Twice-daily dosing	Increased diarrhea versus other regimens

    4. Dual therapy regimens using a PPI plus one antibiotic have eradication rates significantly lower (60 to 85 percent) than the standard regimens.

    5. One-week treatment protocols have ulcer healing rates of 90 percent and H. pylori eradication rates of 77 to >85 percent.

B. Treatment failures. Initial eradication of H. pylori fails in 5 to 12 percent of patients. For patients failing one course of H. pylori treatment, quadruple therapy consisting of a PPI twice daily and bismuth-based triple therapy (Pepto Bismol 2 tablets, tetracycline 500 mg, and high dose metronidazole 500 mg all four times daily) preferably given with meals for 14 days is recommended. Two weeks should be the duration of subsequent courses of treatment.

C. Side effects are reported in up to 50 percent of patients taking one of the triple agent regimens:

    1. The most common side effect is a metallic taste due to metronidazole or clarithromycin.

    2. Metronidazole can cause peripheral neuropathy, seizures, and a disulfiram-like reaction when taken with alcohol.

    3. Tetracycline can induce a photosensitivity reaction. It should not be administered to pregnant women.

    4. Amoxicillin can cause diarrhea or an allergic reaction.

    5. Bismuth side effects are rare. Proton pump inhibitors have no significant documented adverse effects.

D. Treatment of NSAID-related ulcers

    1. When the ulcer is caused by NSAID use, healing of the ulcer is greatly facilitated by discontinuing the NSAID. Acid antisecretory therapy with an H2-blocker or proton pump inhibitor speeds ulcer healing. Proton pump inhibitors are more effective in inhibiting gastric acid production and are often used to heal ulcers in patients who require continuing NSAID treatment.

    2. If serologic or endoscopic testing for H pylori is positive, antibiotic treatment is necessary.

3. **Acute H$_2$-blocker therapy**
   a. **Ranitidine (Zantac)**, 150 mg bid or 300 mg qhs.
   b. **Famotidine (Pepcid)**, 20 mg bid or 40 mg qhs.
   c. **Nizatidine (Axid Pulvules)**, 150 mg bid or 300 mg qhs.
   d. **Cimetidine (Tagamet)**, 400 mg bid or 800 mg qhs.
4. **Proton pump inhibitors**
   a. **Omeprazole (Prilosec)**, 20 mg qd.
   b. **Lansoprazole (Prevacid)**, 15 mg before breakfast qd.
   c. **Esomeprazole (Nexium)** 20-40 mg qd.
   d. **Pantoprazole (Protonix)** 40 mg PO, 20 minuted before the first meal of the day or IV once daily.
   e. **Rabeprazole (AcipHex)** 20 mg/day, 20 to 30 minutes before the first meal of the day.

VI. **Surgical treatment of peptic ulcer disease**
   A. **Indications for surgery** include exsanguinating hemorrhage, >5 units transfusion in 24 hours, rebleeding during same hospitalization, intractability, perforation, gastric outlet obstruction, and endoscopic signs of rebleeding.
   B. **Unstable patients** should receive a truncal vagotomy, oversewing of bleeding ulcer bed, and pyloroplasty.

References: See page 294.

Constipation

Constipation affects about 2% of the population, occurring more frequently in persons older than 65.

I. **Clinical evaluation**
   A. **Diagnostic criteria for constipation (2 or more of the following):**
      1. Fewer than 3 bowel movements/week.
      2. Excessive straining during bowel movements.
      3. A feeling of incomplete evacuation after bowel movements.
      4. Passage of hard or pellet-like stools.
   B. **Clinical evaluation**
      1. The time of onset of constipation, stool frequency and consistency, the degree of straining, or sensation of incomplete evacuation should be sought.
      2. Chronic suppression of the urge to defecate contributes to constipation. The amount of fiber and fluid consumed, obstetric, surgical and drug histories, history of back trauma or neurologic problems should be assessed.
   C. **Secondary causes of constipation**
      1. Fissure in ano, hemorrhoids, fistulas, ischiorectal abscess, colonic neoplasms, hypothyroidism, hypercalcemia, diabetes, Hirschsprung's disease, Parkinson's disease, multiple sclerosis, or cerebrovascular disease may cause constipation.
      2. **Inadequate fiber** intake commonly causes constipation.
      3. **Drugs** that cause constipation include opiate analgesics, aluminum-containing antacids, iron and calcium supplements, antidiarrheals, antihistamines, antidepressants, antiparkinson agents, and calcium channel blockers.
      4. If secondary causes have been excluded, the most likely cause is idiopathic constipation related to a disorder of colorectal motility.
   D. **Physical examination**
      1. A palpable colon with stool in the left lower quadrant may be detected, although the examination is often normal. Gastrointestinal masses should be sought. Perianal inspection may reveal skin excoriation, skin tags, anal fissures, anal fistula, or hemorrhoids.
      2. Rectal examination may reveal a mass or stool. Resting and squeeze sphincter tone should be assessed. When the patient is asked to bear

down as if to defecate, relaxation of anal tone and perineal descent should be palpable. The absence of anal relaxation or inadequate perineal descent, raises the suspicion of obstructive defecation.

E. **Laboratory evaluation.** A complete blood cell count, glucose, calcium, phosphate, thyroid function test, stool examination for ova and parasites, occult blood, and flexible sigmoidoscopy may be indicated to exclude organic causes.

II. Empiric management of constipation

A. **Behavioral modification.** The patient should be encouraged to heed the urge to defecate and not suppress it. Patients should establish a regular pattern of moving their bowels at the same time every day, usually after breakfast. Daily exercise is advised.

B. **Fiber.** The patient should be placed on a diet of 20-30 g of dietary fiber per day. Fiber must be taken with ample fluids.

C. Laxatives and nonessential drugs should be discontinued.

Fiber Preparations		
Preparation	Recommended Dose	Doses/Day
Powder Metamucil (regular) Metamucil (orange flavor or sugar-free) Citrucel (orange flavor or sugar-free) Fiberall Natural Flavor	1 tsp 1 tsp 1 tbsp 1 tsp	1-3 1-3 1-3 1-3
Wafers Metamucil	2	1-3
Tablets Fiberall	1	1-2
Chewable FiberCon	2	1-4

III. Secondary evaluation

A. If dietary measures are unsuccessful, a secondary evaluation should be undertaken.

B. **Colonoscopy or barium enema** is necessary to rule out an organic lesion.

C. **Assessment of colonic transit time**

1. **The Sitzmarks test** consists of administering a Sitzmarks capsule, containing radiopaque markers. A flat-plate film of the abdomen is obtained 5 days after administration.

2. The presence of five or more markers spread out in the colon, suggests slow transit of stool through the colon. If markers are closely clustered in the rectosigmoid segment, this indicates obstructive defecation.

D. **Evaluation of obstructive defecation**

1. **Anorectal manometry.** A pressure probe is placed in the rectum and anus to assesses pressure activity.

2. **Defecography.** Barium is placed in the rectum and the patient bears down during videofluoroscopic imaging.

3. **Electromyograph.** An electrode is placed in the external anal sphincter and myoelectrical activity is measured.

4. **Simulated defecation.** A silicone-filled artificial stool is placed in the rectum. Difficulty in expelling the artificial stool indicates obstructive defecation.

IV. **Treatment of refractory constipation**
   A. **Saline cathartics**, such as magnesium-containing compounds and phosphate enemas, work by an osmotic effect. Magnesium or phosphate overload may occur in renal insufficiency. Long-term use is not recommended. **Magnesium hydroxide** (1-2 tbsp qd-bid) is most commonly used. In refractory cases, a half to 1 glassful of **magnesium citrate** is effective.
   B. **Lactulose** is a hyperosmotic non-absorbable sugar that is often used for long-term management. Its advantages are nonsystemic absorption, minimal toxicity, and safety for prolonged use; 30 mL PO qd-bid. Sorbitol is less expensive than lactulose; the 70% solution is taken as 30 mL qd-bid.
   C. **Lavage solutions (CoLyte, GoLYTELY)** are used for refractory constipation. These agents contain a balanced electrolyte solution. A gallon should be administered in 4 hours to relieve an impaction. Eight to16 oz a day can prevent recurrence.
   D. **Combination therapy** with an osmotic agent combined with a lavage solution may be used for refractory constipation.
   E. **Enemas** may relieve severe constipation. Low-volume tap water enemas or sodium phosphate (Fleet) enemas can be given once a week to help initiate a bowel movement.
   F. **Stool impaction.** A combination of suppositories (glycerin or bisacodyl) and enemas (phosphate) will soften the stool. Digital disimpaction may be necessary should these measures fail.
   G. **Surgery.** When the above measures are not effective, surgical options may include colectomy and ileostomy or an ileoanal pouch.
References: See page 294.

Acute Diarrhea

Acute diarrhea is defined as diarrheal disease of rapid onset, often with nausea, vomiting, fever, and abdominal pain. Most episodes of acute gastroenteritis will resolve within 3 to 7 days.

I.   **Clinical evaluation of acute diarrhea**
   A. The nature of onset, duration, frequency, and timing of the diarrheal episodes should be assessed. The appearance of the stool, buoyancy, presence of blood or mucus, vomiting, or pain should be determined.
   B. Contact with a potential source of infectious diarrhea should be sought.
   C. **Drugs that may cause diarrhea** include laxatives, magnesium-containing compounds, sulfa-drugs, and antibiotics.
II. **Physical examination**
   A. **Assessment of volume status.** Dehydration is suggested by dry mucous membranes, orthostatic hypotension, tachycardia, mental status changes, and acute weight loss.
   B. **Abdominal tenderness**, mild distention and hyperactive bowel sounds are common in acute infectious diarrhea. The presence of rebound tenderness or rigidity suggests toxic megacolon or perforation.
   C. **Evidence of systemic atherosclerosis** suggests ischemia. Lower extremity edema suggests malabsorption or protein loss.
III. **Acute infectious diarrhea**
   A. **Infectious diarrhea** is classified as noninflammatory or inflammatory, depending on whether the infectious organism has invaded the intestinal mucosa.
   B. **Noninflammatory** infectious diarrhea is caused by organisms that produce a toxin (enterotoxigenic E coli strains, Vibrio cholerae). Noninflammatory, infectious diarrhea is usually self-limiting and lasts less than 3 days.
   C. **Blood or mucus** in the stool suggests inflammatory disease, usually caused by bacterial invasion of the mucosa (enteroinvasive E coli, Shigella, Salmonella, Campylobacter). Patients usually have a septic

appearance and fever; some have abdominal rigidity and severe abdominal pain.

D. **Vomiting out of proportion to diarrhea** is usually related to a neuroenterotoxin-mediated food poisoning from Staphylococcus aureus or Bacillus cereus, or rotavirus (in an infant), or Norwalk virus (in older children or adults). The incubation period for neuroenterotoxin food poisoning is less than 4 hours, while that of a viral agent is more than 8 hours.

E. **Traveler's diarrhea** is a common acute diarrhea. Three or four unformed stools are passed/per 24 hours, usually starting on the third day of travel and lasting 2-3 days. Anorexia, nausea, vomiting, abdominal cramps, abdominal bloating, and flatulence may also be present.

F. **Antibiotic-related diarrhea**
   1. Antibiotic-related diarrhea ranges from mild illness to life-threatening pseudomembranous colitis. Overgrowth of Clostridium difficile causes pseudomembranous colitis. Amoxicillin, cephalosporins and clindamycin have been implicated most often, but any antibiotic can be the cause.
   2. Patients with pseudomembranous colitis have high fever, cramping, leukocytosis, and severe, watery diarrhea. Latex agglutination testing for C difficile toxin can provide results in 30 minutes.
   3. **Enterotoxigenic E coli**
      a. The enterotoxigenic E coli include the E coli serotype 0157:H7. Grossly bloody diarrhea is most often caused by E. coli 0157:H7, causing 8% of grossly bloody stools.
      b. Enterotoxigenic E coli can cause hemolytic uremic syndrome, thrombotic thrombocytopenic purpura, intestinal perforation, sepsis, and rectal prolapse.

IV. **Diagnostic approach to acute infectious diarrhea**
   A. An attempt should be made to obtain a pathologic diagnosis in patients who give a history of recent ingestion of seafood (Vibrio parahaemolyticus), travel or camping, antibiotic use, homosexual activity, or who complain of fever and abdominal pain.
   B. Blood or mucus in the stools indicates the presence of Shigella, Salmonella, Campylobacter jejuni, enteroinvasive E. coli, C. difficile, or Yersinia enterocolitica.
   C. Most cases of mild diarrheal disease do not require laboratory studies to determine the etiology. In moderate to severe diarrhea with fever or pus, a stool culture for bacterial pathogens (Salmonella, Shigella, Campylobacter) is submitted. If antibiotics were used recently, stool should be sent for Clostridium difficile toxin.

V. **Laboratory evaluation of acute diarrhea**
   A. **Fecal leukocytes** is a screening test which should be obtained if moderate to severe diarrhea is present. Numerous leukocytes indicate Shigella, Salmonella, or Campylobacter jejuni.
   B. **Stool cultures for bacterial pathogens** should be obtained if high fever, severe or persistent (>14 d) diarrhea, bloody stools, or leukocytes is present.
   C. **Examination for ova and parasites** is indicated for persistent diarrhea (>14 d), travel to a high-risk region, gay males, infants in day care, or dysentery.
   D. **Blood cultures** should be obtained prior to starting antibiotics if severe diarrhea and high fever is present.
   E. **E coli 0157:H7 cultures.** Enterotoxigenic E coli should be suspected if there are bloody stools with minimal fever, when diarrhea follows hamburger consumption, or when hemolytic uremic syndrome is diagnosed.
   F. **Clostridium difficile cytotoxin** should be obtained if diarrhea follows use of an antimicrobial agent.
   G. **Rotavirus antigen test (Rotazyme)** is indicated for hospitalized children <2 years old with gastroenteritis. The finding of rotavirus eliminates the need for antibiotics.

VI. **Treatment of acute diarrhea**
  A. **Fluid and electrolyte resuscitation**
    1. **Oral rehydration.** For cases of mild to moderate diarrhea in children, Pedialyte or Ricelyte should be administered. For adults with diarrhea, flavored soft drinks with saltine crackers are usually adequate.
    2. **Intravenous hydration** should be used if oral rehydration is not possible.
  B. **Diet.** Fatty foods should be avoided. Well-tolerated foods include complex carbohydrates (rice, wheat, potatoes, bread, and cereals), lean meats, yogurt, fruits, and vegetables. Diarrhea often is associated with a reduction in intestinal lactase. A lactose-free milk preparation may be substituted if lactose intolerance becomes apparent.
VII. **Empiric antimicrobial treatment of acute diarrhea**
  A. **Febrile dysenteric syndrome**
    1. If diarrhea is associated with high fever and stools containing mucus and blood, empiric antibacterial therapy should be given for Shigella or Campylobacter jejuni.
    2. Norfloxacin (Noroxin) 400 mg bid **OR**
    3. Ciprofloxacin (Cipro) 500 mg bid.
  B. **Travelers' diarrhea.** Adults are treated with norfloxacin 400 mg bid, ciprofloxacin (Cipro) 500 mg bid, or ofloxacin (Floxin) 300 mg bid for 3 days.
References: See page 294.

Chronic Diarrhea

Diarrhea is considered chronic if it lasts longer than 2 weeks.

I. **Clinical evaluation of chronic diarrhea**
  A. Initial evaluation should determine the characteristics of the diarrhea, including volume, mucus, blood, flatus, cramps, tenesmus, duration, frequency, effect of fasting, stress, and the effect of specific foods (eg, dairy products, wheat, laxatives, fruits).
  B. **Secretory diarrhea**
    1. Secretory diarrhea is characterized by large stool volumes (>1 L/day), no decrease with fasting, and a fecal osmotic gap <40.
    2. **Evaluation of secretory diarrhea** consists of a giardia antigen, Entamoeba histolytica antibody, Yersinia culture, fasting serum glucose, thyroid function tests, and a cholestyramine (Cholybar, Questran) trial.
  C. **Osmotic diarrhea**
    1. Osmotic diarrhea is characterized by small stool volumes, a decrease with fasting, and a fecal osmotic gap >40. Postprandial diarrhea with bloating or flatus also suggests osmotic diarrhea. Ingestion of an osmotically active laxative may be inadvertent (sugarless gum containing sorbitol) or covert (with eating disorders).
    2. **Evaluation of osmotic diarrhea**
      a. Trial of lactose withdrawal.
      b. Trial of an antibiotic (metronidazole) for small-bowel bacterial overgrowth.
      c. Screening for celiac disease (anti-endomysial antibody, antigliadin antibody).
      d. Fecal fat measurement (72 hr) for pancreatic insufficiency.
      e. Trial of fructose avoidance.
      f. Stool test for phenolphthalein and magnesium if laxative abuse is suspected.
      g. Hydrogen breath analysis to identify disaccharidase deficiency or bacterial overgrowth.

D. Exudative diarrhea

1. Exudative diarrhea is characterized by bloody stools, tenesmus, urgency, cramping pain, and nocturnal occurrence. It is most often caused by inflammatory bowel disease, which may be suggested by anemia, hypoalbuminemia, and an increased sedimentation rate.
2. **Evaluation of exudative diarrhea** consists of a complete blood cell count, serum albumin, total protein, erythrocyte sedimentation rate, electrolyte measurement, Entamoeba histolytica antibody titers, stool culture, Clostridium difficile antigen test, ova and parasite testing, and flexible sigmoidoscopy and biopsies.

References: See page 294.

Anorectal Disorders

I. Hemorrhoids

A. Hemorrhoids are dilated veins located beneath the lining of the anal canal. Internal hemorrhoids are located in the upper anal canal. External hemorrhoids are located in the lower anal canal.

B. The most common symptom of internal hemorrhoids is painless rectal bleeding, which is usually bright red and ranges from a few drops to a spattering stream at the end of defecation. If internal hemorrhoids remain prolapsed, a dull aching may occur. Blood and mucus stains may appear on underwear, and itching in the perianal region is common.

Classification of Internal Hemorrhoids		
Grade	Description	Symptoms
1	Non-prolapsing	Minimal bleeding
2	Prolapse with straining, reduce when spontaneously prolapsed	Bleeding, discomfort, pruritus
3	Prolapse with straining, manual reduction required when prolapsed	Bleeding, discomfort, pruritus
4	Cannot be reduced when prolapsed	Bleeding, discomfort, pruritus

C. Management of internal hemorrhoids

1. **Grade 1 and uncomplicated grade 2 hemorrhoids** are treated with dietary modification (increased fiber and fluids).
2. **Symptomatic grade 2 and grade 3 hemorrhoids.** Treatment consists of hemorrhoid banding with an anoscope. Major complications are rare and consist of excessive pain, bleeding, and infection. Surgical hemorrhoidectomy may sometimes be necessary.
3. **Grade 4 hemorrhoids** require surgical hemorrhoidectomy.

D. External hemorrhoids

1. External hemorrhoids occur most often in young and middle-aged adults, becoming symptomatic only when they become thrombosed.
2. External hemorrhoids are characterized by rapid onset of constant burning or throbbing pain, accompanying a new rectal lump. Bluish skin-covered lumps are visible at the anal verge.
3. Management of external hemorrhoids
   a. If patients are seen in the first 48 hours, the entire lesion can be excised in the office. Local anesthetic is infiltrated, and the throm-

bus and overlying skin are excised with scissors. The resulting wound heals by secondary intention.

b. If thrombosis occurred more than 48 hours prior, spontaneous resolution should be permitted to occur.

II. Anal fissures

A. An anal fissure is a longitudinal tear in the distal anal canal, usually in the posterior or anterior midline. Patients with anal fissures complain of perirectal pain which is sharp, searing or burning and is associated with defecation. Bleeding from anal fissures is bright red and not mixed with the stool.

B. Anal fissures may be associated with secondary changes such as a sentinel tag, hypertrophied anal papilla, induration of the edge of the fissure, and anal stenosis. Crohn's disease should be considered if the patient has multiple fissures, or whose fissure is not in the midline.

C. Anal fissures are caused by spasm of the internal anal sphincter. Risk factors include a low-fiber diet and previous anal surgery.

D. Treatment of anal fissures

1. High-fiber foods, warm sitz baths, stool softeners (if necessary), and daily application of 1% hydrocortisone cream to the fissure should be initiated. These simple measures may heal acute anal fissures within 3 weeks in 90% of patients.

2. **Lateral partial internal sphincterotomy** is indicated when 4 weeks of medical therapy fails. The procedure consists of surgical division of a portion of the internal sphincter, and it is highly effective. Adverse effects include incontinence to flatus and stool.

III. Levator ani syndrome and proctalgia fugax

A. Levator ani syndrome refers to chronic or recurrent rectal pain, with episodes lasting 20 minutes or longer. Proctalgia fugax is characterized by anal or rectal pain, lasting for seconds to minutes and then disappearing for days to months.

B. Levator ani syndrome and proctalgia fugax are more common in patients under age 45, and psychological factors are not always present.

C. Levator ani syndrome is caused by chronic tension of the levator muscle. Proctalgia fugax is caused by rectal muscle spasm. Stressful events may trigger attacks of proctalgia fugax and levator ani syndrome.

D. Diagnosis and clinical features

1. Levator ani syndrome is characterized by a vague, indefinite rectal discomfort or pain. The pain is felt high in the rectum and is sometimes associated with a sensation of pressure.

2. Proctalgia fugax causes pain that is brief and self limited. Patients with proctalgia fugax complain of sudden onset of intense, sharp, stabbing or cramping pain in the anorectum.

3. In patients with levator ani syndrome, palpation of the levator muscle during digital rectal examination usually reproduces the pain.

E. Treatment

1. **Levator ani syndrome.** Treatment with hot baths, nonsteroidal anti-inflammatory drugs, muscle relaxants, or levator muscle massage is recommended. EMG-based biofeedback may provide improvement in pain.

2. **Proctalgia fugax.** For patients with frequent attacks, physical modalities such as hot packs or direct anal pressure with a finger or closed fist may alleviate the pain. Diltiazem and clonidine may provided relief.

IV. Pruritus ani

A. Pruritus ani is characterized by the intense desire to scratch the skin around the anal orifice. It occurs in 1% of the population. Pruritus ani may be related to fecal leakage.

B. Patients report an escalating pattern of itching and scratching in the perianal region. These symptoms may be worse at night. Anal hygiene and dietary habits, fecal soiling, and associated medical conditions should be sought.

C. Examination reveals perianal maceration, erythema, excoriation, and lichenification. A digital rectal examination and anoscopy should be performed to assess the sphincter tone and look for secondary causes of pruritus. Patients who fail to respond to 3 or 4 weeks of conservative treatment should undergo further investigations such as skin biopsy and sigmoidoscopy or colonoscopy.

D. Treatment and patient education

1. Patients should clean the perianal area with water following defecation, but avoid soaps and vigorous rubbing. Following this, the patient should dry the anus with a hair dryer or by patting gently with cotton. Between bowel movements a thin cotton pledget dusted with unscented cornstarch should be placed against the anus. A high fiber diet is recommended to regulate bowel movements and absorb excess liquid. All foods and beverages that exacerbate the itching should be eliminated.

2. Topical medications are not recommended because they may cause further irritation. If used, a bland cream such as zinc oxide or 1% hydrocortisone cream should be applied sparingly two to three times a day.

3. Diphenhydramine (Benadryl) or hydroxyzine (Vistaril) may relieve the itching and allow the patient to sleep.

V. Perianal abscess

A. The anal glands, located in the base of the anal crypts at the level of the dentate line, are the most common source of perianal infection. Acute infection causes an abscess, and chronic infection results in a fistula.

B. The most common symptoms of perianal abscess are swelling and pain. Fevers and chills may occur. Perianal abscess is common in diabetic and immunosuppressed patients, and there is often a history of chronic constipation. A tender mass with fluctuant characteristics or induration is apparent on rectal exam.

C. Management of perianal abscess. Perianal abscesses are treated with incision and drainage using a local anesthetic. Large abscesses require regional or general anesthesia. A cruciate incision is made close to the anal verge and the corners are excised to create an elliptical opening which promotes drainage. An antibiotic, such as Zosyn, Timentin, or Cefotetan, is administered.

D. About half of patients with anorectal abscesses will develop a fistula tract between the anal glands and the perianal mucosa, known as a fistula-in-ano. This complication manifests as either incomplete healing of the drainage site or recurrence. Healing of a fistula-in-ano requires a surgical fistulotomy.

References: See page 294.

Neurologic Disorders

Migraine Headache

Migraine is an episodic headache that may occur in up to 17 percent of women and 6 percent of men. Migraine is three times more common in women than men. It tends to run in families, and typically it is a disorder of young, healthy women. Migraine without aura is the most common type, accounting for 80 percent of all migraine sufferers.

I. **Pathophysiology**
   A. Primary neuronal dysfunction leads to a sequence of changes intracranially and extracranially that account for migraine.
   B. Serotonin (released from brainstem serotonergic nuclei) plays an important role in the pathogenesis of migraine; this is probably mediated via its direct action upon the cranial vasculature, through its role in central pain control pathways and through cerebral cortical projections of brainstem serotonergic nuclei.

II. **Clinical manifestations**
   A. Migraine often begins early in the morning but can occur at any time. Nocturnal headaches, which awaken the patient from sleep, are common with cluster headaches, but migraine can also awaken patients.
   B. The headache is lateralized during severe migraine attacks in 60 to 70 percent of patients; bifrontal or global headache occurs in up to 30 percent. Occasionally, other locations are described, including biocciptal headaches. The pain is usually gradual in onset, following a crescendo pattern with gradual but complete resolution. The headache is usually dull, deep, and steady when mild to moderate; it becomes throbbing or pulsatile when severe.
   C. Migraine headaches are often worsened by rapid head motion, sneezing, straining, motion, or physical exertion. Many individuals report photophobia or phonophobia during attacks.
   D. Premonitory symptoms precede a migraine attack by several hours to one or two days. Typical symptoms include fatigue, concentration difficulty, neck stiffness, sensitivity to light or sound, nausea, blurred vision, yawning, or pallor.
   E. Migraine aura is the complex of neurologic symptoms that accompanies migraine headache. An aura presents as a progressive neurologic deficit or disturbance with subsequent complete recovery. Auras are caused by cortical spreading depression occurring in regions of the cortex.
   F. Auras typically occur before the onset of migraine headache, and the headache usually begins simultaneously with or just after the end of the aura phase.
   G. Typical auras may involve any of the following manifestations:
      1. Visual disturbances
      2. Sensory symptoms
      3. Motor weakness
      4. Speech disturbances
   H. Visual disturbances are the most common type of aura, accounting for the majority of the neurologic symptoms associated with migraine. Numbness and tingling of the lips, lower face, and fingers of one hand (cheio-oral) is the second most common type of aura.
      1. The typical visual aura starts with a flickering uncolored zig-zag line in the center of the visual field and gradually progressed toward the periphery of one hemifield, often leaving a scotoma.
   I. Autonomic and sinus symptoms characteristically occur in cluster headaches but are also commonly associated with migraine headache. These

symptoms may include nasal congestion, rhinorrhea, tearing, color and temperature change, and changes in pupil size.

J. Cutaneous allodynia is the perception of pain produced by innocuous stimulation of normal skin. Brushing hair, touching the scalp, shaving, or wearing tight clothes may trigger allodynic symptoms of pain during migraine.

K. **Complications of migraine:**
   1. Chronic migraine
   2. Status migrainosus
   3. Persistent aura without infarction
   4. Migrainous infarction
   5. Migraine-triggered seizure

L. **Precipitating factors**. Migraine headaches may be precipitated by stress, worry, menstruation, oral contraceptives, exertion, fatigue, lack of sleep, hunger, head trauma, and certain foods and beverages containing nitrites, glutamate, aspartate, and tyramine.

M. **Menstrual migraine** is defined as migraine headache that occurs in close temporal relationship to the onset of menstruation; this time period usually encompasses two days before through three days after the onset of menstrual bleeding.

N. **Migraine with aura** is a recurrent disorder manifesting in attacks of reversible focal neurologic symptoms that usually develop gradually over 5 to 20 minutes and last for less than 60 minutes. A headache begins during the aura or follows aura within 60 minutes.

Features of Migraine Headache and Headache Caused by Underlying Disease	
Migraine headache	**Headache caused by serious underlying disease**
History	
• Chronic headache pattern similar from attack to attack • Gastrointestinal symptoms • Aura, especially visual • Prodrome	• Onset before puberty or after age 50 (tumor) • "Worst headache ever" (subarachnoid hemorrhage) • Headache occurring after exertion, sex, or bowel movement (subarachnoid hemorrhage) • Headache on rising in the morning (increased intracranial pressure, tumor) • Personality changes, seizures, alteration of consciousness (tumor) • Pain localized to temporal arteries or sudden loss of vision (giant cell arteritis) • Very localized headache (tumor, subarachnoid hemorrhage, giant cell arteritis)

Migraine headache	Headache caused by serious underlying disease
Physical examination	
• No signs of toxicity • Normal vital signs • Normal neurologic examination	• Signs of toxicity (infection, hemorrhage) • Fever (sinusitis, meningitis, or other infection) • Meningismus (meningitis) • Tenderness of temporal arteries (giant cell arteritis) • Focal neurologic deficits (tumor, meningitis, hemorrhage) • Papilledema (tumor)
Laboratory tests and neuroimaging	
• Normal results	• Erythrocyte sedimentation rate >50 mm/hr (giant cell arteritis) • Abnormalities on lumbar puncture (meningitis, hemorrhage) • Abnormalities on CT or MRI (tumor, hemorrhage, aneurysm)

III. Diagnostic testing
  A. Neuroimaging is not necessary for most patients with migraine. Neuroimaging is recommended in the following patients with nonacute headache:
1. Patients with an unexplained abnormal finding on neurologic examination.
2. Patients with atypical headache features or headaches that do not fulfill the strict definition of migraine or other primary headache disorder (or have some additional risk factor, such as immune deficiency).
3. Patients with sudden severe headache also need neuroimaging because of the suspicion of subarachnoid hemorrhage.
  B. Symptoms which increase the odds of finding an abnormality on neuroimaging:
1. Rapidly increasing headache frequency
2. History of lack of coordination
3. History of localized neurologic signs or numbness or tingling
4. History of headache causing awakening from sleep
  C. A head CT scan (without and with contrast) is sufficient in many patients when neuroimaging is deemed necessary. An MRI is indicated when posterior fossa lesions or cerebrospinal fluid (CSF) leak are suspected. Magnetic resonance angiography (MRA) and mMagnetic resonance venography (MRV) are indicated when arterial or venous lesions are suspected.

IV. Acute treatment of migraine in adults
  A. **Mild analgesics**
1. Some patients with migraine have an optimal response with nonsteroidal antiinflammatory drugs (NSAIDs) or acetaminophen. Acetaminophen and many other analgesics are not advisable, in the patient who requires frequent medication, since they have been associated with rebound headaches.
2. **Nonsteroidal anti-inflammatory drugs** (NSAIDs) with efficacy in migraine therapy include ibuprofen (Advil, 400 to 1200 mg), naproxen (Naprosyn, 750 to 1250 mg), diclofenac (Voltaren, 50 to 100 mg), tolfenamic acid (Clotam Rapid, 200 mg), and aspirin (650 to 1000 mg).
3. Indomethacin (Indocin) is a potent NSAID that is also available in suppository form, which may be helpful for nauseated patients.

Indomethacin suppositories contain 50 mg of the drug; the suppositories may be cut into halves or thirds.
4. Acetaminophen is an effective abortive agent in some patients.
Acetaminophen can be used in combination with NSAIDs. The combination of acetaminophen, aspirin, and caffeine (Excedrin, 2 extra
strength tablets) alleviates headaches.

B. Triptans

1. Triptans inhibit the release of vasoactive peptides, promote
vasoconstriction, and block pain pathways in the brainstem. Triptans
inhibit transmission in the trigeminal nucleus caudalis. Triptans may
also activate 5-HT 1b/1d receptors in descending brainstem pain
modulating pathways.
2. **Preparations and efficacy.** Sumatriptan can be given as a subcutaneous injection, as a nasal spray, or orally. Zolmitriptan is also available
for both nasal and oral use. The others are available for oral use only.
3. **Side effects of subcutaneous sumatriptan** include an injection site
reaction, chest pressure, flushing, weakness, drowsiness, dizziness,
malaise, warmth, and paresthesias. Most of these reactions resolve
spontaneously within 30 minutes. There have been rare reports of
myocardial infarction and sudden death. The most common side effect
of intranasal sumatriptan is an unpleasant taste.
4. **Choice of triptan.** All of the available oral serotonin agonists are
effective and well tolerated. The highest likelihood of consistent
success was found with rizatriptan (10 mg), eletriptan (80 mg), and
almotriptan (12.5 mg). Sumatriptan (Imitrex) offers the most options for
drug delivery.
5. Rizatriptan has the fastest onset of action; the dose must be adjusted
downward in patients who take propranolol since propranolol increases rizatriptan levels by 70 percent. Almotriptan has fewer side
effects than sumatriptan. Patients who do not respond well to one
triptan may respond to another.
6. Triptans should be avoided in patients with familial hemiplegic migraine, basilar migraine, ischemic stroke, ischemic heart disease,
Prinzmetal's angina, uncontrolled hypertension, and pregnancy.
7. Combination with monoamine oxidase inhibitors is contraindicated with
triptans other than eletriptan, frovatriptan (Frova), and naratriptan.
Triptans should not be used within 24 hours of the use of ergotamine
preparations.
8. Eletriptan is metabolized by cytochrome P-450 enzyme CYP3A4.
Therefore, eletriptan should not be used within at least 72 hours of
treatment with other drugs that are potent CYP3A4 inhibitors, such as
ketoconazole, itraconazole, nefazodone, troleandomycin,
clarithromycin, ritonavir, and nelfinavir.

Drugs for Treatment of Migraine and Tension Headache	
Drug	**Dosage**
5-HT₁ Receptor Agonists ("Triptans")	
Rizatriptan (Maxalt)	5- or 10-mg tablet or wafer (MLT); can be re-peated in 2 hours; max 30 mg/day, 15 mg/day in patients on propranolol
Almotriptan (Axert)	12.5 mg at the onset of a migraine. Patients with hepatic or renal impairment should start with 6.25 mg. Max 2 doses per day.

Drug	Dosage
Sumatriptan (Imitrex)	6 mg SC; can be repeated in 1 hour; max 2 injections/day 50 mg PO; can be repeated in 2 hours; max 100 mg 20 mg intranasally; can be repeated after 2 hours; max 40 mg/day Max in combination: two injections or sprays; or one of either plus two tablets
Naratriptan (Amerge)	2.5-mg tablet, can be repeated 4 hours later; max 5 mg/day
Zolmitriptan (Zomig, Zomig-ZMT, Zomig nasal spray)	2.5-5 mg PO; can be repeated in 2 hours. Tablets and orally disintegrating tablets, 2.5, 5 mg. Intranasally 5 mg; can be repeated after 2 hours; max 10 mg/day
Frovatriptan (Frova)	2.5 mg PO, repeat after 2 hours if the headache recurs; max 3 tabs in 24 hours. Longest half-life, slow onset, less effective
Eletriptan (Relpax)	20 or 40 mg, repeated after 2 hours if headache recurs; max 80 mg in 24 hours.
NSAIDs	
Ibuprofen (Motrin)	400-800 mg, repeat as needed in 4 hr
Naproxen sodium (Anaprox DS)	550-825 mg, repeat as needed in 4 hr
Ergot Alkaloids	

Dihydroergotamine
    DHE 45
 	
    Migranal Nasal Spray
	1 mg IM; can be repeated twice at 1-hour intervals (max 3 mg/attack)
	1 spray (0.5 mg)/nostril, repeated 15 minutes later (2 mg/dose; max 3 mg/24 hours)

Ergotamine 1 mg/caffeine 100 mg (Ercaf, Gotamine, Wigraine)	2 tablets PO, then 1 q30min, x 4 PRN (max 6 tabs/attack)
Butalbital combinations	
Aspirin 325 mg, caffeine 40 mg, butalbital 50 mg (Fiorinal)	2 tablets, followed by 1 tablet q4-6h as needed
Isometheptene combination	
Isometheptene 65 mg, acetaminophen 325 mg, dichloralphenazone 100 mg (Midrin)	2 tablets, followed by 1 tablet as needed q4-6h prn

Drug	Dosage
Opioid Analgesics	
Butorphanol (Stadol NS)	One spray in one nostril; can be repeated in the other nostril in 60-90 minutes; the same two-dose sequence can be repeated in 3 to 5 hours

C. Ergots

1. Ergotamine preparations, alone and in combination with caffeine and other analgesics, have been used for the abortive treatment of migraine. Both ergotamine and dihydroergotamine (DHE 45) bind to 5HT 1b/d receptors.

2. Ergotamine
   a. Ergotamine may worsen the nausea and vomiting associated with migraine. Vascular occlusion and rebound headaches have been reported with oral doses. Years of use also may be associated with valvular heart disease.
   b. Ergots should be avoided in patients with coronary artery disease because they cause sustained coronary artery constriction, peripheral vascular disease, hypertension, and hepatic or renal disease. In addition, ergotamine overuse has been associated with an increased risk of cerebrovascular, cardiovascular, and peripheral ischemic complications. Ergotamine should not be used in patients who have migraine with prolonged aura because they may reduce cerebral blood flow.
   c. Ergotamine is the drug of choice in relatively few patients with migraine.

D. Antiemetic

1. Chlorpromazine IV appears to be more effective than placebo in the acute treatment of migraine. IV prochlorperazine also appears to be as effective or more effective than placebo in the acute treatment of migraine.

2. Metoclopramide should be considered a primary agent for acute migraine treatment in emergency departments. In addition, parenteral metoclopramide may be effective when combined with other treatments.

V. Drug choice and sequence

A. Migraine therapy should begin with a triptan for outpatients.

B. Intravenous (IV) metoclopramide (10 mg) or prochlorperazine (10 mg) are suggested for initial treatment of patients who present to the hospital emergency department with severe migraine

VI. Preventive treatment of migraine in adults

A. Indications for prophylactic headache treatment:

1. Recurring migraines that significantly interfere with daily routine, despite acute treatment
2. Contraindication to or failure or overuse of acute therapies
3. Adverse events with acute therapies
4. Patient preference
5. Hemiplegic migraine
6. Basilar type migraine
7. Migraine with prolonged aura
8. Migrainous infarction

B. Antihypertensives

1. **Beta blockers.** Chronic therapy with propranolol reduces the frequency and severity of migraine in 60 to 80 percent of patients. Propranolol is more effective than placebo in the short-term treatment of migraine. Only propranolol and timolol have been approved for

migraine prophylaxis, but metoprolol, nadolol, and atenolol are commonly used.

2. The use of beta blockers may be limited in patients with erectile dysfunction, peripheral vascular disease, Raynaud's syndrome or disease, and in patients with baseline bradycardia or low blood pressure. They must be used cautiously as well asthma, diabetes mellitus, and those with cardiac conduction disturbances or sinus node dysfunction.

3. **Calcium channel blockers** are widely used for migraine prophylaxis. These agents may relieve aura symptoms as well as prevent migraines. Verapamil is frequently a first choice for prophylactic therapy because of a favorable side effect profile.

4. **Antidepressants** are useful for migraine prophylaxis. The tricyclic antidepressants (eg, amitriptyline and clomipramine) and serotonin blockers (eg, pizotifen, mirtazapine) are effective in preventing chronic migraines.

5. The tricyclic antidepressants most commonly used for migraine prophylaxis include amitriptyline, nortriptyline, doxepin, and protriptyline. Amitriptyline is the only tricyclic that has proven efficacy for migraine.

6. Side effects are common with tricyclic antidepressants. Most are sedating, particularly with amitriptyline and doxepin. Therefore, these drugs are usually used at bedtime and started at a low dose. Additional side effects of tricyclics include dry mouth, constipation, tachycardia, palpitations, orthostatic hypotension, weight gain, blurred vision, and urinary retention. Confusion can occur, particularly in the elderly.

C. **Anticonvulsants.** The anticonvulsants sodium valproate, gabapentin, and topiramate are more effective than placebo for reducing the frequency of migraine attacks. Both valproate and topiramate are approved for migraine prophylaxis.

D. **Valproate (Depakote)** decreases headache frequency by approximately 50 percent. Divalproex (valporate and valproic acid)is at least as effective as beta blockers and may be better tolerated. It can cause weight gain and hair loss and is contraindicated in pregnancy.

E. **Gabapentin (Neurontin)**has been found to reduce migraine headache frequency.

F. **Topiramate (Topamax)** is an effective prophylactic therapy.
   1. Significant reductions in migraine frequency occur within the first month at topiramate doses of 100 and 200 mg/day.

Prophylactic treatment of migraine and tension type headache			
Drug	Starting dose	Maximum dose	Special precautions
Calcium channel blockers			
Verapamil	120 mg/day	720 mg/day	3 to 4 weeks required until effective; contraindicated in heart block, hypotension, congestive heart failure, atrial flutter and fibrillation
Nifedipine	30 mg/day	180 mg/day	
Diltiazem	60 mg/day	360 mg/day	
Flunarazine (not approved in U.S.)			

Drug	Starting dose	Maximum dose	Special precautions
Tricyclic antidepressants			
Nortriptyline	10 mg/day	125 mg/day	Contraindicated in urinary retention, glaucoma, bundle branch block; severe anticholinergic effects and weight gain
Amitriptyline	10 mg/day	250 mg/day	
SSRIs			
Fluoxetine (Prozac)	10 mg/day	80 mg/day	Less anticholinergic side effects; generally better tolerated
Paroxetine (Paxil)	10 mg/day	40 mg/day	
Sertraline (Zoloft)	25 mg/day	200 mg/day	
Beta blockers			
Propranolol	60 mg/day	320 mg/day	3 to 4 weeks before effective; contraindicated in asthma, diabetes mellitus, congestive heart failure, heart block; depression, impotence, or hypotension
Nadolol	40 mg/day	240 mg/day	
Timolol	10 mg/day	40 mg/day	
Atenolol	50 mg/day	150 mg/day	
Metoprolol	50 mg/day	300 mg/day	
Anticonvulsants			
Carbamazepine (Tegretol)	100 mg/day	200-600 mg TID	Monitor CBC, LFTs
Valproate (Depakote)	250 mg BID	500 mg TID/QID	Teratogenic
Gabapentin (Neurontin)	100 mg TID or 300 mg QHS	300-800 mg TID	No blood monitoring required
Topiramate (Topamax)	25 mg/day	100 mg BID	Slow titration minimizes adverse events Weight loss common

VII. **Menstrual migraine**
   A. NSAIDs are often used for prophylaxis. Naproxen sodium 550 mg twice daily during the perimenstrual period is one commonly used regimen.
   B. For patients who fail NSAID treatment or have contraindications to NSAIDs, frovatriptan (Frova, 2.5 mg daily or 2.5 mg twice daily) for six days is an alternative.

References: See page 294.

Vertigo

The clinical evaluation of vertigo begins with the patient's description of symptoms and the circumstances in which they occur. Many drugs can cause dizziness. Common nonvestibular causes (eg, hyperventilation, orthostatic hypotension, panic disorder) are often diagnosed.

I. **History and physical examination**
   A. Patients may use the term "dizziness" to describe one or more different sensations. These sensations include vertigo (spinning), light-headedness, unsteadiness and motion intolerance. The onset of symptoms, whether the sensation is constant or episodic, how often episodes occur and the duration of episodes should be assessed. Activities or movements that provoke or worsen a patient's dizziness should be sought as well as activities that minimize symptoms. Rotational vertigo when rolling over in bed is highly suggestive of BPPV.
   B. Vertigo is a sensation of movement of the self or of one's surroundings. Patients may describe vertigo as a sensation of floating, giddiness or disorientation. The duration of vertiginous symptoms and whether head movement provokes symptoms (positional vertigo) or if attacks occur without provocation (spontaneous vertigo) should be assessed.
   C. Hearing loss, tinnitus and aural fullness should be sought. Vision, strength and sensation, coordination, speech and swallowing should be evaluated. Double vision or hemiplegia strongly suggest a central nervous system lesion rather than a peripheral vestibular disorder. History for cardiac disease, migraine, cerebrovascular disease, thyroid disease and diabetes should be sought.

Drugs Associated with Dizziness		
Class of drug	**Type of dizziness**	**Mechanism**
Alcohol	Positional vertigo	Specific-gravity difference in endolymph vs cupula
Intoxication	CNS depression	Disequilibrium Cerebellar dysfunction
Tranquilizers	Intoxication	CNS depression
Anticonvulsants	Intoxication Disequilibrium	CNS depression Cerebellar dysfunction
Antihypertensives	Near faint	Postural hypotension
Aminoglycosides	Vertigo Disequilibrium Oscillopsia	Asymmetric hair-cell loss Vestibulospinal reflex loss Vestibulo-ocular reflex loss

   D. **Physical examination** should evaluate orthostatic blood pressure changes followed by a complete head and neck examination as well as otologic and neurologic examinations. A pneumatic otoscope should be used to confirm normal tympanic membrane mobility. Balance, gait, cerebellar and cranial nerve function, and nystagmus should be evaluated.
   E. **Nystagmus** consists of involuntary eye movements caused by asymmetry of signals from the right and left vestibular systems. Nystagmus of periph-

eral vestibular origin is usually horizontal with a slight or dramatic rotary component. Nystagmus of central origin is usually predominantly vertical.

F. **The Dix-Hallpike test** is particularly helpful to elicit nystagmus associated with BPPV. This maneuver stimulates the posterior semicircular canal, which is the semicircular canal most commonly involved in BPPV.

G. **An audiogram** should be performed if a specific cause of dizziness cannot be found after a thorough history and physical examination. Additional testing may include electronystagmography, auditory evoked brainstem response testing, radiologic imaging of the brain, brainstem and temporal bone and selected blood tests. Auditory evoked brainstem response testing measures the integrity of the auditory system and is useful to screen for acoustic tumors. Magnetic resonance imaging (MRI) should be reserved for patients with unilateral otologic symptoms or neurologic symptoms or those in whom dizziness persists despite appropriate treatment.

II. Benign paroxysmal positional vertigo

A. The most common cause of peripheral vestibular vertigo is BPPV. This condition is characterized by sudden, brief and sometimes violent vertigo after a change in head position. The sensation of vertigo usually lasts for only a few seconds. This form of vertigo is often noticed when a patient lies down, arises or turns over in bed. BPPV does not cause hearing loss, ear fullness or tinnitus. BPPV can occur at any age but is most commonly seen in elderly persons. Although usually unilateral, bilateral BPPV occurs in up to 15 percent of patients. Nystagmus is characteristic of BPPV.

B. BPPV is caused by displacement of otoconia from the utricle or saccule into the posterior semicircular canal. Therefore, when a patient moves the head into a provocative position, the otoconia provoke movement of the endolymphatic fluid inside the semicircular canal, creating a sensation of vertigo.

C. **Treatment of BPPV.** In-office physical therapy, known as repositioning maneuvers, redirects displaced otoconia into the utricle. This form of treatment is effective in 85 to 90 percent of patients.

D. During these exercises, the patient initially sits upright on the edge of a bed or couch. Then the patient rapidly lies down on his side with the affected ear down. Vertigo usually occurs. After the vertigo subsides (or after one minute if no vertigo occurs), the patient rapidly turns in a smooth arc to the opposite side. After vertigo associated with this movement subsides (or after one minute if no vertigo occurs), the patient slowly sits upright. Surgical treatment is reserved for the 2 to 5 percent of cases that fail to respond to nonsurgical treatment.

III. Vestibular neuronitis

A. Vestibular neuronitis is characterized by acute onset of intense vertigo associated with nausea and vomiting that is unaccompanied by any neurologic or audiologic symptoms. The symptoms usually reach their peak within 24 hours and then gradually subside. During the first 24 to 48 hours of a vertiginous episode, severe truncal unsteadiness and imbalance are present.

B. Vestibular neuronitis is presumed to have a viral etiology because it is often associated with a recent history of a flu-like illness. Management of the initial stage of vestibular neuronitis includes bed rest and the use of antiemetics (eg, promethazine [Phenergan]) and vestibular suppressants (eg, diazepam [Valium]). After the patient is able to stand, the brain begins compensating for the acute loss of unilateral vestibular function. The compensation process may be enhanced by performance of vestibular exercises twice per day for eight to 10 weeks.

IV. Ménière's disease

A. Ménière's disease is characterized by fluctuating hearing loss, tinnitus, episodic vertigo and, occasionally, a sensation of fullness or pressure in the ear. Vertigo rapidly follows and is typically severe, with episodes occurring abruptly and without warning. The duration of vertigo is usually several minutes to hours. Unsteadiness and dizziness may persist for days after the episode of vertigo.

B. Diseases with similar symptoms include syphilis, acoustic neuroma and migraine. Isolated episodes of hearing loss or vertigo may precede the characteristic combination of symptoms by months or years.

C. Ménière's disease results from excessive accumulation of endolymphatic fluid (endolymphatic hydrops). As inner-ear fluid pressure increases, symptoms of Ménière's disease develop.

D. Diuretics (eg, triamterene-hydrochlorothiazide [Dyazide, Maxzide]) and a low-salt diet are the mainstays of treatment. This combined regimen reduces endolymphatic fluid pressure. Other preventive measures include use of vasodilators and avoidance of caffeine and nicotine. Acute vertiginous episodes may be treated with oral or intravenous diazepam. Promethazine or glycopyrrolate (Robinul) is effective in the treatment of nausea.

E. Surgical treatments are an option when appropriate prophylactic measures fail to prevent recurrent episodes of vertigo. Surgical procedures used in the treatment of Ménière's disease range from draining excess endolymphatic fluid from the inner ear (endolymphatic shunt) to severing the vestibular nerve (with hearing preservation). In selected cases, a chemical labyrinthectomy may be performed. Chemical labyrinthectomy involves the injection of a vestibulotoxic gentamicin (Garamycin) solution into the middle ear.

Antivertiginous and Antiemetic Drugs		
Classes and agents	Dosage	Comments
Antihistamines		
Dimenhydrinate (Benadryl)	50 mg PO q4-6h or 100-mg supp. q8h	Available without prescription, mild sedation, minimal side effects
Meclizine (Antivert)	25-50 mg PO q4-6h	Mild sedation, minimal side effects
Promethazine (Phenergan)	25-50 mg PO, IM, or suppository q4-6h	Good for nausea, vertigo, more sedation, extrapyramidal effects
Monoaminergic agents		
Amphetamine	5 or 10 mg PO q4-6h	Stimulant, can counteract sedation of antihistamines, anxiety
Ephedrine	25 mg PO q4-6h	Available without prescription
Benzodiazepine		
Diazepam (Valium)	5 or 10 mg PO q6-8h	Sedation, little effect on nausea
Phenothiazine		
Prochlorperazine (Compazine)	5-25 mg PO, IM, or suppository q4-6h	Good antiemetic; extrapyramidal side effects, particularly in young patients

References: See page 294.

Dementia

Dementia is characterized by a general decrease in the level of cognition (especially memory), behavioral disturbances, and interference with daily function and independence. Alzheimer's disease (AD) is the most common form of dementia, accounting for 60 to 80 percent of cases.

I. **Identification of dementia**
   A. The normal cognitive decline associated with aging consists of mild changes in memory and the rate of information processing, which are not progressive and do not affect daily function.
   B. Patients with dementia may have difficulty with one or more of the following:
      1. Learning and retaining new information (eg, trouble remembering events).
      2. Handling complex tasks (eg, balancing a checkbook).
      3. Reasoning (eg, unable to cope with unexpected events).
      4. Spatial ability and orientation (eg, getting lost in familiar places).
      5. Language (eg, word finding).
      6. Behavior.
   C. The date of onset of dementia can often be identified when the patient stopped driving or managing finances. Useful questions are, "When did you first notice the memory loss?" and "How has the memory loss progressed since then?"
   D. The diagnosis of dementia must be distinguished from delirium and depression. Delirium is usually acute in onset with a clouding of the sensorium. Patients with delirium may have fluctuations in their level of consciousness and have difficulty with attention and concentration.
   E. Patients with depression are more likely to complain about memory loss than those with dementia. Patients with depression may have psychomotor slowing and poor effort on testing.
   F. **Mild cognitive impairment (MCI)** is defined by the following features:
      1. Memory complaint, corroborated by an informant.
      2. Objective memory impairment.
      3. Normal general cognitive function.
      4. Intact activities of daily living.
      5. Not demented.
   G. Patients with MCI are at increased risk of dementia. The prevalence of MCI was estimated at 3 to 4 percent.
   H. **Dementia syndromes.** The major dementia syndromes include:
      1. Alzheimer's disease.
      2. Vascular ("multi-infarct") dementia.
      3. Parkinson's disease and related dementias (including Lewy body dementia and progressive supranuclear palsy).
      4. Frontal lobe dementia.
      5. Reversible dementias.
      6. Most elderly patients with chronic dementia have Alzheimer's disease (60 to 80 percent). The vascular dementias account for 10 to 20 percent, and Parkinson's disease 5 percent. Alcohol-related dementia, medication side effects, depression, normal pressure hydrocephalus, and other central nervous system illnesses are responsible for the remainder of the chronic dementias.

DSM-IV Criteria for Dementia

1. Memory impairment
2. At least one of the following:
   - Aphasia
   - Apraxia
   - Agnosia
   - Disturbance in executive functioning
3. The disturbance in 1 and 2 significantly interferes with work, social activities, or relationships
4. Disturbance does not occur exclusively during delirium

Additional criteria for dementia type

Dementia of the Alzheimer's type:
- Gradual onset and continuing cognitive decline
- Not caused by identifiable medical, psychiatric, or neurologic condition

---

Vascular dementia

Focal from history, physical exam, or laboratory findings of a specific medical condition

---

Dementia due to other medical conditions

Evidence from history, physical exam, or laboratory findings of a specific medical condition causing cognitive deficits (HIV disease, head trauma, Parkinson's disease, Huntington's disease, Pick's disease, Creutzfeldt-Jacob)

I. **Alzheimer's disease** is a progressive neurologic disorder that results in memory loss, personality changes, global cognitive dysfunction, and functional impairments. Loss of short-term memory is most prominent early. In the late stages of disease, patients are totally dependent upon others for basic activities of daily living, such as feeding and toileting.
   1. Alzheimer's disease is characterized by cerebral extracellular deposition of amyloid-beta protein, intracellular neurofibrillary tangles, and loss of neurons. The DSM-IV criteria for the diagnosis of Alzheimer's dementia include the following:
      a. The gradual onset and continuing decline of cognitive function from a previously higher level, resulting in impairment in social or occupational function.
      b. Impairment of recent memory (inability to learn new information) and at least one of the following: disturbance of language; inability to execute skilled motor activities in the absence of weakness; disturbances of visual processing; or disturbances of executive function (including abstract reasoning and concentration).
      c. The cognitive deficits are not due to other psychiatric, neurologic, or systemic diseases.
      d. The deficits do not occur exclusively in the setting of delirium.
   2. Behavioral problems are common in Alzheimer's disease; personality changes (progressive passivity to open hostility) may precede the cognitive impairments. Delusions (particularly paranoid) and hallucinations contribute to the behavioral difficulties.
J. **Vascular dementia.** Features that suggest the diagnosis include:
   1. The onset of cognitive deficits associated with a stroke.
   2. Abrupt onset of symptoms followed by stepwise deterioration.
   3. Findings on neurologic examination consistent with prior stroke(s).
   4. Infarcts on cerebral imaging.
K. **Poststroke dementia** develops in 19.3 percent of subjects with stroke. Subjects with stroke have a twofold higher risk of dementia at 10 years.

L. Mixed dementia. Many individuals have mixed features of vascular and Alzheimer's dementia.

M. Reversible dementia. The potentially reversible dementias include the following:

1. **Medication-induced** (eg, analgesics, anticholinergics, psychotropic medications, and sedative-hypnotics).
2. **Alcohol-related** (eg, intoxication, withdrawal).
3. **Metabolic disorders** (eg, thyroid disease, vitamin B12 deficiency, hyponatremia, hypercalcemia, hepatic and renal dysfunction).
4. **Depression.**
5. **Central nervous system neoplasms,** chronic subdural hematomas, chronic meningitis.
6. **Normal pressure hydrocephalus.**
7. **Bismuth exposure** can cause a myoclonic encephalopathy that can be confused with CJD.
8. **Hashimoto's thyroiditis** can cause encephalopathy with myoclonus or choreoathetosis and seizures.
9. **Whipple's disease** is characterized by dementia, supranuclear gaze palsy, oculomasticatory myorhythmia, and myoclonus.

N. Normal pressure hydrocephalus is often considered in patients who present with the triad of gait disturbance, urinary incontinence, and cognitive dysfunction.

1. The Miller Fisher test, consisting of objective gait assessment before and after the removal of 30 mL of spinal fluid, is useful to confirm the diagnosis of normal pressure hydrocephalus. Radioisotope diffusion studies in the cerebrospinal fluid also confirm the diagnosis.

O. Other disorders

1. **Creutzfeldt-Jakob disease** is a rare neurodegenerative disease caused by prions. It presents with a rapidly progressive dementia that is usually fatal within one year. The diagnosis may be suspected on the basis of the rapid onset of cognitive impairment, motor deficits, and seizures. The disease is not treatable, but the disease is potentially transmissible.
2. Other more common infectious disorders that may be associated with dementia include tertiary syphilis and HIV infection.

II. Diagnostic approach

A. History of cognitive and behavioral changes should be assessed. Drugs that impair cognition (eg, analgesics, anticholinergics, psychotropic medications, and sedative-hypnotics) should be sought.

B. Physical examination, including neurologic examination. The work-up may include laboratory and imaging studies should be completed.

C. Mini-Mental State Examination (MMSE) is the most widely used cognitive test for dementia. It tests a broad range of cognitive functions, including orientation, recall, attention, calculation, language manipulation, and constructional praxis. The MMSE includes the following tasks:

1. **Orientation**
   a. What is the date: (year, season, date, day, month) - 5 points
   b. Where are we: (state)(county)(town)(hospital)(floor) - 5 points
2. **Registration**
   a. Name three objects. Ask the patient all three after you have said them. Give one point for each correct answer. Then repeat them until he learns all three. Maximum score - 3 points.
3. **Attention and calculation**
   a. Serial 7s, beginning with 100 and counting backward. One point for each correct, stop after 5 answers. Alternatively, spell WORLD backwards (one point for each letter that is in correct order). Maximum score - 5 points.
   b. Ask for the three objects repeated above. One point for each correct. Maximum score - 3 points.
   c. Show and ask patient to name a pencil and wrist watch - 2 points.

      d. Repeat the following, "No ifs ands or buts." Allow only one trial - 1 point.

      e. Follow a three stage command, "Take a paper in your right hand, fold it in half, and put it on the floor." Score one point for each task executed. Maximum score - 3 points.

      f. On a blank piece of paper write "close your eyes" and ask the patient to read and do what it says - 1 point.

      g. Give the patient a blank piece of paper and ask him to write a sentence. The sentence must contain a noun and verb and be sensible - 1 point.

      h. Ask the patient to copy intersecting pentagons. All ten angles must be present and two must intersect - 1 point.

  4. A total maximal score on the MMSE is 30 points. A score of less than 24 points is suggestive of dementia or delirium. The MMSE has a sensitivity of 87 percent and a specificity of 82 percent. However, the test is not sensitive in cases of mild dementia, and scores are spuriously low in individuals with a low education level, poor motor function, black or Latino ethnicity, poor language skills, or impaired vision.

D. Physical examination and a neurologic examination should seek for focal neurologic deficits that may be consistent with prior strokes, signs of Parkinson's disease (eg, cogwheel rigidity and tremors), gait, and eye movements.

E. Laboratory testing

  1. Screening for B12 deficiency and hypothyroidism is recommended. Routine laboratory studies may include a complete blood count, electrolytes, calcium, glucose, blood urea nitrogen, creatinine, and liver function tests. Screening for neurosyphilis (RPR) is not recommended unless there is a high clinical suspicion of neurosyphilis.

  2. Red blood cell folate should be obtained in ethanol dependence. Ionized serum calcium should be measured in multiple myeloma, prostate cancer, or breast cancer.

F. Neuroimaging. A noncontrast head CT or MRI is recommended for all patients with dementia.

III. Treatment of dementia

A. Cholinesterase inhibitors

  1. Patients with AD have reduced cerebral production of choline acetyl transferase, which leads to a decrease in acetylcholine synthesis and impaired cortical cholinergic function. Cholinesterase inhibitors increase cholinergic transmission by inhibiting cholinesterase at the synaptic cleft.

  2. Four cholinesterase inhibitors, tacrine, donepezil, rivastigmine, and galantamine are currently approved. Tacrine was can cause hepatotoxicity and is rarely used. The choice between the other three agents is based upon cost and patient tolerability because efficacy is similar.

  3. **Donepezil (Aricept)** has relatively little peripheral anticholinesterase activity and is generally well-tolerated. This combined with its once-daily dosing has made it a popular drug in patients with AD. The recommended dose for donepezil is 5 mg per day for 4 weeks, then increasing to 10 mg per day.

      a. Cognition, as measured by the Alzheimer's Disease Assessment Scale (ADAS-cog), and the Clinician's global ratings significantly improved.

      b. There was a small but significant beneficial effect of donepezil for cognition compared with placebo, with a 0.8 point difference in the Mini Mental Status Exam (MMSE) score (95% CI 0.5-1.2).

      c. Donepezil may have some symptomatic benefit in patients with mild cognitive impairment (MCI) who are likely to convert to AD, delaying the clinical diagnosis but not changing the underlying course of the disease.

d. Prolonged treatment with donepezil appears to be safe and effective. Cholinergic side effects (primarily diarrhea, nausea, and vomiting) are transient and generally mild, occurring in about 20 percent of patients.

4. **Rivastigmine (Exelon)** appears to be beneficial for patients with mild-to-moderate AD. Its side-effect profile is related to cholinergic effects, with significant nausea, vomiting, anorexia, and headaches. It should be given with food to minimize nausea. One case of esophageal rupture do to severe vomiting has been reported. Therapy is initiated at 1.5 mg BID with titration every two weeks up to 6 mg BID and, if treatment is interrupted for longer than several days, it should be restarted at the lowest daily dose and then titrated again. Its efficacy appears similar although it may have more gastrointestinal side-effects.

5. **Galantamine (Reminyl)** and appears to be effective in patients with mild-to-moderate AD. Treatment with galantamine (maintenance dose 24 or 32 mg/day) slows the decline in both cognition and activities of daily living compared with placebo in patients with early Alzheimer's disease.

   a. Gastrointestinal symptoms (nausea, vomiting, diarrhea, anorexia, weight loss) are the most common adverse effects of galantamine. Like rivastigmine, galantamine appears to have similar efficacy to donepezil in patients with AD, but may have more gastrointestinal side-effects.

6. **Degree of benefit.** Cholinesterase inhibitors can improve cognitive function in patients with AD, vascular dementia, and diffuse Lewy body disease. However, the average benefit is a small improvement in cognition and activities of daily living.

7. **Administration.** Cholinesterase inhibitors are a symptomatic treatment and not disease-modifying; therefore, the drugs should be given for eight weeks and the patient's response should be reviewed. Treatment is continued if improvement is noted. The medication should be discontinued when a patient progresses to advanced dementia

Cholinesterase Inhibitors for the Treatment of Mild-to-Moderate Alzheimer's Disease

Drug	Dosage	Side effects	Specific cautions
Donepezil (Aricept)	Initial dosage is 5 mg once daily; if necessary, dosage can be increased to 10 mg once daily after 4 to 6 weeks.	Mild side effects, nausea, vomiting, and diarrhea; effects can be reduced by taking with food. Initial agitation in some subsides after a few weeks.	Possible interactions with cimetidine (Tagamet), theophylline, warfarin (Coumadin), and digoxin (Lanoxin).
Rivastigmine (Exelon)	Initial dosage of 1.5 mg bid (3 mg per day) is well tolerated; dosage can be increased as tolerated to maximum of 6 mg twice daily (12 mg per day).	Nausea, vomiting, diarrhea, headaches, dizziness, abdominal pain, fatigue, malaise, anxiety, and agitation; these effects can be reduced by taking rivastigmine with food.	Weight loss Interacting drugs include aminoglycosides and procainamide (Procanbid).

Drug	Dosage	Side effects	Specific cautions
Galantamine (Reminyl)	Initial dosage is 4 mg bid (8 mg per day) for 4 weeks; dosage is then increased to 8 mg twice daily (16 mg per day) for at least 4 weeks. An increase to 12 mg twice daily (24 mg per day) should be considered.	Mild side effects, including nausea, vomiting, and diarrhea; these effects can be reduced by taking galantamine with food. No apparent association with sleep disturbances (which can occur with other cholinergic treatments)	Contraindicated for use in patients with hepatic or renal impairment
Tacrine (Cognex)	Initial dosage is 10 mg four times daily (40 mg per day) for 4 weeks.	High incidence of side effects, including gastrointestinal problems.	Hepatotoxicity is a problem; hence, liver tests should be performed.

IV. Disease-modifying agents

A. Memantine (Namenda) is an N-methyl-D-aspartate (NMDA) receptor antagonist. Glutamate is the principle excitatory amino acid neurotransmitter in cortical and hippocampal neurons. One of the receptors activated by glutamate is the NMDA receptor, which is involved in learning and memory. Excessive NMDA stimulation can be induced by ischemia and lead to excitotoxicity, suggesting that agents that block pathologic stimulation of NMDA receptors may protect against further damage in patients with vascular dementia.

1. Memantine results in a small but statistically significant improvement in ADAS-cog scores compared with placebo (difference between the groups 2 points on a 70 point scale.
2. Memantine appears to be effective in patients with moderate to severe Alzheimer's disease. A 28-week randomized trial in 252 patients with MMSE scores of 3 to 14 (mean approximately 8) at study entry found that memantine significantly reduced deterioration on multiple scales of clinical efficacy.
3. The mechanism of action of memantine is distinct from that of the cholinergic agents; it appears to be neuroprotective. Memantine also appears to have fewer side effects than the cholinergic agents.
4. **Memantine plus cholinesterase inhibitors.** Treatment with memantine plus donepezil results in significantly better outcomes than placebo plus donepezil on measures of cognition, activities of daily living, global outcome, and behavior. Memantine is used in combination with a cholinesterase inhibitor in patients with advanced disease. Since it may be disease-modifying. Memantine should be continued even when there is no clinical improvement.

B. Recommendations

1. Start patients with mild-to-moderate dementia on a cholinesterase inhibitor. Tacrine should not be used. The choice between donepezil, rivastigmine, and galantamine can be based upon cost, individual patient tolerance, and physician experience, as efficacy appears to be similar.
2. In patients with moderate to advanced dementia, add memantine to a cholinesterase inhibitor, or use memantine alone in patients who do not tolerate or benefit from a cholinesterase inhibitor.
3. In patients with severe dementia, cholinesterase inhibitors can be discontinued, but they should be restarted if the patient worsens without the medication. Memantine should be continued even in severe dementia, given the possibility that memantine may be disease modifying.

However, in some patients with advanced dementia medications should be discontinued to maximize quality of life and patient comfort.

4. For delusions and hallucinations, the atypical neuroleptics olanzapine (starting at a dose of 2.5 mg daily, titrating up to a maximum of 5 mg twice a day) or quetiapine (starting at a dose of 25 mg at bedtime, titrating up to a maximum of 75 mg twice a day) are recommended at the lowest effective doses.

5. For depression, avoid tricyclic antidepressants. SSRIs are preferred, but fluoxetine should be avoided because of its long half-life and drug interactions, and avoid paroxetine because it is more anticholinergic than other SSRIs.

6. For agitation and aggression, look for triggers and try to treat those first. Most behavioral symptoms have precipitants (constipation, urinary retention, fear of unrecognized caregivers, etc). Frightening delusions respond to atypical neuroleptics, and agitation may be due to unrecognized depression and responds to SSRIs. If a treatable etiology cannot be found, treat with trazodone starting with 25 mg at bedtime or twice daily and titrating the dose up to 50 to 100 mg twice daily. If this is unsuccessful, an atypical neuroleptic should be used.

References: See page 294.

Endocrinologic and Hematologic Disorders

Type 1 Diabetes Mellitus

Up to 4 percent of Americans have diabetes. The diagnosis of diabetes mellitus is easily established when a patient presents with classic symptoms of hyperglycemia (thirst, polyuria, weight loss, visual blurring), and has a fasting blood glucose concentration of 126 mg/dL or higher, or a random value of 200 mg/dL or higher, and confirmed on another occasion.

I. **Definitions from the 2003 ADA report:**
   Normal. Fasting plasma glucose (FPG) <100 mg/dL.
   Impaired fasting glucose (IFG). Fasting plasma glucose between 100 and 125 mg/dL.
   Diabetes mellitus. FPG at or above 126 mg/dL, a two-hour value in an OGTT (2-h PG) at or above 200 mg/dL, or a random plasma glucose concentration > 200 mg/dL in the presence of symptoms. The diagnosis of diabetes must be confirmed on a subsequent day by measuring any one of the three criteria.

Routine Diabetes Care

History
Review physical activity, diet, self-monitored blood glucose readings, medications
Assess for symptoms of coronary heart disease
Evaluate smoking status, latest eye examination results, foot care

Physical examination
Weight
Blood pressure
Foot examination
Pulse
Sores or callus
Monofilament test for sensation
Insulin injection sites
Refer for dilated retinal examination annually

Laboratory studies
HbA1c every three to six months
Annual fasting lipid panel
Annual urine albumin/creatinine ratio
Annual serum creatinine

Goals of intensive diabetes treatment

Premeal blood glucose level	Postprandial (ie, mealtime) glucose level	Bedtime glucose level	Hemoglobin A_{1c} (HbA$_{1c}$) level
90 to 130 mg/dL	120 to 180 mg/dL	110 to 150 mg/dL	Less than 6.5%

Pharmacokinetics of insulin preparations			
Insulin type	Onset of action	Time to peak effect	Duration of action
Lispro (Humalog), aspart (Novolog), glulisine (Apidra)	5 to 15 min	45 to 75 min	2 to 4 h
Regular insulin	About 30 min	2 to 4 h	5 to 8 h
NPH	About 2 h	6 to 10 h	18 to 28 h
Insulin glargine (Lantus)	About 2 h	No peak	20 to >24 h
Insulin detemir (Levemir)	About 2 h	No peak	6 to 24 h

II. Insulin therapy in type 1 diabetes mellitus

A. The Diabetes Control and Complications Trial (DCCT) demonstrated that improved glycemic control with intensive insulin therapy in patients with type 1 diabetes mellitus led to graded reductions in retinopathy, nephropathy, and neuropathy. Intensive therapy is now considered to be standard therapy for management of type 1 diabetes.

B. The term "intensive insulin therapy" describes treatment with three or more injections per day or with continuous subcutaneous insulin infusion with an insulin pump.

C. Choice of insulin regimen. The basic requirements are a stable baseline dose of insulin (basal insulin) (whether an intermediate or long-acting insulin or given via continuous subcutaneous insulin infusion) plus adjustable doses of pre-meal short-acting insulin (regular) or rapid-acting insulin analogs (lispro, aspart, or glulisine).

Multiple daily insulin injection regimens				
Regimen	Breakfast	Lunch	Dinner	Bedtime
1	R + N		R	N
2	R	R	R	N
3	VRA	VRA	VRA	G
4	VRA + G	VRA	VRA	
5	VRA + G	VRA	VRA + G	

R: regular insulin; N: NPH insulin; VRA: any very-rapid-acting analog (lispro, aspart, or glulisine); G: glargine.

D. Insulin glargine. The time-action profile for insulin glargine has virtually no peak, which makes it a good basal insulin preparation for intensive insulin therapy.

1. The therapeutic advantage of insulin glargine over NPH is modest, with no real advantage with regard to A1C achieved. Lower fasting blood glucose and fewer hypoglycemic episodes occur when insulin glargine was substituted for once or twice daily NPH insulin, but A1C values have generally not been lower in studies comparing glargine and NPH-based regimens.

2. Although many patients can achieve stable basal serum insulin concentrations with a single daily injection of insulin glargine given in

the morning or evening this is not always the case. About 20 percent of patients with type 1 diabetes need twice-daily glargine.

E. **Insulin detemir** is the second available long-acting insulin analog. However, its duration of action appears to be substantially shorter than that of insulin glargine, though still longer than NPH. Like NPH, twice-daily injections appear to be necessary in patients with type 1 diabetes. Glycemic control appears to be similar with insulin detemir and NPH; however, insulin detemir may be associated with slightly less nocturnal hypoglycemia and weight gain. These modest advantages of insulin detemir may be offset by its higher cost.

F. **Rapid-acting insulins** (insulin lispro, aspart, and glulisine) have an onset of action within 5 to 15 minutes, peak action at 30 to 90 minutes, and a duration of action of two to four hours.

G. In patients with type 1 diabetes, rapid-acting insulin has the following advantages when compared to regular insulin:
   1. It decreases the postprandial rise in blood glucose concentration better than regular insulin.
   2. It may modestly reduce the frequency of hypoglycemia in patients with type 1 diabetes.
   3. It is more convenient because it can be injected immediately before meals, whereas regular insulin should be given 30 to 45 minutes before meals. In addition, the action of insulin lispro is not blunted by mixing with NPH insulin just before injection, as is the action of regular insulin.

H. **Designing an MDI insulin regimen.** Most newly diagnosed patients with type 1 diabetes can be started on a total daily dose of 0.2 to 0.4 units of insulin per kg per day, although most will ultimately require 0.6 to 0.7 units per kg per day. Adolescents, especially during puberty, often need more, but the dose can be adjusted upward every few days based upon blood glucose measurements.

I. In designing an MDI regimen, one-half of the total dose should be given as a basal insulin, either as once per day long-acting insulin (glargine or determir) or as twice per day intermediate-acting insulin (NPH). The long-acting insulin can be given either at bedtime or in the morning; the NPH is usually given as two-thirds of the dose in the morning and one-third at bedtime. The remainder of the total daily dose (TDD) is given as short or rapid-acting insulin, divided before meals. The pre-meal dosing is determined by the usual meal size and content. The sliding-scale that is constructed for premeal use usually takes into account the carbohydrate content and the blood glucose levels before the meal. Regimens that use NPH in the morning may not require a pre-lunch dose of short or rapid-acting insulin.

III. **Other management issues**
   A. Consistency. The content and timing of meals, the site of insulin injections, and the timing and frequency of exercise should be consistent.
   B. Blood glucose monitoring. Testing at home should to be done four to seven times daily (before breakfast, mid-morning, before lunch, mid-afternoon, before the evening meal, before bedtime, and occasionally at 3 AM). Additionally, it is useful to test blood glucose levels at intervals after certain meals and before, during and after exercise. Chronic glucose control should be monitored with periodic A1C (hemoglobin A1c or HbA1c) levels.

IV. **Screening for microvascular complications in diabetics**
   A. **Retinopathy.** Diabetic retinopathy and macular degeneration are the leading causes of blindness in diabetes. Adults with diabetes should receive annual dilated retinal examinations beginning at the time of diagnosis.
   B. **Nephropathy.** Diabetes-related nephropathy affects 40% of patients with type 1 disease and 10-20% of those with type 2 disease. Microalbumin may be tested annually by screening with either a specifically sensitive dipstick or a laboratory assay on a spot urine sample, to determine an

albumin-to-creatinine ratio. Abnormal results should be repeated at least two or three times over a three to six month period. Screening can be deferred for five years after the onset of disease in patients with type 1 diabetes because microalbuminuria is uncommon before this time.

C. **Peripheral neuropathy** affects many patients with diabetes and causes nocturnal or constant pain, tingling and numbness. The feet should be evaluated regularly for sensation, pulses and sores.

D. **Autonomic neuropathy** is found in many patients with long-standing diabetes, resulting in diarrhea, constipation, gastroparesis, vomiting, orthostatic hypotension, and erectile or ejaculatory dysfunction.

References: See page 294.

Type 2 Diabetes Mellitus

I. **Degree of glycemic control**
   A. Measurement of hemoglobin A1C (A1C) provides a better estimate of chronic glycemic control than measurements of fasting blood glucose. The Diabetes Control and Complications Trial (DCCT) demonstrated that achieving near normal blood glucose concentrations markedly reduces the risk of microvascular and neurologic complications in type 1 diabetes.
   B. The goal of therapy should be an A1C value of 7.0 percent or less. The goal should be set somewhat higher for older patients. In order to achieve the A1C goal, the glucose goals below are usually necessary:
      1. Fasting glucose 70 to 130 mg/dL
      2. Postprandial glucose (90 to 120 minutes after a meal) <180 mg/dL
   C. Cardiovascular risk factor reduction (smoking cessation, aspirin, blood pressure, reduction in serum lipids, diet, exercise, and, in high-risk patients, an angiotensin converting enzyme inhibitor) should be accomplished for all patients with type 2 diabetes.

II. **Nonpharmacologic treatment**
   A. Diet modification can improve obesity, hypertension, and insulin release and responsiveness.
   B. Regular exercise leads to improved glycemic control due to increased responsiveness to insulin; it can also delay the progression of impaired glucose tolerance to overt diabetes.

III. **Medications for initial therapy**
   A. Sulfonylureas and meglitinides increase insulin release.
   B. Biguanides (metformin) and thiazolidinedione increase insulin responsiveness.
   C. Alpha-glucosidase inhibitors reduce intestinal absorption of carbohydrate and lipase inhibitors reduce the absorption of fat.
   D. **Biguanides.** Metformin (Glucophage) often leads to modest weight reduction and is a reasonable first choice for oral treatment of type 2 diabetes.
      1. **Metformin (Glucophage)** is available as 500 and 850 mg tablets, which should be taken with meals; extended release formulations may be convenient once the dose is adjusted. Metformin should not be given to elderly (>80 years) patients unless renal sufficiency is proven with a direct measure of GFR, or to patients who have renal, hepatic or cardiac disease or drink excess alcohol. Patients who are about to receive intravenous iodinated contrast material (with potential for contrast-induced renal failure) or undergo a surgical procedure (with potential compromise of circulation) should have metformin held.
      2. Initial dosage is 500 mg once daily with the evening meal and, if tolerated, a second 500 mg dose is added with breakfast. The dose can be increased slowly (one tablet every one to two weeks). The usual maximum effective dose is 850 mg twice per day.

Contraindications to metformin therapy

Renal dysfunction
    Serum creatinine level $\geq$1.5 mg/dL in men, $\geq$1.4 mg/dL in women
    Metformin should be temporarily discontinued in patients undergoing radiologic
    studies involving intravascular administration of iodinated contrast materials.
    Treatment may be restarted 48 hours after the procedure when normal renal
    function is documented.
    Treatment should be carefully initiated in patients $\geq$80 years of age after measure-
    ment of
    creatinine clearance demonstrates that renal function is not reduced.
Congestive heart failure that requires pharmacologic therapy
Hepatic dysfunction
Dehydration
Acute or chronic metabolic acidosis (diabetic ketoacidosis)
Known hypersensitivity to metformin

- E. **Sulfonylureas** are moderately effective, lowering blood glucose concentrations by 20 percent and A1C by 1 to 2 percent. Their effectiveness decreases over time.
  1. The choice of sulfonylurea is primarily dependent upon cost, since the efficacy of the available drugs is similar.
- F. **Meglitinides.** Repaglinide (Prandin) and nateglinide (Starlix) are short-acting glucose-lowering drugs that act similarly to the sulfonylureas and have similar or slightly less efficacy in decreasing glycemia. Meglitinides may be used in patients who have allergy to sulfonylureas. However, they are considerably more expensive than sulfonylureas, and have no therapeutic advantage.
  1. **Nateglinide (Starlix)** is hepatically metabolized, with renal excretion of active metabolites. With decreased renal function, the accumulation of active metabolites and hypoglycemia has occurred. Repaglinide is principally metabolized by the liver, with less than 10 percent renally excreted.
- G. **Thiazolidinediones,** rosiglitazone (Avandia) and pioglitazone (Actos), lower blood glucose concentrations by increasing insulin sensitivity. Hepatotoxicity with rosiglitazone and pioglitazone is very rare.
  1. Pioglitazone and rosiglitazone are approved for monotherapy or in combination with metformin, sulfonylurea or insulin. Combination tablets of metformin and rosiglitazone (Avandamet) are available. Thiazolidinediones are similar to metformin as monotherapy. They are associated with more weight gain than metformin, and are considerably more expensive than any of the other oral hypoglycemic drugs.
  2. Thiazolidinediones are reserved for second-line treatment in combination with other anti-diabetic medications where synergistic effects can lower A1C substantially. Fluid retention and precipitation or worsening of heart failure are significant concerns.

Pharmacotherapy of Type 2 Diabetes

Agent	Starting dose	Maximum dose	Comments
Biguanide Metformin (Glucophage)	500 mg daily	850 mg three times daily	Do not use if serum creatinine is greater than 1.4 mg/dL in women or 1.5 mg/dL in men or in the presence of heart failure, chronic obstructive pulmonary disease or liver disease; may cause lactic acidosis
Glyburide/ metformin (Glucovance)	25 mg/250 mg; 2.5 mg/500 mg; 5 mg/500 mg	1 tab qAM-bid	
Sulfonylureas Glipizide (Glucotrol) Glyburide (DiaBeta, Micronase) Glimepiride (Amaryl)	5 mg daily 2.5 mg daily 1 mg daily	20 mg twice daily 10 mg twice daily 8 mg daily	May cause hypoglycemia, weight gain. Maximum dose should be used only in combination with insulin therapy
Thiazolidine-diones Pioglitazone (Actos) Rosiglitazone (Avandia)	15 mg daily 4 mg daily	45 mg per day 4 mg twice daily	Should be used only in patients who have contraindications to metformin
Alpha-glucosidase inhibitor Acarbose (Precose) Miglitol (Glyset)	50 mg tid 50 mg tid	100 mg three times daily 100 mg three times daily	Flatulence; start at low dose to minimize side effects; take at mealtimes
Meglitamide Repaglinide (Prandin) Nateglinide (Starlix)	0.5 mg before meals 120 mg tid before meals or 60 mg tid before meals	4 mg tid-qid 120 mg tid	Take at mealtimes

H. Alpha-glucosidase inhibitors. Because they act by a different mechanism, the alpha-glucosidase inhibitors, acarbose and miglitol, have additive hypoglycemic effects in patients receiving diet, sulfonylurea, metformin, or insulin therapy. This class of drugs is less potent than the sulfonylureas or metformin, lowering A1C by about 0.5 to 1.0 percentage points.
  1. Side effects are flatulence and diarrhea. These agents are not first-line therapy because of low efficacy and poor tolerance.
  2. Acarbose is available as 50 and 100 mg tablets which should be taken with the first bite of each meal. Initiate therapy with 50 mg three times daily. Flatulence, diarrhea, and abdominal discomfort resolve if the dose is decreased. Few patients tolerate more than 300 mg daily.
I. Insulin should be used early in type 2 diabetes. When treated early with insulin, patients with type 2 diabetes can have remissions of at least

several years, during which A1C is normal. A patient who is 20 percent above ideal body weight and has a fasting blood glucose of 180 mg/dL could be started on a total dose of 21 units per day.

IV. **Choosing Initial Therapy**

A. **Metformin** therapy should be started in most patients at the time of diabetes diagnosis, in the absence of contraindications, along with lifestyle intervention. The dose of metformin should be titrated to its maximally effective dose (usually 850 mg twice per day) over one to two months, as tolerated.

B. Metformin should not be given to elderly (>80 years) patients unless renal sufficiency is proven with a direct measure of GFR, or to patients who have renal, hepatic or cardiac disease or drink excess alcohol. Another oral agent (a sulfonylurea or thiazolidinedione) should be used for initial therapy in these patients.

C. **Patients who are underweight**, are losing weight, or are ketotic should be started on insulin. Insulin should be initial therapy for patients presenting with A1C >10 percent, fasting plasma glucose >250 mg/dL, random glucose consistently >300 mg/dL, or ketonuria.

D. **If inadequate control is achieved** (A1C remains >7 percent), another medication should be added within two to three months of initiation of metformin. The choice of the second medication might be insulin, a sulfonylurea, or a thiazolidinedione. Insulin is recommended for patients whose A1C remains >8.5 percent.

E. Further adjustments of therapy should usually be made every three months, based on the A1C result, aiming for levels as close to the nondiabetic range as possible. Values >7 percent suggest the need for further adjustments in the diabetic regimen.

F. The patient should perform self blood glucose monitoring and keep a record of the fasting blood glucose, obtained after meals and at other times during the day, and when hypoglycemia is suspected.

V. **Combination oral therapy for persistent hyperglycemia**

A. **Metformin plus sulfonylureas.** Metformin has an additive hypoglycemic effect when given in combination with a sulfonylurea.

1. A combination tablet **(Glucovance)** is now available in the following glyburide/metformin doses: 1.25 mg/250 mg; 2.5 mg/500 mg; 5 mg/500 mg.

B. **Metformin plus a thiazolidinedione.** Patients who fail initial therapy with metformin may benefit from the addition of a thiazolidinedione such as rosiglitazone or pioglitazone.

C. **Insulin** is a reasonable choice for initial therapy in patients who present with symptomatic or poorly controlled diabetes, and is the preferred second-line medication for patients with A1C >8.5 percent or with symptoms of hyperglycemia despite metformin titration. The dose of insulin may be adjusted every three days, until glycemic targets are achieved.

1. Patients with persistent hyperglycemia despite oral hypoglycemic therapy may stop the oral drug and begin insulin, or may add insulin to oral medication.

2. While NPH has been used commonly at bedtime to supplement oral hypoglycemia drug therapy, insulin glargine may be equally effective for reducing A1C values and may cause less nocturnal hypoglycemia. Although it may be reasonable to administer glargine at bedtime, morning administration may be better.

References: See page 294.

Hypothyroidism

Hypothyroidism is second only to diabetes mellitus as the most common endocrine disorder, and its prevalence may be as high as 18 cases per 1,000 persons in the general population. The disorder becomes increasingly common with advancing age, affecting about 2 to 3 percent of older women.

I. Etiology

A. Primary hypothyroidism

1. The most common cause of hypothyroidism is Hashimoto's (chronic lymphocytic) thyroiditis. Most patients who have Hashimoto's thyroiditis have symmetrical thyroid enlargement, although many older patients with the disease have atrophy of the gland. Anti-thyroid peroxidase (TPO) antibodies are present in almost all patients. Some patients have blocking antibodies to the thyroid-stimulating hormone (TSH) receptor.

2. Hypothyroidism also occurs after treatment of hyperthyroidism by either surgical removal or radioiodine ablation. Less common causes of hypothyroidism include congenital dyshormonogenesis, external radiotherapy, infiltrative diseases, such as amyloidosis, and peripheral resistance to thyroid hormone action.

B. Secondary and central hypothyroidism.
Pituitary and hypothalamic dysfunction can lead to hypothyroidism. Pituitary adenomas, craniopharyngiomas, pinealomas, sarcoidosis, histiocytosis X, metastatic disease, primary central nervous system (CNS) neoplasms (eg, meningioma), and head trauma all may cause hypothyroidism.

C. Transient hypothyroidism.
Subacute thyroiditis is frequently associated with a hyperthyroid phase of 4 to 12 weeks' duration; a 2- to 16-week hypothyroid phase follows, before recovery of thyroid function. Subacute granulomatous (de Quervain's) thyroiditis and subacute lymphocytic (painless) thyroiditis are viral and autoimmune disorders, respectively; the latter condition may occur post partum.

II. Diagnosis

A. Symptoms and signs
of hypothyroidism include fatigue, weight gain, muscle weakness and cramps, fluid retention, constipation, and neuropathy (eg, carpal tunnel syndrome). Severe hypothyroidism may be associated with carotenemia, loss of the lateral aspect of the eyebrows, sleep apnea, hypoventilation, bradycardia, pericardial effusion, anemia, hyponatremia, hyperprolactinemia, hypercholesterolemia, hypothermia, and coma.

B.
In patients with primary hypothyroidism, the thyroid-stimulating hormone (TSH) level is elevated, and free thyroid hormone levels are depressed. In contrast, patients with secondary hypothyroidism have a low or undetectable TSH level.

C.
TSH results have to be interpreted in light of the patient's clinical condition. A low TSH level should not be misinterpreted as hyperthyroidism in the patient with clinical manifestations of hypothyroidism. When symptoms are nonspecific, a follow-up assessment of the free thyroxine (T_4) level can help distinguish between primary and secondary hypothyroidism.

Laboratory Values in Hypothyroidism

TSH level	Free T_4 level	Free T_3 level	Likely diagnosis
High	Low	Low	Primary hypothyroidism
High (>10 µU per mL)	Normal	Normal	Subclinical hypothyroidism with high risk for future development of overt hypothyroidism
High (6 to 10 µU per mL)	Normal	Normal	Subclinical hypothyroidism with low risk for future development of overt hypothyroidism
High	High	Low	Congenital absence of

TSH level	Free T_4 level	Free T_3 level	Likely diagnosis
			T_4-T_3—converting enzyme; amiodarone (Cordarone) effect on T_4-T_3 conversion
High	High	High	Peripheral thyroid hormone resistance
Low	Low	Low	Pituitary thyroid deficiency or recent withdrawal of thyroxine after excessive replacement therapy

Causes of Hypothyroidism

Primary hypothyroidism (95% of cases)
Idiopathic hypothyroidism
Hashimoto's thyroiditis Irradiation of the thyroid subsequent to Graves' disease
Surgical removal of the thyroid
Late-stage invasive fibrous thyroiditis
Iodine deficiency
Drug therapy (eg, lithium, interferon)
Infiltrative diseases (eg, sarcoidosis, amyloidosis, scleroderma, hemochromatosis)

Secondary hypothyroidism (5% of cases)
Pituitary or hypothalamic neoplasms
Congenital hypopituitarism
Pituitary necrosis (Sheehan's syndrome)

III. Treatment of hypothyroidism
  A. Initiating thyroid hormone replacement
  1. Most otherwise healthy adult patients with hypothyroidism require thyroid hormone replacement in a dosage of 1.7 mcg per kg per day, with requirements falling to 1 mcg per kg per day in the elderly. Thus, (Synthroid) in a dosage of 0.10 to 0.15 mg per day is needed to achieve euthyroid status. For full replacement, children may require up to 4 mcg per kg per day.
  2. In young patients without risk factors for cardiovascular disease, thyroid hormone replacement can start close to the target goal. In most healthy young adults, replacement is initiated using levothyroxine in a dosage of 0.075 mg per day, with the dosage increased slowly as indicated by continued elevation of the TSH level.
  3. Levothyroxine (Synthroid) should be initiated in a low dosage in older patients and those at risk for cardiovascular compromise; the usual starting dosage is 0.025 mg per day, increased in increments of 0.025 to 0.050 mg every four to six weeks until the TSH level returns to normal.

Commonly Prescribed Thyroid Hormone Preparations			
Generic Name	Brand Name(s)	Approximate Equivalent Dose	Preparations
Levothyroxine	Synthroid Levothroid Levoxyl Eltroxin	100 mcg	Tablets: 25, 50, 75, 88, 100, 112, 125, 137, 150, 175, 200, 300 mcg

IV. **Monitoring thyroid function**
   A. In patients with an intact hypothalamic-pituitary axis, the adequacy of thyroid hormone replacement can be followed with serial TSH assessments. The TSH level should be evaluated no earlier than four weeks after an adjustment in the levothyroxine dosage. The full effects of thyroid hormone replacement on the TSH level may not become apparent until after eight weeks of therapy.
   B. In patients with pituitary insufficiency, measurements of free T_4 and T_3 levels can be performed to determine whether patients remain euthyroid. TSH or free T_4 levels are monitored annually in most patients with hypothyroidism.
V. **Subclinical Hypothyroidism**
   A. The TSH level can be mildly elevated when the free T_4 and T_3 levels are normal, a situation that occurs most often in women and becomes increasingly common with advancing age. This condition has been termed "subclinical hypothyroidism."
   B. In patients at higher risk for osteoporosis or fractures, the deleterious effects of excessive thyroid hormone can be avoided by withholding replacement until the free T_4 and T_3 levels drop below normal.
References: See page 294.

Thyroiditis

Thyroiditis refers to a group of inflammatory diseases affecting the thyroid gland.

Classification of Thyroiditis	
Histologic classification	Synonyms
Chronic lymphocytic	Chronic lymphocytic thyroiditis, Hashimoto's thyroiditis
Subacute lymphocytic	Subacute lymphocytic thyroiditis: (1) postpartum thyroiditis and (2) sporadic painless thyroiditis
Granulomatous	Subacute granulomatous thyroiditis, de Quervain's thyroiditis
Microbial inflammatory	Suppurative thyroiditis, acute thyroiditis
Invasive fibrous	Riedel's struma, Riedel's thyroiditis

I. **Chronic lymphocytic thyroiditis (Hashimoto's thyroiditis)**
   A. Chronic lymphocytic thyroiditis is the most common inflammatory condition of the thyroid gland and the most common cause of goiter. It is an autoimmune condition.
   B. Chronic lymphocytic thyroiditis is the most common cause of hypothyroidism, and euthyroid persons with Hashimoto's disease develop hypothyroidism at a rate of 5 percent per year. Up to 95 percent of cases of chronic lymphocytic thyroiditis occur in women, usually between 30 and 50 years of age.
   C. **Clinical manifestations**. Hashimoto's thyroiditis is usually asymptomatic. Symptoms of hypothyroidism are present in 20 percent of patients. Physical examination generally reveals a firm, irregular, nontender goiter. The definitive indicator of chronic lymphocytic thyroiditis is the presence of thyroid-specific autoantibodies in the serum. A dominant nodule in a patient with Hashimoto's disease should prompt a fine-needle aspiration biopsy to exclude malignancy.
   D. **Treatment**. Because thyroiditis is usually asymptomatic, many patients do not require treatment. When hypothyroidism is present, treatment with thyroxine (T4) is indicated. Lifetime replacement of levothyroxine is indicated in hypothyroid patients, at a starting dosage of 25 to 50 µg per day, with gradual titration to an average daily dosage of 75 to 150 µg.

II. **Subacute lymphocytic thyroiditis**
   A. Subacute lymphocytic thyroiditis occurs most often in the postpartum period but may also occur sporadically. Antimicrosomal antibodies are present in 50 to 80 percent of patients, while antithyroid peroxidase antibodies are present in nearly all patients. Subacute lymphocytic thyroiditis starts with an initial hyperthyroid phase, followed by subsequent hypothyroidism and, finally, a return to the euthyroid state. In the postpartum patient, thyrotoxicosis usually develops in the first three months following delivery and lasts for one or two months.
   B. Patients usually present with tachycardia, palpitations, heat intolerance, nervousness and weight loss. A small painless goiter is present in 50 percent. T4 and triiodothyronine (T3) levels are initially elevated.
   C. **Treatment**. Acute symptoms of hyperthyroidism are managed with beta blockers. Antithyroid drugs are not indicated. Replacement of thyroid hormone in the hypothyroid phase is indicated if the patient's symptoms are severe. If the hypothyroid phase lasts longer than six months, permanent hypothyroidism is likely.

III. **Subacute granulomatous thyroiditis**
   A. Subacute granulomatous thyroiditis is the most common cause of a painful thyroid gland. It is most likely caused by a viral infection and is generally preceded by an upper respiratory tract infection.
   B. **Clinical manifestations**
      1. Subacute granulomatous thyroiditis presents with acute onset of pain in the thyroid. Symptoms of hypermetabolism may be present, and the ESR usually is markedly elevated. A normal ESR essentially rules out the diagnosis of subacute granulomatous thyroiditis. The thyroid is firm, nodular and tender. Thyrotoxicosis is present in 50 percent of patients. Serum TSH concentrations are low.
      2. **Clinical management**
         a. The acute phase of thyroid pain and thyrotoxicosis may last three to six weeks. Hypothyroidism often ensues and may last weeks to months or may be permanent (in up to 5 percent of patients).
         b. Therapy with antithyroid drugs is not indicated. Therapy with beta blockers may be indicated for the symptomatic treatment of thyrotoxicosis. Nonsteroidal anti-inflammatory drugs are generally effective in reducing mild thyroid pain in patients with mild cases. More severe disease requires a tapering dosage of prednisone (20 to 40 mg per day) given over two to four weeks.

References: See page 294.

Thyrotoxicosis

I. Diagnosis

A. Thyrotoxicosis is characterized by heat intolerance, weight loss or gain, palpitations, anxiety, tachycardia, and tremor with elevated levels of the thyroid hormones thyroxine (T_4) and triiodothyronine (T_3). Hyperthyroidism refers to the more common forms of thyrotoxicosis in which there is overproduction of thyroid hormones, usually due to stimulation of the thyroid by thyroid-stimulating hormone (TSH) receptor autoantibodies (Graves' disease) or toxic multinodular goiter and toxic adenoma.

B. Thyrotoxicosis is confirmed by a low-serum TSH concentration, usually in association with elevations of the serum free T_4 or T_3 concentrations. Mild thyrotoxicosis, sometimes termed "subclinical thyrotoxicosis," is characterized by suppression of TSH levels in association with high-normal serum T_4 and T_3 concentrations. Rare conditions causing TSH-mediated hyperthyroidism (ie, TSH-secreting pituitary tumors) are typically associated with elevated-free T_4 and T_3 concentrations with an elevated or inappropriately normal TSH level. Isolated suppression of TSH can also be seen in patients with severe nonthyroidal illnesses. Consequently, it is usually necessary to measure the serum TSH and free T_4 concentrations to confirm or exclude thyrotoxicosis with absolute certainty.

C. True hyperthyroidism can be distinguished from other causes with a nuclear thyroid scan. An increased glandular concentration of tracer indicates that hyperthyroidism is present. In contrast, decreased tracer uptake is typically present with inflammatory disorders (eg, subacute [de Quervain's], lymphocytic [postpartum, silent, painless], or suppurative thyroiditis) with exogenous thyroid hormones.

D. TSH receptor-stimulating and -binding immunoglobulins are usually detectable in Graves' disease. The erythrocyte sedimentation rate is typically elevated in subacute thyroiditis. Circulating human chorionic gonadotropin is detectable in choriocarcinoma and molar pregnancy.

II. Treatment

A. **Beta-Adrenergic Blocking Agents**

1. Beta-adrenergic blocking agents (beta-blockers) are used to control tremor, palpitations, anxiety, and insomnia. Propranolol (Inderal) offers the advantage of partially inhibiting the peripheral conversion of T_4 to T_3.

Drugs Used in the Treatment of Hyperthyroidism			
Agent	**Name**	**Available Doses**	**Usual Starting Dose**
Beta-blockers			
Propranolol Regular Sustained-release	Inderal Inderal LA	10, 20, 40, 60, 80, 90 mg 60, 80, 120, 160 mg	10-20 mg PO tid* 60-80 mg PO qd
Atenolol	Tenormin	25, 50, 100 mg	25-50 mg PO qd
Metoprolol Regular Extended-release	Lopressor Toprol XL	50, 100 mg 50, 100, 200 mg	25-50 mg PO bid 50-100 mg qd
Thioamides			
Methimazole	Tapazole	5, 10 mg	20-40 mg PO qd

Agent	Name	Available Doses	Usual Starting Dose
Propylthiouracil	PTU	50 mg	50-100 mg PO tid
Iodine			
Saturated solution of potassium iodide	SSKI	50 mg/drop	10 drops PO bid

2. **Thioamide antithyroid drugs**
   a. The thionamide antithyroid drugs are used to treat hyperthyroidism due to Graves' disease and toxic multinodular goiter. Methimazole (Tapazole) can be given on a once-daily dosing schedule. Propylthiouracil PTU, which must be taken more frequently, partially inhibits the peripheral conversion of T_4 to T_3, an effect that may be valuable in patients with severe thyrotoxicosis.
   b. When PTU is used, it can be started at a dose of 50 to 100 mg every 6 to 8 hours. In patients with more severe hyperthyroidism, methimazole, 20 mg three times daily or 30 mg twice daily or PTU 100 to 200 mg every 6 hours, can be used.
   c. Early in the course of treatment, the serum total or free T_4 and T_3 levels can be monitored at 2- to 4-week intervals. TSH becomes a useful parameter later in the course of treatment. Typically, the antithyroid drug dosage can be decreased once hyperthyroidism is controlled.
   d. For patients with Graves' disease, a 9- to 12-month course of therapy is appropriate before tapering the agent off to determine whether TSH-receptor stimulatory activity has subsided. For patients with toxic adenomas and toxic multinodular goiter, antithyroid medication is strictly a temporary measure until radioiodine treatment or surgery is employed.
   e. Fever, rash, and pruritus occur in approximately 5% of treated patients. Agranulocytosis occurs in approximately 2 of 1000 thionamide treated patients. PTU-associated hepatotoxicity is rare but can progress to acute hepatic failure and death. Methimazole-associated hepatotoxicity is usually milder. Hematologic and liver function test should be monitored.
3. **Radioactive iodine.** Radiation therapy with radioisotopes of iodine treatment is appropriate for the definitive treatment of Graves' disease, toxic adenoma, toxic multinodular goiter, and TSH-secreting pituitary adenomas. The principal side effect is hypothyroidism, which occurs in the majority of cured patients, necessitating lifelong follow-up.
4. Iodine in the form of a saturated solution of potassium iodide or Lugol's solution blocks the release of hormone from the gland and can be used (1) as short-term therapy to prepare patients for surgery, (2) as an adjunct to accelerate recovery after radioiodine treatment, or (3) as one component of polypharmacy for patients in thyrotoxic crisis. Aspirin, nonsteroidal anti-inflammatory agents, and glucocorticoids can be used to relieve pain.
5. Surgery is an appropriate treatment for hyperthyroidism in patients with toxic adenomas or toxic multinodular goiters who are younger than 20 years or whose glands are large enough to cause local symptoms or a cosmetic problem.

B. **Specific conditions**
   1. **Graves' disease**
      a. In patient with mild Graves' disease and thyrotoxicosis, there is a 30 to 40% probability of remission after a course of antithyroid drug therapy. Treatment is usually started with methimazole, which is then adjusted in increments of 5 to 10 mg per dose and continued

until the free T_4 and T_3 levels return to normal. The minimal dose required to maintain euthyroidism is continued for 9 months to 1 year. Treatment is then tapered off to determine if hyperthyroidism recurs. If it does, patients should proceed with treatment with radioactive iodine.

    b. Graves' disease appearing with moderate thyrotoxicosis and no significant complications is usually treated with radioactive iodine. However, many patients do not desire a permanent therapy and may request antithyroid medication.

  2. Toxic multinodular goiter and toxic adenoma. For hyperthyroidism due to toxic multinodular goiter, radioactive iodine is generally the treatment of choice, although occasional surgery should be considered for cosmesis or relief of compressive symptoms. Patients younger than 20 years of age with a toxic adenoma should undergo surgery. In older patients, radioactive iodine may be used.

C. Special circumstances

  1. Mild (subclinical) thyrotoxicosis is diagnosed when the serum TSH concentration is very low or undetectable without elevations of the serum T_4 or T_3 concentrations. These patient may have no symptoms or signs of thyrotoxicosis. For individuals with nonspecific symptoms, a 3-month trial of antithyroid drug therapy may be useful.

  2. Thyrotoxic crisis or storm is characterized by marked sympathomimetic and hypermetabolic effects of thyroid hormone excess. It typically develops in the setting of Graves' disease. Patients may develop high fever, atrial tachyarrhythmias, congestive heart failure, nausea and vomiting, diarrhea, delirium, psychosis, or seizures. Therapy includes antipyretics, beta blockers, high-dose PTU, iodinated contrast agents, and glucocorticoids.

References: See page 294.

Obesity

Evaluation of the obese patient should include determination of the body mass index (BMI), the distribution of fat based upon the waist circumference, and investigations for comorbid conditions such as diabetes mellitus, dyslipidemia, hypertension, and heart disease. Anti-obesity drugs can be useful adjuncts to diet and exercise for obese subjects with a BMI greater than 30 kg/m².

I. Goals of therapy and criteria for success

  A. Weight loss should exceed 2 kg during the first month of drug therapy (1 pound per week), fall more than 5 percent below baseline by three to six months, and remain at this level to be considered effective. A weight loss of 5 to 10 percent can significantly reduce the risk factors for diabetes and cardiovascular disease.

  B. Weight loss of 10 to 15 percent is considered a very good response and weight loss exceeding 15 percent is considered an excellent response. This degree of weight loss may lower blood pressure and serum lipid concentrations, increase insulin sensitivity, and reduce hyperglycemia.

II. Practice guidelines

  A. Counsel all obese patients (BMI $\geq$30 kg/m²) on diet, lifestyle, and goals for weight loss.

  B. Pharmacologic therapy may be offered to those who have failed to achieve weight loss goals through diet and exercise alone. Bariatric surgery should be considered for patients with BMI >40 kg/m² who have failed diet and exercise (with or without drug therapy) and who have obesity-related co-morbidities (hypertension, impaired glucose tolerance, diabetes mellitus, dyslipidemia, sleep apnea).

C. Noradrenergic sympathomimetic drugs:

  1. Stimulate the release of norepinephrine or inhibit its reuptake into nerve terminals

  2. Block norepinephrine and serotonin reuptake (sibutramine)

    3. May increase blood pressure

    4. Sympathomimetic drugs reduce food intake by causing early satiety.

  D. Sibutramine (Meridia) is a specific inhibitor of norepinephrine, serotonin and to a lesser degree dopamine reuptake into nerve terminals. It inhibits food intake. Sibutramine result is weight loss of about 9.5 percent.

    1. Sympathomimetic drugs can increase blood pressure. Sibutramine may increase systolic and diastolic blood pressure increased on average by 1 to 3 mmHg, and pulse increases by four to five beats per minute. Thus, sibutramine should be given cautiously to subjects receiving other drugs that may increase blood pressure.

    2. Sibutramine produces a significant overall weight loss and significant increase in both systolic and diastolic blood pressure.

    3. **Sibutramine should be avoided in:**

      a. Patients with a history of coronary heart disease, congestive heart failure, cardiac arrhythmia, or stroke.

      b. Patients receiving a monoamine oxidase inhibitor or selective serotonin reuptake inhibitor (risk of serotonin syndrome).

      c. Patients taking erythromycin and ketoconazole (sibutramine is metabolized by the cytochrome P450 enzyme system [isozyme CYP3A4])

    4. Sibutramine is available in 5, 10, and 15 mg tablets. The recommended starting dose is 10 mg daily, with titration up or down based upon the response. Doses above 15 mg daily are not recommended.

    5. Phentermine leads to more weight loss than placebo. Weight loss slowed during the drug-free periods in the intermittently-treated patients, but accelerated when treatment was resumed.

III. Drugs that alter fat digestion

  A. Orlistat (Xenical) inhibits pancreatic lipases. As a result, ingested fat is not completely hydrolyzed to fatty acids and glycerol, and fecal fat excretion is increased.

  B. Pharmacology. Orlistat does not alter the pharmacokinetics of digoxin, phenytoin, warfarin, glyburide, oral contraceptives, alcohol, furosemide, captopril, nifedipine, or atenolol. However, absorption of fat-soluble vitamins may be decreased by orlistat.

Anorectic Medication for Obesity Treatment

Medication	Schedule	Trade Name(s)	Dosage (mg)	Common Use
Phentermine	IV		8, 15, 30	Initial dose: 8-15 mg/d Higher dose: 15 mg bid or 30 mg q AM
		Adipex-P	37.5	Initial dose: ½ tablet/d Higher dose: ½ tablet bid or 37.5-mg tablet q AM
		Fastin	30	1 capsule q AM
Phentermine resin	IV	Ionamin	15, 30	Initial dose: 15 mg/d Higher dose: 15 mg bid or 30 mg q AM

Medication	Sche dule	Trade Name(s)	Dosage (mg)	Common Use
Diethylpro-pion	IV	Tenuate Tenuate Dospan (sustained-release form)	25 75	25 mg tid 75 mg qd
Sibutramine	IV	Meridia	5, 10, 15	Initial dose: 5-10 mg/d Higher dose: 15-25 mg/d
Orlistat	IV	Xenical	120	Initial dose: 1 capsule with a fatty meal qd; bid; or tid

- C. **Efficacy.** The mean weight loss due to orlistat is 2.89 kg. Weight loss at one year varies from 8.5 to 10.2 percent.
- D. **Side effects.** Orlistat is generally well-tolerated. Major side effects are intestinal borborygmi and cramps, flatus, fecal incontinence, oily spotting, and flatus with discharge occur in 15 to 30 percent. These gastrointestinal complaints are usually mild and subside after the first several weeks of treatment.
- E. Absorption of vitamins A and E and beta-carotene may be slightly reduced. Vitamin supplements should be given to patients treated with this drug.
- F. Orlistat is available in 120 mg capsules. The recommended dose is 120 mg three times daily.

IV. **Diabetes drugs**
- A. Metformin is a biguanide that is approved for the treatment of diabetes mellitus. Patients receiving metformin lose 1 to 2 kg.
- B. Although metformin does not produce enough weight loss (5 percent) to qualify as a "weight-loss drug," it is very useful for overweight individuals at high risk for diabetes.

V. **Recommendations**
- A. **Diet and lifestyle**
  1. All patients who are overweight (BMI $\geq$27 kg/m^2) or obese (BMI $\geq$30 kg/m^2), should receive counseling on diet, lifestyle, and goals for weight loss.
  2. Patients with a BMI of 25 to 29.9 kg/m^2 who have an increased waist circumference (>40 inches in men or >35 inches in women) or those with a BMI 27 to 30 kg/m^2 with comorbidities deserve the same consideration for obesity intervention as those with BMI >30 kg/m^2.
- B. **Pharmacotherapy**
  1. For patients who have failed to achieve weight loss goals through diet and exercise alone, pharmacologic therapy should be initiated.
  2. For obese patients with elevated blood pressure, cardiovascular disease, or dyslipidemia, orlistat is first line pharmacologic therapy.
  3. For otherwise healthy obese patients, sibutramine should be given because of the efficacy and easy tolerability of this agent.
  4. For patients with type 2 diabetes, in addition to lifestyle modifications, metformin should be prescribed both for glycemic control and for weight reduction. If the patient has coexisting hypertension, sibutramine should not be used. Orlistat is recommended if further weight reduction is needed.
- C. **Bariatric surgery**
  1. For patients with BMI $\geq$40 kg/m^2 who have failed diet and exercise (with or without drug therapy) or for patients with BMI >35 kg/m^2 and obesity-related co-morbidities (hypertension, impaired glucose tolerance,

diabetes mellitus, dyslipidemia, sleep apnea), bariatric surgery is recommended.

References: See page 294.

Hematologic and Rheumatologic Disorders

Anemia

The prevalence of anemia is about 29 to 30 cases per 1,000 females of all ages and six cases per 1,000 males under the age of 45 Deficiencies of iron, vitamin B12 and folic acid are the most common causes.

I. **Clinical manifestations.** Severe anemia may be tolerated well if it develops gradually. Patients with an Hb of less than 7 g/dL will have symptoms of tissue hypoxia (fatigue, headache, dyspnea, light-headedness, angina). Pallor, syncope and tachycardia may signal hypovolemia and impending shock.

II. **History and physical examination**
   A. The evaluation should determine if the anemia is of acute or chronic onset, and clues to any underlying systemic process should be sought. A history of drug exposure, blood loss, or a family history of anemia should be sought.
   B. Lymphadenopathy, hepatic or splenic enlargement, jaundice, bone tenderness, neurologic symptoms or blood in the feces should be sought.

III. **Laboratory evaluation**
   A. **Hemoglobin and hematocrit** serve as an estimate of the RBC mass.
   B. **Reticulocyte count** reflects the rate of marrow production of RBCs. Absolute reticulocyte count = (% reticulocytes/100) × RBC count. An increase of reticulocytes to greater than 100,000/mm^3 suggests a hyperproliferative bone marrow.
   C. **Mean corpuscular volume (MCV)** is used in classifying anemia as microcytic, normocytic or macrocytic.

Normal Hematologic Values			
Age of patient	Hemoglobin	Hematocrit (%)	Mean corpuscular volume (pm^3)
One to three days	14.5-22.5 g per dL	45-67	95-121
Six months to two years	10.5-13.5 g per dL	33-39	70-86
12 to 18 years (male)	13.0-16.0 g per dL	37-49	78-98
12 to 18 years (female)	12.0-16.0 g per dL	36-46	78-102
>18 years (male)	13.5-17.5 g per dL	41-53	78-98
>18 years (female)	12.0-16.0 g per dL	36-46	78-98

IV. Iron deficiency anemia

A. Iron deficiency is the most common cause of anemia. In children, the deficiency is typically caused by diet. In adults, the cause should be considered to be a result of chronic blood loss until a definitive diagnosis is established.

B. Laboratory results

1. The MCV is normal in early iron deficiency. As the hematocrit falls below 30%, hypochromic microcytic cells appear, followed by a decrease in the MCV.

2. A serum ferritin level of less than 10 ng/mL in women or 20 ng/mL in men is indicative of low iron stores. A serum ferritin level of more than 200 ng/mL indicates adequate iron stores.

C. Treatment of iron deficiency anemia

1. Ferrous salts of iron are absorbed much more readily and are preferred. Commonly available oral preparations include ferrous sulfate, ferrous gluconate and ferrous fumarate (Hemocyte). All three forms are well absorbed. Ferrous sulfate is the least expensive and most commonly used oral iron supplement.

Oral Iron Preparations			
Preparation	Elemental iron (%)	Typical dosage	Elemental iron per dose
Ferrous sulfate	20	325 mg three times daily	65 mg
Ferrous sulfate, exsiccated (Feosol)	30	200 mg three times daily	65 mg
Ferrous gluconate	12	325 mg three times daily	36 mg
Ferrous fumarate (Hemocyte)	33	325 mg twice daily	106 mg

2. For iron replacement therapy, a dosage equivalent to 150 to 200 mg of elemental iron per day is recommended.

3. Ferrous sulfate, 325 mg of three times a day, will provide the necessary elemental iron for replacement therapy. Hematocrit levels should show improvement within one to two months.

4. Depending on the cause and severity of the anemia, replacement of low iron stores usually requires four to six months of iron supplementation. A daily dosage of 325 mg of ferrous sulfate is necessary for maintenance therapy.

5. Side effects from oral iron replacement therapy are common and include nausea, constipation, diarrhea and abdominal pain. Iron supplements should be taken with food; however, this may decrease iron absorption by 40 to 66 percent. Changing to a different iron salt or to a controlled-release preparation may also reduce side effects.

6. For optimum delivery, oral iron supplements must dissolve rapidly in the stomach so that the iron can be absorbed in the duodenum and upper jejunum. Enteric-coated preparations are ineffective since they do not dissolve in the stomach.

7. Causes of resistance to iron therapy include continuing blood loss, ineffective intake and ineffective absorption. Continuing blood loss may be overt (eg, menstruation, hemorrhoids) or occult (e.g., gastrointestinal malignancies, intestinal parasites, nonsteroidal anti-inflammatory drugs).

V. Vitamin B12 deficiency anemia

A. Since body stores of vitamin B12 are adequate for up to five years, deficiency is generally the result of failure to absorb it. Pernicious anemia, Crohn's disease and other intestinal disorders are the most frequent causes of vitamin B12 deficiency.

B. Symptoms are attributable primarily to anemia, although glossitis, jaundice, and splenomegaly may be present. Vitamin B12 deficiency may cause decreased vibratory and positional sense, ataxia, paresthesias, confusion, and dementia. Neurologic complications may occur in the absence of anemia and may not resolve completely despite adequate treatment. Folic acid deficiency does not cause neurologic disease.

C. Laboratory results

1. A macrocytic anemia usually is present, and leukopenia and thrombocytopenia may occur. Lactate dehydrogenase (LDH) and indirect bilirubin typically are elevated.
2. Vitamin B12 levels are low. RBC folate levels should be measured to exclude folate deficiency.

D. Treatment of vitamin B12 deficiency anemia. Intramuscular, oral or intranasal preparations are available for B12 replacement. In patients with severe vitamin B12 deficiency, daily IM injections of 1,000 mcg of cyanocobalamin are recommended for five days, followed by weekly injections for four weeks. Hematologic improvement should begin within five to seven days, and the deficiency should resolve after three to four weeks.

Vitamin B12 and Folic Acid Preparations	
Preparation	Dosage
Cyanocobalamin tablets	1,000 μg daily
Cyanocobalamin injection	1,000 μg weekly
Cyanocobalamin nasal gel (Nascobal)	500 μg weekly
Folic acid (Folvite)	1 mg daily

VI. Folate deficiency anemia

A. Folate deficiency is characterized by megaloblastic anemia and low serum folate levels. Most patients with folate deficiency have inadequate intake. Lactate dehydrogenase (LDH) and indirect bilirubin typically are elevated, reflecting ineffective erythropoiesis and premature destruction of RBCs.

B. RBC folate and serum vitamin B_{12} levels should be measured. RBC folate is a more accurate indicator of body folate stores than is serum folate, particularly if measured after folate therapy has been initiated.

C. Treatment of folate deficiency anemia

1. A once-daily dosage of 1 mg of folic acid given PO will replenish body stores in about three weeks.
2. Folate supplementation is also recommended for women of childbearing age to reduce the incidence of fetal neural tube defects. Folic acid should be initiated at 0.4 mg daily before conception. Prenatal vitamins contain this amount. Women who have previously given birth to a child with a neural tube defect should take 4 to 5 mg of folic acid daily.

References: See page 294.

Low Back Pain

Approximately 90 percent of adults experience back pain at some time in life, and 50 percent of persons in the working population have back pain every year.

I. Evaluation of low back pain

A. A comprehensive history and physical examination can identify the small percentage of patients with serious conditions such as infection, malignancy, rheumatologic diseases and neurologic disorders.

B. The history and review of systems include patient age, constitutional symptoms and the presence of night pain, bone pain or morning stiffness. The patient should be asked about the occurrence of visceral pain, claudication, numbness, weakness, radiating pain, and bowel and bladder dysfunction.

History and Physical Examination in the Patient with Acute Low Back Pain

History
Onset of pain (eg, time of day, activity)
Location of pain (eg, specific site, radiation of pain)
Type and character of pain (sharp, dull)
Aggravating and relieving factors
Medical history, including previous injuries
Psychosocial stressors at home or work
"Red flags": age greater than 50 years, fever, weight loss
Incontinence, constipation
Physical examination
Informal observation (eg, patient's posture, expressions, pain behavior)
Physical examination, with attention to specific areas as indicated by the history
Neurologic evaluation
Back examination
    Palpation
    Range of motion or painful arc
    Stance
    Gait
    Mobility (test by having the patient sit, lie down and stand up)
    Straight leg raise test

C. Specific characteristics and severity of the pain, a history of trauma, previous therapy and its efficacy, and the functional impact of the pain on the patient's work and activities of daily living should be assessed.

D. The most common levels for a herniated disc are L4-5 and L5-S1. The onset of symptoms is characterized by a sharp, burning, stabbing pain radiating down the posterior or lateral aspect of the leg, to below the knee. Pain is generally superficial and localized, and is often associated with numbness or tingling. In more advanced cases, motor deficit, diminished reflexes or weakness may occur.

E. **If a disc herniation** is responsible for the back pain, the patient can usually recall the time of onset and contributing factors, whereas if the pain is of a gradual onset, other degenerative diseases are more probable than disc herniation.

F. Rheumatoid arthritis often begins in the appendicular skeleton before progressing to the spine. Inflammatory arthritides, such as ankylosing spondylitis, cause generalized pain and stiffness that are worse in the morning and relieved somewhat throughout the day.

G. **Cauda equina syndrome.** Only the relatively uncommon central disc herniation provokes low back pain and saddle pain in the S1 and S2 distributions. A central herniated disc may also compress nerve roots of the cauda equina, resulting in difficult urination, incontinence or impotence. If bowel or bladder dysfunction is present, immediate referral to a specialist is required for emergency surgery to prevent permanent loss of function.

II. Physical and neurologic examination of the lumbar spine

A. **External manifestations of pain**, including an abnormal stance, should be noted. The patient's posture and gait should be examined for sciatic list, which is indicative of disc herniation. The spinous processes and interspinous ligaments should be palpated for tenderness.

B. **Range of motion** should be evaluated. Pain during lumbar flexion suggests discogenic pain, while pain on lumbar extension suggests facet disease. Ligamentous or muscular strain can cause pain when the patient bends contralaterally.

C. **Motor, sensory and reflex function** should be assessed to determine the affected nerve root level. Muscle strength is graded from zero (no evidence of contractility) to 5 (motion against resistance).

D. **Specific movements and positions that reproduce the symptoms** should be sought. The upper lumbar region (L1, L2 and L3) controls the iliopsoas muscles, which can be evaluated by testing resistance to hip flexion. While seated, the patient should attempt to raise each thigh. Pain and weakness are indicative of upper lumbar nerve root involvement. The L2, L3 and L4 nerve roots control the quadriceps muscle, which can be evaluated by manually trying to flex the actively extended knee. The L4 nerve root also controls the tibialis anterior muscle, which can be tested by heel walking.

Indications for Radiographs in the Patient with Acute Low Back Pain

History of significant trauma
Neurologic deficits
Systemic symptoms
Temperature greater than 38°C (100.4°F)
Unexplained weight loss
Medical history
   Cancer
   Corticosteroid use
   Drug or alcohol abuse
Ankylosing spondylitis suspected

Waddell Signs: Nonorganic Signs Indicating the Presence of a Functional Component of Back Pain

Superficial, nonanatomic tenderness
Pain with simulated testing (eg, axial loading or pelvic rotation)
Inconsistent responses with distraction (eg, straight leg raises while the patient is sitting)
Nonorganic regional disturbances (eg, nondermatomal sensory loss)
Overreaction

Differential Diagnosis of Acute Low Back Pain

Disease or condition	Patient age (years)	Location of pain	Quality of pain	Ae fa
Back strain	20 to 40	Low back, buttock, posterior thigh	Ache, spasm	In be
Acute disc herniation	30 to 50	Low back to lower leg	Sharp, shooting or burning pain, paresthesia in leg	De cs tir
Osteoarthritis or spinal stenosis	>50	Low back to lower leg; often bilateral	Ache, shooting pain, "pins and needles" sensation	In ci c
Spondylolisthesis	Any age	Back, posterior thigh	Ache	In be
Ankylosing spondylitis	15 to 40	Sacroiliac joints, lumbar spine	Ache	M
Infection	Any age	Lumbar spine, sacrum	Sharp pain, ache	V
Malignancy	>50	Affected bone(s)	Dull ache, throbbing pain; slowly progressive	In c

Location of Pain and Motor Deficits in Association with Nerve Root Involvement

Disc level	Location of pain	Motor deficit
T12-L1	Pain in inguinal region and medial thigh	None
L1-2	Pain in anterior and medial aspect of upper thigh	Slight weakness in quadriceps; slightly diminished suprapatellar reflex
L2-3	Pain in anterolateral thigh	Weakened quadriceps; diminished patellar or suprapatellar reflex
L3-4	Pain in posterolateral thigh and anterior tibial area	Weakened quadriceps; diminished patellar reflex
L4-5	Pain in dorsum of foot	Extensor weakness of big toe and foot
L5-S1	Pain in lateral aspect of foot	Diminished or absent Achilles reflex

E. **The L5 nerve root** controls the extensor hallucis longus, which can be tested with the patient seated and moving both great toes in a dorsiflexed position against resistance. The L5 nerve root also innervates the hip abductors, which are evaluated by the Trendelenburg test. This test requires the patient to stand on one leg; the physician stands behind the patient and puts his or her hands on the patient's hips. A positive test is characterized by any drop in the pelvis and suggests L5 nerve root pathology.

F. **Cauda equina syndrome** can be identified by unexpected laxity of the anal sphincter, perianal or perineal sensory loss, or major motor loss in the lower extremities.

G. **Nerve root tension signs** are evaluated with the straight-leg raising test in the supine position. The physician raises the patient's legs to 90 degrees. If nerve root compression is present, this test causes severe pain in the back of the affected leg and can reveal a disorder of the L5 or S1 nerve root.

H. **The most common sites for a herniated lumbar disc** are L4-5 and L5-S1, resulting in back pain and pain radiating down the posterior and lateral leg, to below the knee.

I. **A crossed straight-leg raising test** may suggest nerve root compression. In this test, straight-leg raising of the contralateral limb reproduces more specific but less intense pain on the affected side. In addition, the femoral stretch test can be used to evaluate the reproducibility of pain. The patient lies in either the prone or the lateral decubitus position, and the thigh is extended at the hip, and the knee is flexed. Reproduction of pain suggests upper nerve root (L2, L3 and L4) disorders.

J. **Laboratory tests**
   1. Evaluation may include a complete blood count, determination of erythrocyte sedimentation rate.
   2. **Radiographic evaluation**. Plain-film radiography is rarely useful in the initial evaluation of patients with acute-onset low back pain. Plain-film radiographs are normal or equivocal in more than 75 percent of patients with low back pain. Views of the spine uncover useful information in fewer than 3 percent of patients. Anteroposterior and lateral

radiographs should be considered in patients who have a history of trauma, neurologic deficits, or systemic symptoms.

3. **Magnetic resonance imaging and computed tomographic scanning**
   a. Magnetic resonance imaging (MRI) and computed tomographic (CT) scanning often demonstrate abnormalities in "normal" asymptomatic people. Thus, positive findings in patients with back pain are frequently of questionable clinical significance.
   b. MRI is better at imaging soft tissue (eg, herniated discs, tumors). CT scanning provides better imaging of bone (eg, osteoarthritis). MRI has the ability to demonstrate disc damage. MRI or CT studies should be considered in patients with worsening neurologic deficits or a suspected systemic cause of back pain such as infection or neoplasm.

4. **Bone scintigraphy** or bone scanning, can be useful when radiographs of the spine are normal, but the clinical findings are suspicious for osteomyelitis, bony neoplasm or occult fracture.

5. **Physiologic assessment**. Electrodiagnostic assessments such as needle electromyography and nerve conduction studies are useful in differentiating peripheral neuropathy from radiculopathy or myopathy.

III. Management of acute low back pain

A. **Pharmacologic therapy**
   1. The mainstay of pharmacologic therapy for acute low back pain is acetaminophen or a nonsteroidal anti-inflammatory drug (NSAID). If no medical contraindications are present, a two- to four-week course of medication at anti-inflammatory levels is suggested.
   2. Naproxen (Naprosyn) 500 mg, followed by 250 mg PO tid-qid prn [250, 375,500 mg].
   3. Naproxen sodium (Aleve) 200 mg PO tid prn.
   4. Naproxen sodium (Anaprox) 550 mg, followed by 275 mg PO tid-qid prn.
   5. Ibuprofen (Motrin, Advil) 800 mg, then 400 mg PO q4-6h prn.
   6. Diclofenac (Voltaren) 50 mg bid-tid or 75 mg bid.
   7. Gastrointestinal prophylaxis, using a histamine H_2 antagonist or misoprostol (Cytotec), should be prescribed for patients who are at risk for peptic ulcer disease.
   8. Celecoxib (Celebrex) are NSAIDs with selective cyclo-oxygenase-2 inhibition. These agents have fewer gastrointestinal side effects.
   9. Celecoxib (Celebrex) is given as 200 mg qd or 100 mg bid.
   10. For relief of acute pain, short-term use of a narcotic may be considered.

B. **Rest.** Two to three days of bed rest in a supine position may be recommended for patients with acute radiculopathy.

C. **Physical therapy modalities**
   1. Superficial heat, ultrasound (deep heat), cold packs and massage are useful for relieving symptoms in the acute phase after the onset of low back pain.
   2. No convincing evidence has demonstrated the long-term effectiveness of lumbar traction and transcutaneous electrical stimulation.

D. **Aerobic exercise** has been reported to improve or prevent back pain. Exercise programs that facilitate weight loss, trunk strengthening and the stretching of musculotendinous structures appear to be most helpful. Exercises should promote the strengthening of muscles that support the spine.

E. **Trigger point injections** can provide extended relief for localized pain sources. An injection of 1 to 2 mL of 1 percent lidocaine (Xylocaine) without epinephrine is usually administered. Epidural steroid injection therapy has been reported to be effective in patients with lumbar disc herniation.

F. **Indications for herniated disc surgery.** Most patients with a herniated disc may be effectively treated conservatively. Indications for referral

include the following: (1) cauda equina syndrome, (2) progressive neuro-logic deficit, (3) profound neurologic deficit and (4) severe and disabling pain refractory to four to six weeks of conservative treatment.
References: See page 294.

Osteoarthritis

Approximately 40 million Americans of are affected by osteoarthritis, and 70 to 90 percent of Americans older than 75 years have at least one involved joint. The prevalence of osteoarthritis ranges from 30 to 90 percent.

Clinical Features of Osteoarthritis	
Symptoms Joint pain Morning stiffness lasting less than 30 minutes Joint instability or buckling Loss of function	**Pattern of joint involvement** **Axial:** cervical and lumbar spine **Peripheral:** distal interphalangeal joint proximal interphalangeal joint first carpometacarpal joints, knees, hips
Signs Bony enlargement at affected joints Limitation of range of motion Crepitus on motion Pain with motion Malalignment and/or joint deformity	

I. **Clinical evaluation**
   A. **Pathogenesis.** Osteoarthritis is caused by a combination of mechanical, cellular, and biochemical processes leading to changes in the composition and mechanical properties of the articular cartilage and degenerative changes and an abnormal repair response.
   B. The typical patient with osteoarthritis is middle-aged or elderly and complains of pain in the knee, hip, hand or spine. The usual presenting symptom is pain involving one or only a few joints. Joint involvement is usually symmetric. The patient usually has pain, stiffness, and some limitation of function. Pain typically worsens with use of the affected joint and is alleviated with rest. Morning stiffness lasting less than 30 minutes is common. (morning stiffness in rheumatoid arthritis lasts longer than 45 minutes.)
   C. Patients with osteoarthritis of the hip may complain of pain in the buttock, groin, thigh or knee. Hip stiffness is common, particularly after inactivity. Involvement of the apophyseal or facet joints of the lower cervical spine may cause neck symptoms, and involvement of the lumbar spine may cause pain in the lower back. Patients may have radicular symptoms, including pain, weakness and numbness.
   D. The physical examination should include an assessment of the affected joints, surrounding soft tissue and bursal areas. Joint enlargement may become evident. Crepitus, or a grating sensation in the joint, is a late manifestation.
   E. Laboratory work may include erythrocyte sedimentation rate and rheumatoid factor.
   F. Radiographic findings consistent with osteoarthritis include presence of joint space narrowing, osteophyte formation, pseudocyst in subchondral bone, and increased density of subchondral bone. The absence of radiographic changes does not exclude the diagnosis of osteoarthritis. Radiographs are recommended for patients with trauma, joint pain at night, progressive joint pain, significant family history of inflammatory arthritis, and children younger than 18 years.

Distinction Between Rheumatoid Arthritis and Osteoarthritis		
Feature	Rheumatoid arthritis	Osteoarthritis
Primary joints affected	Metacarpophalangeal Proximal interphalangeal	Distal interphalangeal Carpometacarpal
Heberden's nodes	Absent	Frequently present
Joint characteristics	Soft, warm, and tender	Hard and bony
Stiffness	Worse after resting (eg, morning stiffness)	Worse after effort
Laboratory findings	Positive rheumatoid factor Elevated ESR and C reactive protein	Rheumatoid factor negative Normal ESR and C reactive protein

II. Treatment of osteoarthritis

A. **Analgesics.** Acetaminophen at doses of up to 4 g/day is the drug of choice for pain relief. Hepatotoxicity is primarily seen only in patients who consume excessive amounts of alcohol. Combination analgesics (eg, acetaminophen with aspirin) increase the risk for renal failure.

1. Opioid analgesics, such as codeine, oxycodone, or propoxyphene may be beneficial for short-term use.
2. Tramadol (Ultram) alone or in combination with acetaminophen are useful when added to an NSAID or COX-2 inhibitor. The combination of tramadol and acetaminophen (37.5 mg/325 mg) is roughly equivalent to 30 mg codeine and 325 mg of acetaminophen.

B. **Nonsteroidal anti-inflammatory drugs** (NSAIDs) are indicated in patients with OA who fail to respond to acetaminophen. NSAIDs are more efficacious than acetaminophen. Gastrointestinal symptoms were more frequent with use of nonselective NSAIDs than with acetaminophen. Nonacetylated salicylates (salsalate, choline magnesium trisalicylate), sulindac, and perhaps nabumetone appear to have less renal toxicity. The nonacetylated salicylates and nabumetone (Relafen) have less antiplatelet activity. Low-dose ibuprofen (less than 1600 mg/day) may have less serious gastrointestinal toxicity.

C. **COX-2 inhibitors** have a 200 to 300 fold selectivity for inhibition of COX-2 over COX-1. Celecoxib (Celebrex) is available.

1. Selective COX-2 inhibitors are an option for patients with a history of peptic ulcer, gastrointestinal bleeding, or gastrointestinal intolerance to NSAIDs (including salicylates). These agents are contraindicated in cardiovascular disease or with multiple risk factors for atherosclerotic coronary heart disease. An alternative approach is the use of a nonselective NSAID and misoprostol or a proton pump inhibitor. Selective COX-2 and nonselective NSAIDs should be avoided in renal disease, congestive heart failure, cirrhosis, and volume depletion. Celecoxib (Celebrex) dosage is 100 mg twice daily and 200 mg once daily.

D. **Adverse effects.** NSAID use is often limited by toxicity. Among the side effects that can occur are:

1. Rash and hypersensitivity reactions.
2. Abdominal pain and gastrointestinal bleeding.

3. Impairment of renal, hepatic, and bone marrow function, and platelet aggregation.
4. Central nervous system dysfunction in the elderly.
5. NSAIDs are contraindicated in patients with active peptic ulcer disease. Non-specific COX inhibitors should be avoided in patients with a history of peptic ulcer disease. Specific COX-2 inhibitors are preferred in these individuals.
6. Non-specific COX-2 inhibitors must be used with caution in patients on warfarin. NSAID-induced platelet dysfunction can increase the risk of bleeding. Specific COX-2 inhibitors can be used in this setting.
7. Patients with intrinsic renal disease, congestive heart failure, and those receiving diuretic therapy are at risk for developing reversible renal failure while using an NSAID, resulting in an elevation in the plasma creatinine. Nonacetylated salicylates and sulindac (Clinoril) in low doses appear to relatively spare renal prostaglandin synthesis and can be used in these settings.
8. NSAIDs may interfere with the control of hypertension, usually resulting in a modest rise in blood pressure of 5 mm Hg.
9. Some patients with diminished cardiac function may develop overt congestive heart failure when given NSAIDs.
10. NSAIDs can be safely used in combination with low-dose aspirin (81 to 325 mg/day) that is prescribed for cardiovascular protection. NSAIDs should be avoided in patients with aspirin sensitivity.

Dosage of nonsteroidal anti-inflammatory drugs (NSAIDs)				
Agent	Brand name(s)	Dosing	Daily use	Specific benefits
Salicylates				
Aspirin		BID-QID	500-4000 mg	Titrate dose by serum levels
Choline magnesium trisalicylate	Trilisate	BID-QID	975-3600 mg	Decreased GI toxicity, titrate dose by serum levels
Salsalate	Disalcid, Salflex, Monogesic	BID-QID	975-3600 mg	Decreased GI toxicity, titrate dose by serum levels

Agent	Brand name(s)	Dosing	Daily use	Specific benefits
Short half-life NSAID				
Fenoprofen calcium	Nalfon	TID-QID	900-2400 mg	Generally fewer side effects
Ibuprofen	Motrin, Advil, Midol, Nuprin	TID-QID	600-3600 mg	
Indometha-cin	Indocin	TID-QID	75-200 mg	Excellent efficacy if tolerated
Ketoprofen	Orudis	TID-QID	75-300 mg	Dialyzable
Meclofena-mate so-dium	Meclomen	TID-QID	150-400 mg	
Tolmetin	Tolectin	TID-QID	600-2000 mg	
Intermediate half-life NSAID				
Diclofenac	Cataflam, Voltaren	BID-QID	100-200 mg	
Etodolac	Lodine	BID-QID	400-1200 mg	
Flurbipro-fen	Ansaid	BID-QID	100-300 mg	
Naproxen	Naproxyn, Napron X	BID-TID	500-1500 mg	
Naproxen-sodium	Anaprox, Aleve	BID-TID	550-1650 mg	
Sulindac	Clinoril	BID	150-1000 mg	Decreased renal pros-taglandin effect
Diflunisal	Dolobid	BID	500-1000 mg	Most uricosuric NSAID
Long half-life NSAID				
Nabumet-one	Relafen	QD-BID	1000-2000 mg	Decreased GI side effects
Oxaprozin	Daypro	QD-BID	600-1800 mg	

Agent	Brand name(s)	Dosing	Daily use	Specific benefits
Piroxicam	Feldene	QD	10-20 mg	

Cyclooxygenase-2 inhibitor			
Celecoxib (Celebrex)	100 mg twice daily or 200 mg daily for osteoarthritis 100 to 200 mg twice daily for rheumatoid arthritis	100 mg 200 mg	

E. Choice of NSAID

1. None of the available NSAIDs is more effective than any other. It is preferable to use a NSAID on a periodic basis in patients with noninflammatory OA since the presence and intensity of symptoms usually vary with time; a short-acting agent is ideal in this setting. Continuous therapy with a long-acting agent is indicated if this regimen does not provide adequate symptom control.

2. A short-acting NSAID is generally used initially. An over-the-counter agent (ibuprofen or naproxen) is a reasonable choice. If there is inadequate control with the initial dose, then the dose should be gradually increased toward the maximum for that drug. If one NSAID is not effective after two to four weeks on a maximal dosage, then another NSAID or nonacetylated salicylate should be tried. If there is a history of gastroduodenal disease, a specific COX-2 inhibitor is preferred

3. **Misoprostol (Cytotec)** can also be used as prophylaxis for the development of upper gastrointestinal bleeding in patients who receive nonspecific COX-2 inhibitors. Misoprostol dose is 100 μg twice daily.

F. Intraarticular corticosteroid injections

may be appropriate in patients with OA who have one or several joints that are painful despite the use of a NSAIDs and in patients with monoarticular or pauciarticular inflammatory osteoarthritis in whom NSAIDs are contraindicated. Intraarticular corticosteroids are effective for short-term pain relief.

1. Common corticosteroid suspensions used for intraarticular injection include triamcinolone acetonide, hexacetonide, and Depo-Medrol:
   a. 10 mg for small joints (interphalangeal, metacarpophalangeal and metatarsophalangeal joints).
   b. 20 mg for medium-sized joints (wrists, elbows, ankles).
   c. 40 mg for larger joints (shoulders, knees, hips).
   d. Corticosteroid injections in a weight-bearing joint should be limited to three to four per year.

G. Intraarticular hyaluronic acid derivatives

are more efficacious than intraarticular placebo. However, the magnitude of the benefit is modest.

H. Joint irrigation

may be warranted in patients with inflammatory symptoms who are refractory to NSAIDs or intraarticular corticosteroid injections.

I. Colchicine

may be a reasonable treatment option in patients with inflammatory OA who have symptoms that are unresponsive to nonpharmacologic interventions and NSAIDs.

J. Arthroscopic debridement.

Patients who will benefit from arthroscopic lavage and debridement have predominantly mechanical symptoms.

K. Surgical intervention

should be considered in patients with severe symptomatic OA who have failed to respond to medical management (including arthroscopic procedures), and who have marked limitations in activities of daily living. Total joint arthroplasty replacement provides

marked pain relief and functional improvement in patients with severe hip or knee OA.
L. The risk of NSAID-induced renal and hepatic toxicity is increased in older patients and in patients with preexisting renal or hepatic insufficiency. Choline magnesium trisalicylate (Trilisate) and salsalate (Disalcid) cause less renal toxicity. Liver function tests and serum hemoglobin, creatinine and potassium measurements should be performed initially and after six months of treatment.

References: See page 294.

Gout

Gout comprises a heterogeneous group of disorders characterized by deposition of uric acid crystals in the joints and tendons. Gout has a prevalence of 5.0 to 6.6 cases per 1,000 men and 1.0 to 3.0 cases per 1,000 women.

I. **Clinical features**
   A. **Asymptomatic hyperuricemia** is defined as an abnormally high serum urate level, without gouty arthritis or nephrolithiasis. Hyperuricemia is defined as a serum urate concentration greater than 7 mg/dL. Hyperuricemia predisposes patients to both gout and nephrolithiasis, but therapy is generally not warranted in the asymptomatic patient.
   B. **Acute gout** is characterized by the sudden onset of pain, erythema, limited range of motion and swelling of the involved joint. The peak incidence of acute gout occurs between 30 and 50 years of age. First attacks are monoarticular in 90 percent. In more than one-half of patients, the first metatarsophalangeal joint is the initial joint involved, a condition known as podagra. Joint involvement includes the metatarsophalangeal joint, the instep/forefoot, the ankle, the knee, the wrist and the fingers.
   C. **Intercritical gout** consists of the asymptomatic phase of the disease following recovery from acute gouty arthritis.
   D. **Recurrent gouty arthritis.** Approximately 60 percent of patients have a second attack within the first year, and 78 percent have a second attack within two years.
   E. **Chronic tophaceous gout.** Tophi are deposits of sodium urate that are large enough to be seen on radiographs and may occur at virtually any site. Common sites include the joints of the hands or feet, the helix of the ear, the olecranon bursa, and the Achilles tendon.

II. **Diagnosis**
   A. Definitive diagnosis of gout requires aspiration and examination of synovial fluid for monosodium urate crystals. Monosodium urate crystals are identified by polarized light microscopy.
   B. If a polarizing microscope is not available, the characteristic needle shape of the monosodium urate crystals, especially when found within white blood cells, can be identified with conventional light microscopy. The appearance resembles a toothpick piercing an olive.

III. **Treatment of gout**
   A. **Asymptomatic hyperuricemia.** Urate-lowering drugs should not be used to treat patients with asymptomatic hyperuricemia. If hyperuricemia is identified, associated factors such as obesity, hypercholesterolemia, alcohol consumption and hypertension should be addressed.
   B. **Acute gout**
      1. NSAIDs are the preferred therapy for the treatment of acute gout. Indomethacin (Indocin), ibuprofen (Motrin), naproxen (Naprosyn), sulindac (Clinoril), piroxicam (Feldene) and ketoprofen (Orudis) are effective. More than 90 percent of patients have a resolution of the attack within five to eight days.

Drugs Used in the Management of Acute Gout

Drug	Dosage	Side effects/comments
NSAIDS		
Indomethacin (Indocin) Naproxen (Naprosyn) Ibuprofen (Motrin) Sulindac (Clinoril) Ketoprofen (Orudis)	25 to 50 mg four times daily 500 mg two times daily 800 mg four times daily 200 mg two times daily 75 mg four times daily	Contraindicated with peptic ulcer disease or systemic anticoagulation; side effects include gastropathy, nephropathy, liver dysfunction, and reversible platelet dysfunction; may cause fluid overload in patients with heart failure
Corticosteroids		
Oral	Prednisone, 0.5 mg per kg on day 1, taper by 5.0 mg each day thereafter	Fluid retention; impaired wound healing
Intramuscular	Triamcinolone acetonide (Kenalog), 60 mg intramuscularly, repeat in 24 hours if necessary	May require repeat injections; risk of soft tissue atrophy
Intra-articular	Large joints: 10 to 40 mg Small joints: 5 to 20 mg	Preferable route for monoarticular involvement
ACTH	40 to 80 IU intramuscularly; repeat every 8 hours as necessary	Repeat injections are commonly needed; requires intact pituitary-adrenal axis; stimulation of mineralocorticoid release may cause volume overload
Colchicine	0.5 to 0.6 mg PO every hour until relief or side effects occur, or until a maximum dosage of 6 mg is reached	Dose-dependent gastrointestinal side effects; improper intravenous dosing has caused bone marrow suppression, renal failure and death

2. **Corticosteroids**
   a. **Intra-articular, intravenous, intramuscular or oral corticosteroids** are effective in acute gout. In cases where one or two joints are involved, intra-articular injection of corticosteroid can be used.
   b. **Intramuscular triamcinolone acetonide** (60 mg) is as effective as indomethacin in relieving acute gouty arthritis. Triamcinolone acetonide is especially useful in patients with contraindications to NSAIDs.
   c. **Oral prednisone** is an option when repeat dosing is anticipated. Prednisone, 0.5 mg per kg on day 1 and tapered by 5 mg each day is very effective.
3. **Colchicine** is effective in treating acute gout; however, 80 percent of patients experience gastrointestinal side effects, including nausea,

vomiting and diarrhea. Intravenous colchicine is available but is highly toxic and not recommended.

C. **Treatment of intercritical gout**

1. Prophylactic colchicine (from 0.6 mg to 1.2 mg) should be administered at the same time urate-lowering drug therapy is initiate. Colchicine should be used for prophylaxis only with concurrent use of urate-lowering agents. Colchicine is used for prophylaxis until the serum urate concentration is at the desired level and the patient has been free from acute gouty attacks for three to six months.

2. **Urate-lowering agents**
   a. After the acute gouty attack is treated and prophylactic therapy is initiated, sources of hyperuricemia should be eliminated to lower the serum urate level without the use of medication.
   b. Medications that may aggravate the patient's condition (eg, diuretics) should be discontinued; purine-rich foods and alcohol consumption should be curtailed, and the patient should gradually lose weight, if obese.

Purine Content of Foods and Beverages

High
  Avoid: Liver, kidney, anchovies, sardines, herring, mussels, bacon, codfish, scallops, trout, haddock, veal, venison, turkey, alcoholic beverages
Moderate
  May eat occasionally: Asparagus, beef, bouillon, chicken, crab, duck, ham, kidney beans, lentils, lima beans, mushrooms, lobster, oysters, pork, shrimp, spinach

---

3. **24-hour urine uric acid excretion measurement** is essential to identify the most appropriate urate-lowering medication and to check for significant preexisting renal insufficiency.
   a. Uricosuric agents should be used in most patients with gout because most are "underexcretors" of uric acid. Inhibitors of uric acid synthesis are more toxic and should be reserved for use in "overproducers" of urate (urine excretion >800 mg in 24 hours).
   b. Urate-lowering therapy should not be initiated until the acute attack has resolved, since they may exacerbate the attack.

Urate-Lowering Drugs for the Treatment of Gout and Hyperuricemia

Drug	Dosage	Indications	Side effects/comments
Probene-cid (Bene-mid)	Begin with 250 mg twice daily, gradually titrating upward until the serum urate level is <6 mg per dL; maximum: 3 g per day	Recurrent gout may be combined with allopurinol in resistant hyperuricemia	Uricosuric agent; creatinine clearance must be >60 mL per minute; therapeutic effect reversed by aspirin therapy; avoid concurrent daily aspirin use; contraindicated in urolithiasis; may precipitate gouty attack at start of therapy; rash or gastrointestinal side effects may occur

Drug	Dosage	Indications	Side effects/comments
Allopurinol (Zyloprim)	Begin with 50 to 100 mg daily, gradually titrating upward until the serum urate level is <6 mg per dL; typical dosage: 200 to 300 mg daily	Chronic gouty arthritis; secondary hyperuricemia related to the use of cytolytics in the treatment of hematologic malignancies; gout complicated by renal disease or renal calculi	Inhibits uric acid synthesis; side effects include rash, gastrointestinal symptoms, headache, urticaria and interstitial nephritis; rare, potentially fatal hypersensitivity syndrome

4. **Probenecid (Benemid)** is the most frequently used uricosuric medication. Candidates for probenecid therapy must have hyperuricemia attributed to undersecretion of urate (ie, <800 mg in 24 hours), a creatinine clearance of >60 mL/minute and no history of nephrolithiasis. Probenecid should be initiated at a dosage of 250 mg twice daily and increased as needed, up to 3 g per day, to achieve a serum urate level of less than 6 mg per dL. Side effects include precipitation of an acute gouty attack, renal calculi, rash, and gastrointestinal problems.

5. **Allopurinol (Zyloprim)** is an inhibitor of uric acid synthesis. Allopurinol is initiated at a dosage of 100 mg per day and increased in increments of 50 to 100 mg per day every two weeks until the urate level is <6 mg per dL. Side effects include rash, gastrointestinal problems, headache, urticaria and interstitial nephritis. A hypersensitivity syndrome associated with fever, bone marrow suppression, hepatic toxicity, renal failure and a systemic hypersensitivity vasculitis is rare.

References: See page 294.

Dermatologic and Allergic Disorders

Acne Vulgaris

Acne vulgaris affects over 17 million Americans, and 85 percent of the adolescent population experiences acne

I. **Classification of acne**
   A. Type 1. Mainly comedones with an occasional small inflamed papule or pustule; no scarring present.
   B. Type 2. Comedones and more numerous papules and pustules (mainly facial); mild scarring.
   C. Type 3. Numerous comedones, papules, and pustules, spreading to the back, chest, and shoulders, with an occasional cyst or nodule; moderate scarring.
   D. Type 4. Numerous large cysts on the face, neck, and upper trunk; severe scarring.

II. **Diagnostic evaluation**
   A. History should exclde polycystic ovary syndrome (PCOS), the most common cause of hyperandrogenism, which is characterized by menstrual irregularity, hirsutism, acne, ovarian cysts, insulin resistance, and acanthosis nigricans. Women with acne and oligomenorrhea should be evaluated for PCOS.
   B. The sudden appearance of acne with virilization suggests an adrenal or ovarian tumor; patients with Cushing's disease or syndrome and adult onset congenital adrenal hyperplasia may also have acne vulgaris. Evidence of virilization includes a deepening voice, decreased breast size, clitoromegaly, alopecia, oligomenorrhea, and hirsutism. Imaging studies of the adrenal glands and ovaries, and/or hormonal evaluation may be required.
   C. **Medications known to causes of acne** include ACTH, androgens, azathioprine, barbiturates, bromides, corticosteroids, cyclosporine, disulfiram, halogens, iodides, isoniazid, lithium, phenytoin, psoralens, thiourea, and vitamins B2, B6, and B12.
   D. **Physical examination** should focus upon the type and location of lesions, scarring, keloids, and postinflammatory pigmentary changes. Hirsutism or virilization should prompt further laboratory and imaging studies.

III. **Treatment of comedonal acne**
   A. Noninflammatory comedones typically develop in the preteen and early teenage years; there are no inflammatory lesions since P. acne colonization has not yet occurred. Treatment of abnormal follicular keratinization is most effective for comedonal acne.
   B. **Topical retinoids** (tretinoin, adapalene, tazarotene) are the initial drugs of choice for comedonal acne. These agents halt the progression of comedones to inflammatory lesions by normalizing follicular keratinization.
   C. **Tazorotene** does not share the same systemic side effects as oral isotretinoin, but it is still contraindicated in pregnancy.
   D. Tretinoin can cause cutaneous irritation; this may be minimized by starting with the lowest strength preparation (0.025 percent cream) and then increasing the potency. The ascending order of potency is as follows: 0.025 percent cream; 0.01 percent gel; 0.05 percent cream; 0.025 percent gel; 0.1 percent cream; and 0.05 percent solution. A microencapsulated form of 0.1 percent tretinoin gel is less irritating. Reduced irritation has been noted with a polyolprepolymer-2 base.

Treatment of Acne

Medication	Dose	Partial list of preparations	Adverse effects
Topical retinoids			
Tretinoin (Retin-A)	Usually twice daily	0.025 percent cream 0.01 percent gel 0.05 percent cream 0.025 percent gel 0.1 percent cream 0.05 percent solution	Local irritation; photosensitivity (use sunscreen)
Adapalene (Differin)	daily or twice daily	0.1 percent gel	Local irritation (slightly less than tretinoin); photosensitivity (use sunscreen)
Tazarotene (Tazorac)	daily	0.05 percent gel 0.1 percent gel	Local irritation; photosensitivity (use sunscreen); contraindicated in pregnancy, nursing
Benzoyl peroxide	daily or twice daily	2.5, 5, and 10 percent gels, lotions 5 percent solution + 3 percent erythromycin 6 and 10 percent gel + glycolic acid	Local irritation; can bleach hair and clothing
Topical antibiotics			
Metronidazole (Metrogel)	twice daily	1 percent cream 0.75 percent gel	
Clindamycin (Cleocin)	twice daily	10 mg/mL gel 10 mg/mL lotion 10 mg/mL topical solution	
Erythromycin (Erycette)	twice daily	1.5 percent solution 2 percent solution 2 percent gel 2 percent ointment 2 percent pledgets	
Azelaic acid (Azelex)	twice daily	20 percent cream	

Medication	Dose	Partial list of preparations	Adverse effects
Oral antibiotics			
Tetracycline	500 mg twice daily (or 250 mg twice daily)		Contraindicated in pregnancy and in children under age 12 due to tooth discoloration
Doxycycline	100 mg twice daily		Phototoxicity; esophageal ulceration
Minocycline	50 to 100 mg twice daily		Vertigo; pseudotumor; tooth discoloration
Erythromycin	250 to 750 mg twice daily		Gastrointestinal complaints
Oral retinoid			
Isotretinoin (Accutane)	0.5 mg/kg, increasing to 1 mg/kg, total dose 120 to 150 mg/kg over 20 weeks		Teratogenicity (absolutely contraindicated in pregnancy, nursing); mucocutaneous effects; hypertriglyceridemia; depression; bone marrow suppression

E. **Adapalene** produces less cutaneous irritation than tretinoin. However, both drugs increase photosensitivity; they should be applied at bedtime with concurrent use of sunscreen in the morning.

F. **Gels** have a drying effect; they may be useful in patients with oily skin. Creams and lotions are moisturizing. Solutions are drying but they cover large areas. Most topical medications are applied twice daily, although once daily or alternate day therapy can be used.

G. **Salicylic acid and azelaic acid** also exhibit comedolytic activity. These preparations are useful for patients who are unable to tolerate the topical retinoids. Salicylic acid is available in a number of nonprescription solutions (0.5 and 2 percent), cleansers, and soaps. Azelaic acid is an antimicrobial agent that reduces cutaneous pigmentation.

H. **Comedo extraction** can be a useful adjunct to topical therapy in patients with resistant comedones. Excise the roof or enlarge the opening of the comedo with an 18-gauge needle or no. 11 blade. Apply pressure with a comedo extractor.

IV. **Mild to moderate inflammatory acne** responds to benzoyl peroxide, a topical antibiotic, or a combination of the two drugs. Combination therapy is more effective than monotherapy for inflammatory lesions.

A. **Benzoyl peroxide** has both antibacterial and comedolytic properties. It is usually applied twice daily, although when combined with a topical retinoid, benzoyl peroxide is typically applied in the morning and the retinoid at night to limit irritation and photosensitivity.

   1. Benzoyl peroxide is available in 2.5, 5, and 10 percent gels and lotions, as a 5 percent solution in combination with 3 percent erythromycin, and as a 6 and 10 percent gel in combination with glycolic acid. Liquids and creams are less irritating than gels, these agents can cause bleaching of the hair and clothing.

B. **Topical antibiotics** are added to eliminate P. acnes and suppress inflammation in papular and inflammatory acne. Topical antibiotics may promote the appearance of resistant strains of P. acne; resistance is diminished by combination use with benzoyl peroxide.

   1. Topical antibiotics are available in gels, solutions, and lotions. Erythromycin and clindamycin are most frequently used. All topical antibiotics rarely cause skin irritation. Topical tetracycline can cause yellow staining of the skin and clothing.

V. **Moderate to severe inflammatory acne.** A sequential topical regimen of combination benzoyl peroxide-erythromycin in the morning and topical tretinoin in the evening is often effective. Patients with severe disease should be treated with oral antibiotics or oral isotretinoin in addition to topical therapy. Hormonal therapy may be useful in some women.

A. Oral antibiotics improve inflammatory acne by inhibiting the growth of P. acnes. The tetracyclines also have direct antiinflammatory properties; they inhibit the neutrophil chemotaxis and granuloma formation. Systemic antibiotics may induce vaginal candidiasis, decrease the efficacy of concomitantly administered oral contraceptive pills, and cause gastrointestinal distress.

B. Tetracycline is the preferred oral antibiotic due to its low cost and high efficacy. It is initiated at a dose of 500 mg twice daily, although 250 mg twice daily may also be effective. Absorption is inhibited by food, dairy products, antacids, and iron; it must be taken on an empty stomach. Tetracycline is contraindicated during pregnancy and in children younger than 12 years of age due to its ability to discolor the enamel of developing teeth.

C. Doxycycline and minocycline are more lipid soluble than tetracycline and can therefore be used in lower doses (100 mg twice daily and 50 to 100 mg twice daily, respectively); an extended release formulation of minocycline is also available (45 to 135 mg once daily). Either drug can be taken with meals. Minocycline or doxycycline may be prescribed in those who fail therapy with tetracycline.

   1. **Doxycycline** may be photosensitizing, and must be swallowed with ample fluids in order to avoid the development of esophageal ulcerations.

   2. **Minocycline** does not cause the phototoxicity seen with both tetracycline and doxycycline, but can cause vertigo, pseudotumor cerebri, tooth discoloration, and a lupus-like syndrome.

D. Erythromycin may be administered as 250 mg to 1500 mg daily in two divided doses. However, it has less antiinflammatory activity than the tetracyclines, and P. acnes often develop resistance, and intolerable gastrointestinal side effects are common.

E. **Isotretinoin (Accutane)** is a 13-cis retinoic acid that is useful for severe acne. It acts by reducing sebum secretion, an effect that lasts for up to one year after cessation of therapy.

   1. The primary indications for therapy with oral isotretinoin include:
      a. Severe nodulocystic acne
      b. Acne that improves less than 50 percent after six months of treatment with oral antibiotics
      c. Relapsing acne
      d. Scarring acne
      e. Acne that causes undue psychological distress

   2. Treatment is initiated at a daily dose of 0.5 mg/kg and increased to 1 mg/kg, administered in two divided doses with food, with a total treatment course of 120 to 150 mg/kg over 4 to 7 months (usual duration of treatment 20 weeks).

   3. A micronized formulation of isotretinoin offers the advantage of once daily dosing and does not need to be taken with food.

   4. The FDA has imposed restrictions on who may prescribe and distribute isotretinoin. Isotretinoin causes both spontaneous abortions and severe life-threatening congenital malformations. Mucocutaneous side effects include cheilitis, dry skin, desquamation, photosensitivity, and pruritus.

   5. Arthralgias, myalgias, hyperostosis, pseudotumor cerebri, decreased night vision, corneal opacities, hepatotoxicity, bone marrow suppression, and hypervitaminosis A may occur. Hypertriglyceridemia occurs in up to 45 percent. There is a possible association with depression and suicide.

F. **Hormonal and corticosteroid therapy.** Therapy with estrogen or an antiandrogen is an alternative to systemic isotretinoin in women with acne that is unresponsive to other methods of treatment.

1. Women with concomitant hirsutism or menstrual irregularity should have a gynecologic and hormonal evaluation.
2. Glucocorticoids are indicated for those with excessive adrenal androgen production, such as in classical congenital adrenal hyperplasia. For those with nonclassical (late-onset) congenital adrenal hyperplasia, oral contraceptives rather than glucocorticoids are used.
3. Oral contraceptives, particularly those preparations with a low androgenic progestin, are indicated for women with excessive ovarian androgen production (eg, PCOS).
4. Oral contraceptives with a low androgenic progestin may also be useful in some women with normal menses and no evidence of excess androgen production. A triphasic combination pill with norgestimate and ethinylestradiol (Ortho tri-cyclen) has been approved to treat acne vulgaris.
5. Newer oral contraceptives with anti-androgenic properties are being proposed as preferred therapies for women with acne. These include oral contraceptives that contain cyproterone or drospirenone plus an estrogen. Less costly oral contraceptives should be tried before more expensive preparations are prescribed.
6. Antiandrogens act at the peripheral receptor level to decrease sebum production. Spironolactone is most frequently used at a dose of 50 to 150 mg daily. Serum potassium and blood pressure should be monitored.

Androgenic activity of progestins in oral contraceptive pills	
Level of activity	**Brand name**
High	Norgestrel LoOvral Levonorgestrel Nordette Levelen Triphasil Trilevlen
Middle	Norethindrone Genora 1/35 OrthoNovum 1/35 Norinyl 1/35 Ortho 1/11 TriNorinyl Ortho 7/7/7 Modicon Brevicon Ovcon 35 Norethindrone acetate Loestrin 1/20 Loestrin 1.5/30
Low	Ethynodiol Demulen 1/35 Norgestimate Ortho-Cyclen Ortro-Tricyclen Desogestrel Desogen Ortho-Cept Drospirenone Yasmin

References: See page 294.

Contact Dermatitis

Contact dermatitis is an extremely common in the pediatric age group. There are two major forms of contact dermatitis: irritant and allergic. Common causes of irritant contact dermatitis include overbathing, drooling, prolonged contact with moisture and feces in the diaper, and bubble baths.

I. Clinical evaluation
  A. Contact dermatitis usually first appears in infants 2-6 months of age. Infants and children have rashes on the shoulders, chest, abdomen, and back. Infants usually also have a rash on the face, scalp and around the ears. Children older than 18 months old tend to have rashes on the neck and antecubital and popliteal fossae. Contact dermatitis usually resolves by puberty, but it sometimes recurs at times of stress.
  B. Acute lesions are itchy, red, edematous papules and small vesicles, which may progress to weeping and crusting lesions. Chronic rubbing and scratching may cause lichenification and hyperpigmentation.
  C. Patch testing is useful for evaluation of persistent, localized reactions. It also may be useful in patients who have atopic dermatitis and experience a flare or persistence of disease despite appropriate therapy.

II. Treatment of contact dermatitis
  A. **Moisture.** Avoidance of excessive bathing, hand washing, and lip licking is recommended. Showers or baths should be limited to no more than 5 minutes. After bathing, patients should apply a moisturizer (Aquaphor, Eucerin, Vaseline) to noninflamed skin.
  B. **Contact with irritants**
    1. Overuse of soap should be discouraged. Use of nonirritating soaps (eg, Dove, Ivory, Neutrogena) should be limited to the axilla, groin, hands, and feet.
    2. Infants often have bright red exudative contact dermatitis (slobber dermatitis) on the cheeks, resulting from drooling. A corticosteroid will usually bring improvement.
  C. **Topical corticosteroids**
    1. Corticosteroid ointments maintain skin hydration and maximize penetration. Corticosteroid creams may sting when applied to acute lesions.
    2. Mid- and low-potency topical corticosteroids are used twice daily for chronic, atopic dermatitis. High-potency steroids may be used for flare-ups, but the potency should be tapered after the dermatitis is controlled.
    3. Use of high-potency agents on the face, genitalia and skinfolds may cause epidermal atrophy ("stretch marks"), rebound erythema, and susceptibility to bruising.

Commonly Used Topical Corticosteroids	
Preparation	Size
Low-Potency Agents	
Hydrocortisone ointment, cream, 1, 2.5% (Hytone)	30 g
Mild-Potency Agents	
Alclometasone dipropionate cream, ointment, 0.05% (Aclovate)	60 g
Triamcinolone acetonide cream, 0.1% (Aristocort)	60 g
Fluocinolone acetonide cream, 0.01% (Synalar)	60 g

Preparation	Size
Medium-Potency Agents	
Triamcinolone acetonide ointment (Aristocort A), 0.1%	60 g
Betamethasone dipropionate cream (Diprosone), 0.05%	45 g
Mometasone cream 0.1% (Elocon)	45 g
Fluocinolone acetonide ointment, 0.025% (Synalar)	60 g
Hydrocortisone butyrate 0.1% cream, ointment (Locoid)	45 g
Betamethasone valerate cream, 0.1% (Valisone)	45 g
Hydrocortisone valerate cream, ointment, 0.2% (Westcort)	60 g
High-Potency Agents	
Amcinonide ointment, 0.1% (Cyclocort)	60 g
Betamethasone dipropionate ointment (Diprosone) 0.05%	45 g
Fluocinonide cream, ointment, 0.05% (Lidex)	60 g

4. **Allergic reactions to topical corticosteroids** may occur.
Mometasone (Elocon) is the least likely to cause an allergic reaction.
D. **Antihistamines,** such as diphenhydramine or hydroxyzine (Atarax), are somewhat useful for pruritus and are sedating. Nonsedating antihistamines, such as cetirizine (Zyrtec), loratadine (Claritin) and fexofenadine (Allegra), are helpful.
E. **Systemic corticosteroids** are reserved for severe, widespread reactions to poison ivy, or for severe involvement of the hands, face, or genitals. Prednisone, 1-2 mg/kg, is given PO and tapered over 10-18 days.
References: See page 294.

Common Skin Diseases

I. **Alopecia Areata**
   A. Alopecia areata is characterized by asymptomatic, noninflammatory, non-scarring areas of complete hair loss, most commonly involving the scalp, but the disorder may involve any area of hair-bearing skin.
   B. Auto-antibodies to hair follicles are the most likely cause. Emotional stress is sometimes a precipitating factor. The younger the patient and the more widespread the disease, and the poorer the prognosis.
   C. Regrowth of hair after the first attack takes place in 6 months in 30% of cases, with 50% regrowing within 1 year, and 80% regrowing within 5 years. Ten to 30% of patients will not regrow hair; 5% progress to total hair loss.
   D. Lesions are well defined, single or multiple round or oval areas of total hair loss. Typical "exclamation point" hairs (3-10 mm in size with a tapered, less pigmented proximal shaft) are seen at the margins.
   E. **Differential diagnosis** includes tinea capitis, trichotillomania, secondary syphilis, and lupus erythematosus.
   F. A VDRL or RPR test for syphilis should be obtained. A CBC, SMAC, sedimentary rate, thyroid function tests, and antinuclear antibody should

be completed to screen for pernicious anemia, chronic active hepatitis, thyroid disease, lupus erythematosus, and Addison's disease.

G. **Therapy.** Topical steroids, intralesional steroids, and topical minoxidil may be somewhat effective.

1. Intralesional glucocorticoid injection is the most common therapy for limited involvement. Triamcinolone in a dosage of 10 mg per mL, is the preferred agent.

2. Topical therapy may be beneficial when it is combined with minoxidil, anthralin or injected steroids.

3. Topical minoxidil, 5 percent solution, is 40% effective in stimulating hair growth on the scalp, eyebrows and beard area. Minoxidil solution is applied twice daily and stimulates hair growth within 12 weeks.

4. Anthralin cream is commonly used in children. New hair growth may occur within two to three months after initiation of topical anthralin therapy. In one study, 25 percent of patients had cosmetically acceptable results by six months. Side effects of anthralin include redness, itching and scaling. Removal of the cream after application for 20 to 60 minutes is often recommended. However, overnight application has been shown to be well tolerated by some patients.

5. The investigational technique called topical immunotherapy, or contact sensitization, may be effective.

II. Scabies

A. Scabies is an extremely pruritic eruption usually accentuated in the groin, axillae, navel, breasts and finger webs, with sparing the head.

B. Scabies is spread by skin to skin contact. The diagnosis is established by finding the mite, ova, or feces in scrapings of the skin, usually of the finger webs or genitalia.

C. Treatment of choice for nonpregnant adults and children is lindane (Kwell), applied for 12 hours, then washed off.

D. Elimite, a 5% permethrin cream, applied liberally head to toe and rinsed off in 12 hours, is more effective but more expensive than lindane (Kwell).

E. Treatment should be given to all members of an infected household simultaneously. Clothing and sheets must be washed on the day of treatment.

III. Acne Rosacea

A. This condition commonly presents in fair-skinned individuals and is characterized by papules, erythema, and telangiectasias.

B. Initial treatment consists of doxycycline or tetracycline. Once there has been some clearing, topical metronidazole gel (Metro-gel) can prevent remission. Sunblock should be used because sunlight can exacerbate the condition.

IV. Drug Eruptions

A. Drug eruptions may be type I, type II, type III, or type IV immunologic reactions. Cutaneous drug reactions may start within 7 days of initiation of the drug or within 4-7 days after the offending drug has been stopped.

B. The cutaneous lesions usually become more severe and widespread over the following several days to 1 week and then clear over the next 7-14 days.

C. Lesions most often start first and clear first from the head and upper extremities to the trunk and lower legs. Palms, soles, and mucous membranes may be involved.

D. Most drug reactions appear as a typical maculopapular drug reaction. Tetracycline is associated with a fixed drug eruption. Thiazide diuretics have a tendency for photosensitivity eruptions.

E. **Treatment of drug eruptions**

1. Oral antihistamines are very useful. Diphenhydramine (Benadryl), 25-50 mg q4-6h. Soothing, tepid water baths in Aveeno or corn starch or cool compresses are useful.

2. **Severe signs and symptoms.** A 2-week course of systemic steroids (prednisone starting at 60 mg/day and then tapering) will usually stop the symptoms.

F. Erythema Multiforme
1. Erythema multiforme presents as dull red macules or papules on the back of hands, palms, wrists, feet, elbows and knees. The periphery is red and the center becomes blue or darker red, hence the characteristic target or iris lesion.
2. The rash is most commonly a drug reaction caused by sulfa medications or phenytoin (Dilantin). It is also seen as a reaction to herpes simplex virus infections, mycoplasma, and Hepatitis B.
3. Erythema multiforme major or Steven's Johnson syndrome is diagnosed when mucous membrane or eye involvement is present.
4. Prednisone 30-60 mg/day is often given with a 2-4 week taper.
5. For HSV-driven erythema multiforme, acyclovir may be helpful. Ophthalmologic consultation is obtained for ocular involvement.

V. Pityriasis Rosea
A. Pityriasis rosea is an acute inflammatory dermatitis characterized by self-limited lesions distributed on the trunk and extremities. A viral cause is hypothesized. It is most common between the ages of 10 and 35.
B. **Clinical manifestations**
1. The initial lesion, called the "herald patch," can appear anywhere on the body, and is 2-6 cm in size, and begins a few days to several weeks before the generalized eruption. The hands, face, and feet are usually spared.
2. The lesions are oval, and the long axes follow the lines of cleavage. Lesions are 2 cm or less, pink, tan, or light brown. The borders of the lesions have a loose rim of scales, peeling peripherally, called the "collarette." Pruritus is usually minimal.
C. **Differential diagnosis.** Secondary syphilis (a VDRL is indicated for atypical rashes), drug eruptions, viral exanthems, acute papular psoriasis, tinea corporis.
D. **Treatment.** Topical antipruritic emollients (Caladryl) relieve itching. Ultraviolet therapy may be used. The disease usually resolves in 2-14 weeks and recurrences are unusual.

References: See page 294.

Seborrheic Dermatitis

Seborrheic dermatitis is a chronic inflammatory skin disorder generally confined to areas of the head and trunk. When seborrheic dermatitis occurs in the neonatal period, it usually disappears by six to 12 months of age. Seborrheic dermatitis usually occurs after puberty. Pityrosporum ovale, a yeast, has been implicated in this condition.

I. Clinical Manifestations
A. Seborrheic dermatitis typically is symmetric, and common sites of involvement are the scalp margin, eyebrows, eyelashes, mustache and beard. Other common sites are the forehead, the nasolabial folds, the external ear canals, the postauricular creases, and the trunk.
B. Seborrheic dermatitis causes dandruff, a fine, powdery white scale on the scalp. More severe seborrheic dermatitis is characterized by erythematous plaques with powdery or greasy scale.
C. **Treatment of Scalp and Beard Areas**
1. Seborrheic dermatitis is often effectively treated by shampooing daily or every other day with antidandruff shampoos containing 2.5 percent selenium sulfide or 1 to 2 percent pyrithione zinc. Ketoconazole shampoo may also be used. Topical terbinafine solution, 1 percent, has also been shown to be effective.
2. If the scalp is covered with diffuse, dense scale, the scale may first be removed by applying mineral oil or olive oil and washing. An alternative is coal tar-keratolytic combination or phenol-saline solution.

3. Extensive scale with associated inflammation may be treated by moistening the scalp and then applying fluocinolone, 0.01 percent in oil, to the entire scalp, covering overnight with a shower cap and shampooing in the morning. Corticosteroid solutions, lotions or ointments may be used once or twice daily.

4. As a substitute for daily washing, fluocinolone, 0.01 percent in oil, may be used as a scalp pomade. Other options include a moderate- to mid-potency topical corticosteroid in an ointment. After initial control is attained, fluocinolone, 0.01 percent shampoo (FS Shampoo), can be used as an alternative to or in addition to fluocinolone, 0.01 percent in oil (Derma-Smoothe/FS), for maintenance.

D. Treatment of the Face. Ketoconazole cream, 2 percent, may be applied once or twice daily. Hydrocortisone cream 1 percent once or twice daily will reduce erythema and itching.

E. Treatment of the Body. Seborrhea of the trunk may be treated with zinc or coal tar shampoos or by washing with zinc soaps. Additionally, topical ketoconazole cream, 2 percent, and/or a topical corticosteroid cream, lotion or solution may be applied once or twice daily.

F. Treatment of Severe Seborrhea. An occasional patient with severe seborrhea that is unresponsive to topical therapy may be a candidate for isotretinoin therapy. Treatment with daily doses of isotretinoin as low as 0.1 to 0.3 mg per kg may result in improvement in severe seborrhea.

References: See page 294.

Dermatophyte (Tinea) Infections

Dermatophytes are the most common type of fungi that cause infection of the skin and nails. Patients often refer to dermatophyte infections of the body or scalp as "ringworm". Three types of superficial fungi/dermatophytes account for the majority of infections: Epidermophyton, Trichophyton, and Microsporum. Dermatophyte infections affect individuals who are healthy, but people with compromised immune systems are particularly susceptible.

I. Tinea capitis

A. Tinea capitis, dermatophyte infection of the scalp, occurs almost always in small children. A clinical diagnosis of tinea capitis in adults is often incorrect, and frequently turns out to be seborrheic dermatitis or syphilis.

B. Black dot tinea capitis, caused by Trichophyton tonsurans, is the form predominantly seen. Tinea capitis is most often an endothrix infection; nonfluorescent arthroconidia are located within the hair shaft.

C. Clinical features. The infection begins with an erythematous, scaling, well-demarcated patch on the scalp that spreads centrifugally for a few weeks or months, ceases to spread, and persists indefinitely. The inflammation subsides, and the hairs within the patch break off a millimeter or two above the level of the scalp. The hair stubs take on a frosted appearance. In a few cases the lesions change abruptly to become boggy, elevated, tender nodules (kerion).

D. Diagnosis

1. **Black dot tinea capitis (BDTC)** is largely a disease of childhood. All ethnic groups may be infected, but African-American children are particularly susceptible. Spread is usually from child to child contact. Fomites (shared hats, combs, brushes, barrettes, rollers, etc) may play an important role. Asymptomatic carriers in the household may also be involved.

2. **Clinical features.** BDTC usually begins as an asymptomatic, erythematous, scaling patch on the scalp, which slowly enlarges. Lesions may be single or multiple. Hairs within the patches break off flush with the scalp; detritus within the follicular opening formerly occupied by the hair appears as a black dot. In some cases inflammation is prominent, and the lesions can resemble pyoderma or discoid lupus erythematosus. Painful lymphadenopathy can also occur. Left

untreated, scarring with permanent alopecia can occur and the disease can last indefinitely. Patches of tinea corporis may appear on glabrous skin, and the nails are sometimes involved. A sudden transition to kerion may occur.

3. **Diagnosis** of BDTC is made by performing KOH examination of spores on the hair shaft. The infected hairs of BDTC do not fluoresce green under Woods Light. Diagnosis can be confirmed by culture on Sabouraud's medium.

4. **Treatment.** Griseofulvin remains the drug of choice, although oral therapy with terbinafine or itraconazole are effective alternatives for resistant cases or for patients who are allergic to griseofulvin; oral fluconazole also seems to have similar efficacy to griseofulvin. A meta-analysis suggested that terbinafine is at least as effective as griseofulvin for treating tinea capitis due to Trichophyton infections, while griseofulvin appears to be superior to terbinafine for treating tinea capitis due to Microsporum infections.

   a. **Griseofulvin treatment** schedules are as follows:
      (1) Adults: 250 mg ultramicrosize by mouth twice daily for 6 to 12 weeks. A few cases of the black dot type may require 250 mg three times daily.
      (2) Children: 20 to 25 mg/kg of body weight for 6 to 12 weeks.

   b. **Terbinafine (Lamisil) treatment** schedules are based on weight:
      (1) 10 to 20 kg: 62.5 mg daily for four weeks
      (2) 20 to 40 kg: 125 mg daily for four weeks
      (3) Above 40 kg: 250 mg daily for four weeks

   c. **Itraconazole (Sporanox)** can be used in children as continuous therapy at a dose of 3 to 5 mg/kg daily for four to six weeks or as pulse therapy at a dose of 5 mg/kg daily for one week each month for two to three months.

   d. Topical treatment of tinea capitis is futile and a common cause of treatment failure.

   e. Identification of asymptomatic carriers and household fomites is an important part of the management of black dot tinea capitis. Culture on Sabouraud's medium of hairs and scalp dander (collected by brushing the area with a tooth brush) facilitates carrier identification. Carriers should be treated with selenium sulfide shampoo.

   f. **Kerion** responds best by treating the underlying fungal disorder.

II. Tinea pedis

A. Tinea pedis (athlete's foot) is the most common dermatophyte infection. It is often accompanied by tinea manuum, onychomycosis (tinea unguium), or tinea cruris (dermatophyte infection of the hands, nails, or groin).

B. Tinea pedis presents in two readily distinguishable clinical forms, acute and chronic. Both are contagious, contracted by contact with arthro-spores shed by infected individuals onto the floor.

C. **Acute tinea pedis**

1. **Clinical features.** Attacks of acute tinea pedis are self-limited, intermittent, and recurrent. They often follow activities that cause the feet to sweat. Acute tinea pedis begins with the appearance of intensely pruritic, sometimes painful, erythematous vesicular or bullous lesions between the toes and on the soles, frequently extending up the instep. The disease may be unilateral or bilateral. Secondary staphylococcal infections with lymphangitis often complicate the picture.

2. Secondary eruptions at distant sites may occur simultaneously due to an immunologic reaction to the fungus. This is a sterile vesicular eruption that often occurs on the palms and fingers, referred to as an "id" reaction. This improves as the primary infection is treated.

D. **Diagnosis** should be confirmed by KOH examination of scrapings from the lesions. The roof of a vesicle is a good place to look. Culture on Sabouraud's medium is helpful in difficult cases.

E. Chronic tinea pedis
  1. **Clinical features.** Chronic tinea pedis is the most common form of tinea pedis encountered in practice. Untreated it usually persists indefinitely. The disease begins with slowly progressive pruritic, erythematous lesions between the toes, especially in the fourth digital interspace. Interdigital fissures are often present. Extension onto the sole follows and later onto the sides or even the top of the foot ("moccasin ringworm"). The border between involved and uninvolved skin is usually quite sharp, and the normal creases and markings of the skin (dermatogliphs) tend to accumulate scale. In many cases the palms and flexor aspects of the fingers may be involved (tinea manuum). Mycotic nail dystrophy (onychomycosis) is also often present.
  2. **Treatment.** Tinea pedis can usually be treated with a topical antifungal cream for four weeks; interdigital tinea pedis may only require one week of therapy.
  3. Some prescription agents have a broader spectrum of action and may be administered once instead of twice daily, but generally all of the creams are equally effective.
  4. Patients with chronic disease or extensive disease may require oral antifungal therapy with griseofulvin (250 to 500 mg of microsize twice daily), terbinafine (250 mg daily), or itraconazole (200 mg daily). Terbinafine is more effective than griseofulvin, while the efficacy of terbinafine and itraconazole are similar. Nail involvement is another indication for oral therapy. Secondary infection should be treated with oral antibiotics.
  5. **Pediatric dosing options:**
     a. **Griseofulvin** 10 to 15 mg/kg daily or in divided doses
     b. **Terbinafine (Lamisil):**
        (1) 10 to 20 kg: 62.5 mg daily
        (2) 20 to 40 kg: 125 mg daily
        (3) Above 40 kg: 250 mg daily
     c. **Itraconazole** 5 mg/kg daily
     d. **Fluconazole** 6 mg/kg daily
     e. Other adjunctive therapies include use of foot powder to prevent maceration, treatment of shoes with antifungal powders, and avoidance of occlusive footwear.

Topical Antifungal Agents

Drug	Dose	How supplied
Terbinafine (Lamisil)	QD to BID	Cream 1%: 15g, 30g Gel 1%: 5g, 15g, 30g
Clotrimazole (Lotrimin)	BID	Cream 1%: 15g, 30g, 45g, 90g Lotion 1%: 30mL Solution 1%: 10mL, 30mL
Econazole (Spectazole)	QD (BID for candidiasis)	Cream 196: 15g, 30g, 85g
Sulconazole (Exelderm)	QD to BID	Cream 1%: 15g, 30g, 60g Solution 1%: 30mL

Drug	Dose	How supplied
Oxiconazole (Oxistat)	QD to BID	Cream 1%: 15g, 30g, 60g Lotion 1%: 30mL
Naftifine (Naftin)	QD (cream), BID (gel)	Cream 1%: 15g, 30g, 60g Gel 1%: 20g, 40g, 60g
Ciclopirox (Loprox)	BID	Cream 1%: 15g, 30g, 90g Lotion 1%: 30mL, 60mL
Ketoconazole (Nizoral)	QD	Cream 2%: 15g, 30g, 60g
Miconazole (Monistat-Derm)	BID	Cream 2%: 15g, 30g, 56.7g, 85g
Tolnaftate (Tinactin)	BID	Cream 1% : 15g, 30g Gel 1%: 15g Powder 1%: 45g, 90g Topical aerosol: liquid (1%): 59.2mL, 90mL, 120mL powder (1%):56.7g, 100g, 105g, 150g Solution 1%: 10 mL

Oral Antifungal Agents

Terbinafine (Lamisil):
For fingernails — 250 mg daily by mouth for 6 weeks
For toenails — 250 mg daily by mouth for 12 weeks

Itraconazole (Sporanox):
Fixed dosage
For fingernails — 200 mg daily by mouth for 8 weeks
For toenails — 200 mg daily by mouth for 12 weeks
Pulse therapy
For fingernails — 400 mg daily by mouth for one week per month for two months
For toenails — 400 mg daily by mouth for one week per month for three months

III. Tinea corporis
   A. Tinea corporis begins as a pruritic circular or oval erythematous scaling lesion that spreads centrifugally. Central clearing follows, while the active advancing border, a few millimeters wide, retains its red color and is slightly raised. The lesion is shaped like a ring.
   B. Extensive presentations suggest an underlying immunologic disorder, such as diabetes mellitus or HIV infection.
   C. Tinea corporis can also occur in outbreaks among athletes who have skin-to-skin contact, such as wrestlers (tinea corporis gladiatorum).
   D. **Treatment.** Tinea corporis usually responds well to the daily application of topical antifungals. For adults with extensive cases or with folliculitis,

or in patients who are severely immunocompromised, a systemic agent is preferable.

E. Appropriate systemic agents include oral terbinafine, fluconazole, and itraconazole; all of these agents appear to have greater efficacy and fewer side effects than oral griseofulvin, however griseofulvin is less expensive. Reasonable regimens in adults include: terbinafine 250 mg daily for one to two weeks; fluconazole 150 mg once weekly for two to four weeks; itraconazole 200 mg daily for one to two weeks; griseofulvin 250 mg three times daily for two weeks.

F. Patients with tinea corporis gladiatorum should be treated with an oral agent for ten to 15 days along with restricted participation in sports.

IV. **Tinea cruris** (jock itch) is a special form of tinea corporis involving the crural fold. The most common cause is T rubrum. A few cases are caused by E floccosum and occasionally T mentagrophytes.

A. Tinea cruris is far more common in men than women. The disease often begins after physical activity that results in copious sweating, and the source of the infecting fungus is usually the patient's own tinea pedis.

B. Tinea cruris begins with a macular erythematous patch high on the inner aspect of one or both thighs, opposite the scrotum. It spreads centrifugally, with partial central clearing and a slightly elevated, erythematous, sharply demarcated border that may show tiny vesicles.

C. **Diagnosis.** KOH examination of scales scraped from the lesion will show the segmented hyphae and arthrospores. Highest yields are obtained from material taken from the active border of the lesion. Cultures on Sabouraud's medium can also be used to confirm the diagnosis.

D. **Treatment.** Topical antifungal treatment is usually effective. Failure to treat concomitant tinea pedis usually results in prompt recurrence. Lesions resistant to topical medications can be treated with griseofulvin by mouth, 250 mg three times daily for 14 days, or any of the other systemic agents.

References: See page 294.

Paronychia, Herpetic Whitlow, and Ingrown Toenails

I. **Paronychia**

A. Paronychia is an inflammation involving the lateral and posterior fingernail folds. Predisposing factors include overzealous manicuring, nail biting, diabetes mellitus, and frequent immersion in water. Paronychia also is associated with antiretroviral therapy for HIV infection.

B. Paronychia may be either acute or chronic. Acute paronychia is caused by staphylococcus aureus, and it is characterized by the onset of pain and erythema of the posterior or lateral nail folds, with development of a superficial abscess. Chronic paronychia represents an eczematous condition.

C. **Treatment**

1. **Acute paronychia.** Therapy of acute paronychia includes local care (warm compresses or soaks for 20 minutes, three times per day) and antibiotic therapy. An antistaphylococcal agent such as dicloxacillin (250 mg TID) or cephalexin (Keflex) [500 mg BID to TID]) for seven to ten days is the preferred therapy. An alternative is erythromycin 333 mg TID or azithromycin (Zithromax [500 mg on day one, followed by 250 mg per day for four days]). incision and drainage is necessary if an abscess is present.

2. **Chronic paronychia.** Patients should be advised to keep their hands as dry as possible and to use gloves for all wet work. Patients should avoid irritant or allergen exposure. Chronic paronychia is an eczematous process, and Candida infection is a secondary phenomenon.

Thus, the treatment should be a topical corticosteroid, such as triamcinolone 0.1% ointment.

Comparison of Acute and Chronic Paronychia		
Features	**Acute**	**Chronic**
Clinical appearance	Red, hot, tender nail folds, with or without abscess	Swollen, tender, red (not as red as acute), boggy nail fold; fluctuance rare
People at high risk	People who bite nails, suck fingers, experience nail trauma (manicures)	People repeatedly exposed to water or irritants (e.g., bartenders, housekeepers, dishwashers)
Pathogens	Staphylococcal aureus, streptococci, Pseudomonas, anaerobes	Candida albicans (95 percent), atypical mycobacteria, gram-negative rods
Treatment	Warm soaks, oral antibiotics (clindamycin [Cleocin] or amoxicillin-clavulanate potassium [Augmentin]); spontaneous drainage, if possible; surgical incision and drainage	Avoidance of water and irritating substances; use of topical steroids and antifungal agents; surgery

II. Herpetic Whitlow
A. Herpetic whitlow (herpes simplex virus infection of the finger) occurs as a complication of primary oral or genital herpes infection via a break in the skin. It also occurs in medical personnel who have contact with oral secretions. Herpetic whitlow is characterized by erythema, swelling, pain, and vesicular or pustular lesions.
B. The diagnosis of herpetic whitlow is suspected by an exposure history as well as the presence of vesicles. Tzanck smear reveals multinucleated giant cells.
C. Treatment consists of oral acyclovir (Zovirax [400 mg TID]) for ten days A topical antibiotic cream, such as bacitracin, may help to prevent secondary bacterial infection.

III. Ingrown Toenail
A. Ingrown toenails occur when the lateral nail plate pierces the lateral nail fold. The great toenail is most commonly affected. Signs and symptoms include pain, edema, exudate, and granulation tissue. Predisposing factors include poorly fitting shoes, excessive trimming of the lateral nail plate (pincer nail deformity), and trauma.

B. Treatment
1. The lateral nail plate should be allowed to grow well beyond the lateral nail fold before trimming horizontally. Patients should wear well-fitting shoes.
2. **Mild-to-moderate lesion**
   a. Mild-to-moderate lesions are characterized by minimal to moderate pain, little erythema, and no discharge.
   b. Place a cotton wedging or dental floss underneath the lateral nail plate to separate the nail plate from the lateral nail fold, thereby relieving pressure.
   c. Soak the affected foot in warm water for 20 minutes, three times per day.

3. **Moderate-to-severe lesion**
   a. Moderate-to-severe lesions are characterized by substantial erythema and pustular discharge. Treatment consists of the following:
      (1) Anesthetize the area with lidocaine 1% without epinephrine.
      (2) Using nail-splitting scissors or a hemostat, insert the instrument under the nail plate and remove the involved nail wedge with nail clippers or scissors.
      (3) Remove any granulation tissue with a curette and/or silver nitrate sticks.
      (4) Dilute hydrogen peroxide 1:1 with tap water and cleanse the site 2 or 3 times a day, followed by application of either bacitracin or mupirocin ointment.
4. **Recurrent ingrown toenail.** For patients who suffer recurrent ingrown toenails, consider permanent nail ablation of the lateral nail horn with phenol.

References: See page 294.

Bacterial Infections of the Skin

Bacterial skin infections most commonly include cellulitis, impetigo, and folliculitis.

I. **Cellulitis**
   A. Cellulitis is a painful, erythematous infection of the dermis and subcutaneous tissues that is characterized by warmth, edema, and advancing borders. Cellulitis commonly occurs near breaks in the skin, such as surgical wounds, trauma, tinea infections, or ulcerations. Patients may have a fever and an elevated white blood cell count. The most common sites of cellulitis are the legs and digits, followed by the face, feet, hands, torso, neck, and buttocks.
   B. In otherwise healthy adults, isolation of an etiologic agent is difficult and unrewarding. If the patient has diabetes, an immunocompromising disease, or persistent inflammation, blood cultures or aspiration of the area of maximal inflammation may be useful.
   C. Empiric treatment of infection in patients without diabetes:
      1. **Penicillinase-resistant penicillin:** Dicloxacillin (Pathocil) 40 mg/kg/day in 4 divided doses for 7-12 days; adults: 500 mg qid or
      2. **First-generation cephalosporin:** Cephalexin (Keflex) 50 mg/kg/day PO in 4 divided doses for 7-10 days; adults: 500 mg PO qid or
      3. **Amoxicillin-clavulanate (Augmentin)** 500 mg tid or 875 mg bid for 7-10 days.
      4. **Azithromycin (Zithromax)** 500 mg on day 1, then 250 mg PO qd for 4 days.
      5. **Erythromycin ethylsuccinate** 40 mg/kg/day in 3 divided doses for 7-10 days; adults: 250-500 mg qid.
      6. Limited disease can be treated orally, but more extensive disease requires parenteral therapy. Marking the margins of erythema with ink is helpful in following the progression or regression of cellulitis.
      7. Outpatient therapy with injected ceftriaxone (Rocephin) provides 24 hours of parenteral coverage and may be an option for some patients.

Descriptions of Bacterial Skin Infections	
Disease	**Description**
Carbuncle	A network of furuncles connected by sinus tracts

Disease	Description
Cellulitis	Painful, erythematous infection of deep skin with poorly demarcated borders
Erysipelas	Fiery red, painful infection of superficial skin with sharply demarcated borders
Folliculitis	Papular or pustular inflammation of hair follicles
Furuncle	Painful, firm or fluctuant abscess originating from a hair follicle
Impetigo	Large vesicles and/or honey-crusted sores

  D. Antibiotics should be maintained for at least three days after the resolution of acute inflammation. Adjunctive therapy includes cool compresses; appropriate analgesics for pain; tetanus immunization; and immobilization and elevation of the affected extremity.
  E. A parenteral second- or third-generation cephalosporin (with or without an aminoglycoside) should be considered in patients who have diabetes, immunocompromised patients, those with unresponsive infections, or in young children. The patient may also require a plain radiograph of the area or surgical debridement to evaluate for gas gangrene, osteomyelitis, or necrotizing fasciitis.
  F. **Periorbital cellulitis** is caused by the same organisms that cause other forms of cellulitis and is treated with warm soaks, oral antibiotics, and close follow-up. Children with periorbital or orbital cellulitis often have underlying sinusitis. If the child is febrile and appears toxic, blood cultures should be performed and lumbar puncture considered.
  G. **Orbital cellulitis** occurs when the infection passes the orbital septum and is manifested by proptosis, orbital pain, restricted eye movement, visual disturbances, and concomitant sinusitis. This ocular emergency requires intravenous antibiotics, otorhinolaryngology, and ophthalmologic consultation.

II. **Erysipelas**
  A. Erysipelas usually presents as an intensely erythematous infection with clearly demarcated raised margins and lymphatic streaking. Common sites are the legs and face.
  B. Erysipelas is caused almost exclusively by beta-hemolytic streptococcus and thus can be treated with oral or intravenous penicillin, or this infection may be treated the same as cellulitis. Adjunctive treatment and complications are the same as for cellulitis.

III. **Impetigo**
  A. Impetigo is most commonly seen in children aged two to five years and is classified as bullous or nonbullous. The nonbullous type predominates and presents with an erosion (sore), cluster of erosions, or small vesicles or pustules that have a honey-yellow crust. Impetigo usually appears in areas where there is a break in the skin, such as a wound, herpes simplex infection, or angular cheilitis.
  B. The bullous form of impetigo presents as a large thin-walled bulla (2 to 5 cm) containing serous yellow fluid. It often ruptures leaving a denuded area. Both forms of impetigo are primarily caused by S. aureus with Streptococcus usually being involved in the nonbullous form.
  C. An oral antibiotic with activity against S. aureus and group A beta-hemolytic streptococcus is warranted in nonlocalized cases.
    1. Azithromycin (Zithromax) for five days and cephalexin (Keflex) for 10 days have been shown to be effective and well-tolerated.
    2. Dicloxacillin (Pathocil), 500 mg PO qid for 2 weeks.

3. Oxacillin (Prostaphlin) 1-2 gm IV q4-6h.
4. Cephalexin (Keflex) 250-500 mg PO qid.
5. Amoxicillin-clavulanate (Augmentin) 500 mg tid or 875 mg bid for 7-10 days.
6. Broad-spectrum fluoroquinolones have also been shown to be effective for treating skin and soft tissue infections. These medications have excellent skin penetration and good bioavailability.

IV. Folliculitis

A. The most common form is superficial folliculitis that manifests as a tender or painless pustule that heals without scarring. Multiple or single lesions can appear on any skin bearing hair including the head, neck, trunk, buttocks, and extremities. *S. aureus* is the most likely pathogen. Topical therapy with erythromycin, clindamycin (Cleocin T gel), mupirocin (Bactroban), or benzoyl peroxide can be administered to accelerate the healing process.

B. **Staphylococci** will occasionally invade the deeper portion of the follicle, causing swelling and erythema. These lesions are painful and may scar. This inflammation of the entire follicle or the deeper portion of the hair follicle is called deep folliculitis. Oral antibiotics are usually used and include first-generation cephalosporins, penicillinase-resistant penicillins, macrolides, and fluoroquinolones.

C. Gram-negative folliculitis usually involves the face and affects patients with a history of long-term antibiotic therapy for acne. Pathogens include Klebsiella, Enterobacter, and Proteus species. It can be treated as severe acne with isotretinoin (Accutane).

V. Furuncles and Carbuncles

A. **Furuncles** and carbuncles occur as a follicular infection progresses deeper and extends out from the follicle. Commonly known as an abscess or boil, a furuncle is a tender, erythematous, firm or fluctuant mass of walled-off purulent material, arising from the hair follicle. The pathogen is usually S. aureus. Typically, the furuncle will develop into a fluctuant mass and eventually open to the skin surface.

B. **Carbuncles** are an aggregate of infected hair follicles that form broad, swollen, erythematous, deep, and painful masses that usually open and drain through multiple tracts. Fever and malaise, are commonly associated with these lesions. With both of these lesions, gentle incision and drainage is indicated when lesions "point" (fluctuant). The wound may be packed (usually with iodoform gauze) to encourage further drainage. In severe cases, parenteral antibiotics such as cloxacillin (Tegopen), or a first-generation cephalosporin, such as cefazolin (Ancef), are required.

References: See page 294.

Psoriasis

Approximately 1 percent of the population is affected by psoriasis. The typical clinical findings of erythema and scaling are the result of hyperproliferation and abnormal differentiation of the epidermis, plus inflammatory cell infiltrates and vascular changes.

I. Clinical Manifestations

A. Plaque type psoriasis usually presents in young adults with symmetrically distributed plaques involving the scalp, extensor elbows, knees, and back. The plaques are erythematous with sharply defined, raised margins. A thick silvery scale is usually present. The lesions can range from less than 1 cm to more than 10 cm in diameter. The plaques typically are asymptomatic, although some patients complain of pruritus. Inspection may reveal pitting of the nail plates and involvement of intertriginous areas, such as the umbilicus and intergluteal cleft.

B. **Clinical course.** Most patients with psoriasis tend to have the disease for life. However, there may be marked variability in severity over time, and remissions at some stage are seen in 25 percent of cases. Pruritus may be severe and arthritis can be disabling.

C. **Diagnosis.** The diagnosis of psoriasis is made by physical examination and in some cases skin biopsy. The scalp, umbilicus, intergluteal cleft, and nails should be examined.

II. Treatment

A. **Topical emollients.** Keeping psoriatic skin soft and moist minimizes itching. The most effective are ointments such as petroleum jelly or thick creams.

B. **Topical corticosteroids**

1. Topical corticosteroids remain the mainstay of topical psoriasis treatment despite the development of newer agents.

2. In the scalp, potent steroids in an alcohol solution (eg, fluocinonide 0.05 percent) are frequently indicated. On the face and intertriginous areas, a low-potency cream (eg, hydrocortisone 1 percent) should be used.

3. For thick plaques on extensor surfaces, potent steroid ointments (eg, betamethasone 0.05 percent) with added occlusion by tape or plastic wrap may be required.

4. The typical regimen consists of twice-daily application of topical corticosteroids. Generics include, in order of increasing potency, hydrocortisone (Hytone) 1 percent, triamcinolone (Aristocort) 0.1 percent, fluocinonide (Lidex) 0.05 percent, and betamethasone dipropionate (Diprosone) 0.05 percent.

5. Betamethasone valerate in a foam (Luxiq) has superior efficacy for scalp psoriasis.

Types of Psoriasis, Associated Findings and Treatment Options

Type of psoriasis	Clinical features	Differential diagnosis	Treatment options
Plaque-type psoriasis	Red, thick, scaly lesions with silvery scale	Atopic dermatitis, irritant dermatitis, cutaneous T-cell lymphoma, pityriasis rubra pilaris, seborrheic dermatitis	Localized: topical therapy with corticosteroids, calcipotriene (Dovonex), coal tars, anthralin (Anthra-Derm) or tazarotene (Tazorac). Generalized: phototherapy, systemic agents, combination therapy
Guttate psoriasis	Teardrop-shaped, pink to salmon, scaly plaques; usually on the trunk, with sparing of palms and soles	Pityriasis rosea, secondary syphilis, drug eruption	Ultraviolet B phototherapy, natural sunlight
Pustular psoriasis, localized	Erythematous papules or plaques studded with pustules; usually on palms or soles (palmoplantar pustular psoriasis)	Pustular drug eruption, dyshidrotic eczema, subcorneal pustular dermatosis	Same as for plaque-type psoriasis

Type of psoria-sis	Clinical features	Differential diag-nosis	Treatment options
Pustular psoria-sis, generalized	Same as localized with a more general involvement; may be associated with systemic symptoms such as fever, malaise and diarrhea	Pustular drug eruption, subcorneal pustular dermatosis	Systemic therapy and/or hospitalization usually required
Erythrodermic psoriasis	Severe, intense, generalized erythema and scaling covering entire body; often associated with systemic symptoms; may or may not have had preexisting psoriasis	Drug eruption, eczematous dermatitis, mycosis fungoides, pityriasis rubra pilaris	Systemic therapy and/or hospitalization usually required

C. **Calcipotriol**
  1. Calcipotriol (Dovonex) has become an established therapy in psoriasis. Calcipotriol affects the growth of keratinocytes via its action at the level of vitamin D receptors. Calcipotriol is at least as effective as potent topical corticosteroids. Skin irritation is the main adverse effect. Topical calcipotriol may be used as an alternative to topical steroid therapy. Twice-daily application is indicated. Other than skin irritation, side effects are usually minimal; the risk of hypercalcemia is low. However, topical calcipotriol is more expensive than potent steroids.
  2. **Tazarotene (Tazorac)** is a topical retinoid that appears to be safe and effective for the treatment of mild to moderate plaque psoriasis. Once-daily administration of tazarotene gel, 0.05 or 0.1 percent, compared favorably with topical fluocinonide.
D. **Methotrexate**
  1. Methotrexate is usually administered in an intermittent low-dose regimen, such as once weekly. Administration can be oral, intravenous, intramuscular, or subcutaneous; the usual dose range is between 7.5 mg and 25 mg per week.
  2. Folic acid, 1 mg daily, protects against some of the common side effects seen with low-dose MTX such as stomatitis. Monitoring for bone marrow suppression and hepatotoxicity are necessary.
E. **Retinoids.** Systemic retinoids (derivatives of Vitamin A) are indicated in patients with severe psoriasis. The retinoid of choice in psoriasis is acitretin (Soriatane). The usual dose of acitretin is 50 mg daily. Monitoring for hypertriglyceridemia and hepatotoxicity are required with retinoid therapy. Side effects include cheilitis and alopecia. Acitretin is teratogenic and is only indicated in men and in women of nonreproductive potential.
F. **Cyclosporine** is effective in patients with severe psoriasis. Usual doses are in the range of 3 to 5 mg/kg per day orally. Improvement is generally observed within four weeks. Renal toxicity and hypertension are common.
G. **Alefacept (Amevive)**, the first biologic agent for treatment of psoriasis, is fairly effective in moderate to severe disease. Alefacept must be given parenterally (once a week).

References: See page 294.

Allergic Rhinitis

Allergic rhinitis is characterized by paroxysms of sneezing, rhinorrhea, nasal obstruction, and itching of the eyes, nose, and palate. It is also frequently associated with postnasal drip, cough, irritability, and fatigue. Allergic rhinitis is classified as seasonal if symptoms occur at a particular time of the year, or perennial if symptoms occur year round.

I. **Pathophysiology**
   A. Common allergens causing seasonal allergic rhinitis are tree, grass, and weed pollens, and fungi. Dust mites, cockroaches, animal proteins, and fungi are frequently associated with perennial rhinitis.
   B. Perennial allergic rhinitis is associated with nasal symptoms, which occur for more than nine months of the year. Perennial allergic rhinitis usually reflects allergy to indoor allergens like dust mites, cockroaches, or animal dander.
   C. Nine to 40 percent of the population may have some form of allergic rhinitis. The prevalence of allergic rhinitis has a bimodal peak in the early school and early adult years, and declines thereafter.

II. **Clinical manifestations**
   A. The intense nasal itching that occurs in allergic rhinitis is associated with nose rubbing, pushing the tip of the nose up with the hand (the "allergic salute"), and a transverse nasal crease.
   B. Adults and older children frequently have clear mucus. Young children have persistent rhinorrhea and often snort, sniff, cough, and clear their throats. Mouth breathing is common. Allergic rhinitis occurs in association with sinusitis, asthma, eczema and allergic conjunctivitis.

III. **Evaluation**
   A. **Nasal examination.** The nasal mucosa frequently displays a pale bluish hue or pallor along with turbinate edema. In nonallergic or vasomotor rhinitis, the nasal turbinates are erythematous and boggy.
   B. **Identification of allergens.** For patients in whom symptoms are not well controlled with medications and in whom the cause of rhinitis is not evident from the history, skin testing may provide an in vivo assessment of IgE antibodies.
   C. **Skin tests.** Immediate hypersensitivity skin testing is a quick, inexpensive, and safe way to identify the presence of allergen specific IgE.

IV. **Management of allergic rhinitis (rhinosinusitis)**
   A. **Allergen identification and avoidance.** The history frequently identifies involvement of pollens, molds, house dust mites and insects, such as fleas and cockroaches, or animal allergens
   B. **Allergen avoidance measures:**
      1. Maintaining the relative humidity at 50 percent or less to limit house dust mite and mold growth and avoiding exposure to irritants, such as cigarette smoke.
      2. Air conditioners decrease concentrations of pollen, mold, and dust mite allergens in indoor air.
      3. Avoiding exposure to the feces of the house dust mite is facilitated by removing carpets and furry pets, and washing bedding in hot water once weekly.
      4. HEPA filters may help reduce animal allergens. Ordinary vacuuming and dusting have little effect.
   C. **Pharmacologic treatment**
      1. Nasal decongestant sprays are not recommended in the treatment of allergic rhinitis. Tachyphylaxis develops after three to seven days, rebound nasal congestion results, and continued use causes rhinitis medicamentosa.
      2. **Intranasal corticosteroids.** Topical intranasal steroid therapy is presently the most effective single maintenance therapy for allergic rhinitis and causes few side effects. Topical nasal steroids are more

effective than cromolyn and second generation antihistamines. Most studies show no effect on growth at recommended doses.

a. The addition of antihistamine or antihistamine-decongestant combination to nasal corticosteroids offers little additional clinical benefit.

b. Topical nasal steroids are available in both aqueous and freon-propelled preparations. The aqueous preparations may be particularly useful in patients in whom freon preparations cause mucosal drying, crusting, or epistaxis. Rarely, nasal steroids are associated with nasal septal perforation.

c. As needed use appears to be almost as effective as daily use in patients with episodic symptoms.

d. The preparations requiring once-daily dosing are preferred. These include triamcinolone, budesonide, fluticasone, or mometasone. Mometasone is approved for use in children older than two years. For children, mometasone (Nasonex) is the preferred as first-line therapy. Budesonide and fluticasone propionate are approved for use in children older than six years.

Drugs for Allergic Rhinitis

Drug	Trade name	Dose
Corticosteroid Nasal Sprays		
Triamcinolone	Nasacort	Two sprays qd
Budesonide	Rhinocort AQ	Two sprays qd
Fluticasone	Flonase	Two sprays qd
Mometasone	Nasonex	Two sprays qd
Beclomethasone	Beconase Vancenase Beconase AQ Vancenase AQ	One spray two to qid One spray bid-qid One to two sprays bid One to two sprays bid
Flunisolide	Nasalide	Two sprays bid
Oral H$_1$-receptor Blockers		
Citrizine	Zyrtec Zyrtec-D	5 or 10 mg once/d Cetirizine 5 mg, pseudoephedrine 120 mg; 1 tablet bid
Desloratadine	Clarinex	5 mg once/d
Fexofenadine	Allegra	60 mg bid or 180 mg once/d
Loratadine	Claritin Claritin Reditabs Alavert Claritin-D	10 mg once/d Loratadine 5 mg, pseudoephedrine 120 m; 1 tab qAM
Leukotriene Modifier		
Montelukast	Singulair	10 mg once/d

D. Antihistamines

1. Antihistamines are clearly less effective than topical nasal steroids. Antihistamines typically reduce itching, sneezing, and rhinorrhea, but may not completely eliminate the symptoms of nasal congestion.

2. Two second-generation antihistamines are currently available in syrup for young children. Cetirizine (Zyrtec) is approved for children >6 months of age. Loratadine (Claritin) is approved for use in children >2 years of age and is available over the counter. Second-generation antihistamines and nasal corticosteroids are not approved for children under two and three years of age, respectively. Rondec (carbinoxamine maleate-pseudoephedrine) drops are approved for children one month and older.

3. In relieving symptoms, second-generation drugs are less efficacious than corticosteroids and equally or more efficacious than cromolyn. The addition of antihistamines to topical nasal steroids may be useful in patients with concomitant allergic conjunctivitis. Oral antihistamine combinations that contain the decongestant, pseudoephedrine, provide better symptom relief than that associated with antihistamine alone.

4. **Adverse effects.**
   a. First-generation antihistamines easily cross the blood brain barrier and cause sedation, making them relatively less desirable. Sedation occurs uncommonly with second-generation antihistamines other than cetirizine and azelastine.
   b. Metabolites of second-generation antihistamines, such as the metabolite of terfenadine, fexofenadine (Allegra), and desloratadine (Clarinex) are classified as "third-generation antihistamines." These compounds avoid potential cardiotoxic effects of the second-generation compounds.
   c. Cetirizine, fexofenadine, desloratadine, and loratadine have not been associated with QT prolongation. However, coadministration with P450-active drugs increases loratadine levels. In addition, licorice ingestion prolongs QT-intervals and may potentially have additive effects.

5. Second-generation antihistamines may be preferable in patients with mild symptoms, or those preferring pills over nose sprays, especially if allergic conjunctivitis is also present. Cetirizine (Zyrtec) is reserved for those who fail loratadine (Claritin) or fexofenadine (Allegra), as cetirizine has sedative properties.

E. **Cromolyn and nedocromil** decrease allergic inflammation by inhibiting mast cell mediator release. Cromolyn, but not nedocromil, is available in the United States. Cromolyn is less effective than topical nasal steroids.

F. **Allergen immunotherapy**
   1. Allergen immunotherapy involves the subcutaneous administration of increasing doses of therapeutic vaccines of allergens.
   2. **Efficacy.** Allergen immunotherapy to tree, grass and ragweed pollens, Alternaria mold and house dust mite is efficacious in allergic rhinitis. Immunotherapy should be considered in patients in whom pharmacotherapy and avoidance of allergens have failed to resolve symptoms.

References: See page 294.

Allergic Conjunctivitis

Allergic conjunctivitis is estimated to affect 20 percent of the population on an annual basis. Allergic conjunctivitis is associated with itching, tearing, redness, burning, photophobia, and mucus discharge.

I. **Pathophysiology**
   A. Allergic conjunctivitis has an average age of onset of 20 years of age, and is principally a disease of young adults. Symptoms tend to decrease with age.
   B. **Acute allergic conjunctivitis** is an acute, hypersensitivity reaction caused by environmental exposure to allergens. It is characterized by intense episodes of itching, hyperemia, tearing, chemosis, and eyelid edema. It resolves in less than 24 hours.
   C. **Seasonal allergic conjunctivitis** (SAC) is also known as allergic conjunctivitis. It is frequently associated with rhinitis. It occurs in the spring and late summer, and it is caused by exposure to pollen, grasses, and ragweed.
   D. **Perennial allergic conjunctivitis** (PAC) is a mild, chronic, allergic conjunctivitis related to environmental exposure to year-round allergens such as dust mites and mold.
   E. Acute allergic conjunctivitis, seasonal allergic conjunctivitis (SAC), and perennial allergic conjunctivitis (PAC) are referred to as "allergic conjunctivitis," and result from allergens.

II. **Clinical evaluation**
   A. Allergic conjunctivitis is frequently associated with atopy, allergic rhinitis, skin allergies, and asthma.
   B. **Signs and symptoms of allergic conjunctivitis** include itching, tearing, conjunctival edema, hyperemia, eyelid edema, watery discharge, burning, and photophobia. Symptoms are usually bilateral. The differential diagnosis includes infectious conjunctivitis, blepharitis, and dry eye.
   C. Acute allergic conjunctivitis occurs rapidly upon exposure to an allergen, such as cat dander. Symptoms can be severe and debilitating but resolve quickly, usually within 24 hours of removal of the allergen. Seasonal allergic conjunctivitis typically has a less dramatic onset; it will have a more predictable and chronic course that corresponds to the ragweed (late summer and early fall), grass (summer), and pollen (spring) seasons.
   D. **Laboratory findings.** The diagnosis of allergic conjunctivitis is usually made clinically; therefore, laboratory testing is not typically performed.

III. **Treatment of allergic conjunctivitis**
   A. Avoidance of the allergen is recommended. Preventive steps to reduce symptoms of SAC include limiting outdoor exposure during high "counts" of pollen and ragweed, use of air conditioning, and keeping windows closed. For those with PAC, prevention includes replacement of old pillows and mattresses, covers for pillows and mattresses, frequent washing of beddings, reducing humidity, and frequent vacuuming and dusting. Old curtains or drapes should be removed. When the allergen is animal dander, the animal may need to be removed from the home.
   B. In all types of allergic conjunctivitis, patients should not rub their eyes because that can cause mast cell degranulation. Patients should use topical antihistamines, frequent artificial tears, and cool compresses.
   C. **Mast cell stabilizers**
      1. Mast cell stabilizers include Crolom (cromolyn 4.0 percent), Opticrom (cromolyn), and Alomide (lodoxamide). These drugs are particularly useful for allergic conjunctivitis. Dosing is four times per day. Since the onset of action is 5 to 14 days after therapy has been initiated, these medicines are not useful for acute conjunctivitis. These drops cause burning and stinging.

    2. These drugs are well tolerated, non-toxic, and can be used in contact lens wearers. However disadvantages include delayed onset of action, maintenance therapy, and multiple daily dosing.

D. Antihistamines

    1. Oral antihistamines and combinations of antihistamines plus decongestants include Allegra (fexofenadine, 60 mg bid or tab ER: 180 mg qd), Allegra D (fexofenadine plus pseudoephedrine, 1 tab bid), Claritin (loratadine, 10 mg qd), Claritin-D (loratadine plus pseudoephedrine, 1 tab qd), and Zyrtec (cetirizine, 5-10 mg qd) or Zyrtec-D (cetirizine plus pseudoephedrine, 1 tab bid).

    2. The full effect of oral administration of antihistamines occurs hours after initiating therapy. Since oral antihistamine use is associated with drying of mucosal membranes, the use of oral antihistamines may worsen allergic symptoms. This effect is not observed with topical antihistamines.

    3. Topical antihistamines include Emadine (emedastine) and Livostin (levocabastine), which are used as one drop up to 4 times daily. The advantages of topical antihistamine usage include a more rapid onset of action and reduced drowsiness and dry eyes. Emadine and Livostin are topical, highly specific, H1-receptor antagonists, and their onset of action is within minutes.

    4. Topical, antihistamine/vasoconstrictor combinations have been shown to be effective. Examples of such combination drugs include Naphcon-A (naphazoline/pheniramine), Vasocon-A (naphazoline/pheniramine), OcuHist (naphazoline/pheniramine), and Opcon-A (naphazoline/pheniramine). Dosing is up to four times daily. However, chronic use can lead to rebound hyperemia.

    5. Olopatadine (Patanol) is a combination antihistamine and mast cell stabilizer. It is the most commonly prescribed drug for allergic conjunctivitis. The H1-receptor selectivity is superior to that of other antihistamines. Patanol is very safe and effective. Side effects include stinging and headache. Dosing is two to four times daily of the 0.1% drops.

E. Corticosteroids

    1. Topical corticosteroid use should only be used for short "pulse therapy" when antihistamines and mast cell stabilizers provide inadequate therapy. Side effects from corticosteroids include cataract formation, elevated intraocular pressure (IOP), glaucoma, and secondary infections. Ocular steroids should only be administered by ophthalmologists.

    2. Prednisolone and dexamethasone have the greatest risk of raising IOP. "Soft" steroids are a group of topical corticosteroids that have a greatly reduced risk of causing increased IOP, since they undergo rapid inactivation upon penetration of the cornea. These drugs include Pred Mild (prednisolone), FML (fluorometholone), HMS (medrysone), Lotemax (loteprednol), and Vexol (rimexolone). They are administered two to four times per day for two weeks.

F. Treatment recommendations

    1. Acute allergic conjunctivitis

        a. Topical antihistamine/vasoconstrictors are usually sufficient in treating short exacerbations of symptoms. Combination drugs include Naphcon-A (naphazoline/pheniramine), Vasocon-A (naphazoline/pheniramine), OcuHist (naphazoline/pheniramine), and Opcon-A (naphazoline/pheniramine). Dosing is up to four times daily. Chronic use (greater than two weeks) can lead to rebound hyperemia.

        b. For frequent attacks of acute allergic conjunctivitis (occurring more than two days per month), mast cell stabilizers can be added. Olopatadine (Patanol), a combination drug consisting of an antihistamine and mast cell stabilizer, is a good agent for treating more frequent attacks. It can be used up to four times per day.

    c. If these are ineffective, oral antihistamines may be helpful. Oral antihistamines and combinations of antihistamines plus decongestants include Allegra (fexofenadine, 60 mg bid or tab ER: 180 mg qd), Allegra D (fexofenadine plus pseudoephedrine, 1 tab bid), Claritin (loratadine, 10 mg qd), Claritin-D (loratadine plus pseudoephedrine, 1 tab qd), and Zyrtec (cetirizine, 5-10 mg qd) or Zyrtec-D (cetirizine plus pseudoephedrine, 1 tab bid). Frequent use of artificial tears is recommended while using oral antihistamines.

2. Seasonal allergic conjunctivitis and perennial allergic conjunctivitis

    a. **Olopatadine (Patanol)** should be initiated two weeks before the onset of symptoms is anticipated. Patanol, a combination mast cell stabilizer and antihistamine, has become the first-line drug of choice in treating SAC and PAC. It is approved for children older than five years of age and adults. Dosing is two to four times daily.

    b. Oral antihistamines may be helpful; however, these agents cause decreased tear production. These patients are frequently using oral antihistamines for systemic symptoms; therefore, artificial tears should be used.

    c. A short two-week course of topical steroids can be helpful in resistant cases. Pred Mild (prednisolone), FML (fluorometholone), HMS (medrysone), Lotemax (loteprednol), or Vexol (rimexolone) are administered two to four times per day for two to three weeks.

References: See page 294.

Gynecologic Disorders

Screening for Cervical Cancer

Cervical cancer screening should be started three years after the onset of sexual activity, but no later than age 21. The basis of this recommendation is that high grade cervical intraepithelial lesions (HSIL) are almost entirely related to acquisition of human papillomavirus (HPV) infection through genital skin to skin contact and these lesions usually do not occur until three to five years after exposure to HPV. HSIL is a precursor to cervical cancer.

I. **Screening interval**
   A. Cervical cancer screening should be started three years after the onset of sexual activity, but no later than age 21.
   B. The American Cancer Society recommends that initial cervical screening should be performed annually if conventional cervical cytology smears (Pap) are used and every two years with liquid-based cytology tests until age 30. The screening interval can then be increased to every two to three years in women with three or more consecutive normal cytology results who are $\geq$30 years old.
   C. The American College of Obstetricians and Gynecologists recommends annual screening for women younger than 30 years of age regardless of testing method (conventional or liquid-based cytology). Women aged 30 and over who have had three negative smears, no history of CIN II/III, and are not immunocompromised or DES exposed in utero may extend the interval between tests to two to three years. Women aged 30 and over may also consider the option of a combined cervical cytology and HPV test. Women who test negative by both tests should not be screened more frequently than every three years.
   D. Exceptions. Women at increased risk of CIN, such as those with in utero DES exposure, immunocompromise, or a history of CIN II/III or cancer, should continue to be screened at least annually. More frequent surveillance should also be considered in women whose smears do not contain endocervical cells or are partially obscured.
E. **Discontinuing screening**
   1. The United States Preventive Services Task Force stated screening may stop at age 65 if the woman has had recent normal smears and is not at high risk for cervical cancer.
   2. The American Cancer Society guideline stated that women age 70 or older may elect to stop cervical cancer screening if they have had three consecutive satisfactory, normal/negative test results and no abnormal test results within the prior 10 years.
   3. Cervical cancer screening is not recommended in women who have had total hysterectomies for benign indications (presence of CIN II or III excludes benign categorization). Screening of women with CIN II/III who undergo hysterectomy may be discontinued after three consecutive negative results have been obtained. However, screening should be performed if the woman acquires risk factors for intraepithelial neoplasia, such as new sexual partners or immunosuppression.

Bethesda 2001 Pap Smear Report

Interpretation Result
Negative for intraepithelial lesion or malignancy
Infection (Trichomonas vaginalis, Candida spp., shift in flora suggestive of bacterial vaginosis, Actinomyces spp., cellular changes consistent with Herpes simplex virus)
Other Non-neoplastic Findings:
  Reactive cellular changes associated with inflammation (includes typical repair) radiation, intrauterine contraceptive device (IUD)
  Glandular cells status post-hysterectomy
  Atrophy
Other
  Endometrial cells (in a woman $\geq$40 years of age)
Epithelial Cell Abnormalities
  Squamous Cell
    Atypical squamous cells
      -of undetermined significance (ASC-US)
      -cannot exclude HSIL (ASC-H)
    Low-grade squamous intraepithelial lesion (LSIL) encompassing: HPV/mild dysplasia/CIN 1
    High-grade squamous intraepithelial lesion (HSIL) encompassing: moderate and severe dysplasia, CIS/CIN 2 and CIN 3 with features suspicious for invasion (if invasion is suspected)
    Squamous cell carcinoma
  Glandular Cell
    Atypical
      -Endocervical cells (not otherwise specified or specify in comments)
      -Glandular cell (not otherwise specified or specify in comments)
      -Endometrial cells (not otherwise specified or specify in comments)
      -Glandular cells (not otherwise specified or specify in comments)
    Atypical
      -Endocervical cells, favor neoplastic
      -Glandular cells, favor neoplastic
    Endocervical adenocarcinoma in situ
    Adenocarcinoma (endocervical, endometrial, extrauterine, not otherwise specified (not otherwise specified)
Other Malignant Neoplasms (specify)

Management of the Abnormal Papanicolaou Smear

Result	Action
Specimen adequacy	
Satisfactory for evaluation	Routine follow-up
Unsatisfactory for evaluation	Repeat smear
No endocervical cells	Follow-up in one year for low-risk women with a previously normal smear; repeat in 4-6 months for high-risk women

Result	Action
Atypical cells	
Atypical squamous cells of undetermined significance (ASC-US)	HPV testing with referral to colposcopy if positive for high-risk HPV type; if negative for high-risk HPV type, then repeat cytology in 12 months
Special circumstances	Postmenopausal women with atrophic epitheliium may be treated with topical estrogen followed by repeat cervical cytology one week after completing treatment
ASC-H	Immediate referral to colposcopy
Atypical glandular cells (AGS)	Immediate referral to colposcopy with sampling of the endocervical canal. Women over age 35 and any woman with unexplained vaginal bleeding should also have an endometrial biopsy
Intraepithelial neoplasia	
High grade	Immediate referral for colposcopy
Low grade	Immediate referral for colposcopy, except adolescents and postmenopausal women
Endometrial cells	Endometrial biopsy in selected cases
Other malignant cells	Referral to a gynecologic oncologist

References: See page 294.

Atypical Squamous Cells on Cervical Cytology

Atypical squamous cells are commonly caused by self-limited disease, which resolves spontaneously. The risk of invasive cancer in patients with atypical squamous cells is low, 0.1 to 0.2%. However, 5 to 17% of patients with atypical squamous cells and 24 to 94% of those with ASC-high grade will have precancerous lesions at biopsy, therefore, further evaluation is necessary to determine if high-grade dysplasia is present.

I. **Evaluation of atypical squamous cells of undetermined significance (ASC-US).**
   A. Reflex HPV testing with triage of women with high risk HPV types to colposcopy is the recommended approach. Reflex testing refers to concurrent collection of cytology and HPV samples with actual testing for HPV only if indicated by abnormal cytology results.
      1. If liquid-based cytology is used, reflex HPV testing can be performed on the same specimen. If a conventional Papanicolaou (Pap) smear is obtained, a second specimen is collected for HPV DNA testing. If high risk subtypes are found, colposcopy is performed.

Risk of cervical cancer with human papilloma virus
High-risk (oncogenic or cancer-associated) types Common types: 16, 18, 31, 33, 35, 39, 45, 51, 52, 56, 58, 59, 68, 69, 82
Low-risk (non-oncogenic) types Common types: 6, 11, 40, 42, 43, 44, 54, 61, 72, 81

Management of women with combined test screening	
Results of cytology/HPV	**Recommended follow-up**
Negative / Negative	Routine screening in 3 years
Negative / Positive	Repeat combined test in 6 to 12 months
ASCUS / Negative	Repeat cytology in 12 months
ASCUS / Positive	Colposcopy
Greater than ASCUS / Positive or negative	Colposcopy

B. **Special circumstances and populations**
  1. **Pregnant women** with ASC are managed in the same way as nonpregnant women, except endocervical sampling is not performed.
  2. **Infection or reactive changes.** When an infectious organism is identified or suggested, the patient should be contacted to determine if she is symptomatic. Antibiotic therapy is indicated for symptomatic infections, as well as some asymptomatic infections. After treatment of the infection, women with high risk HPV types are referred to colposcopy.
  3. **Atrophic epithelium** (a normal finding in postmenopausal women) is often characterized by nuclear enlargement, which meets one of the pathologic criteria for ASC. Administration of estrogen (eg, 0.3 mg conjugated estrogen applied as vaginal cream nightly for four weeks [1/8th of the applicator]) causes atypical atrophic, but not dysplastic, epithelium to mature into normal squamous epithelium. Hormonal therapy given for vaginal atrophy should be followed by repeat cervical cytology one week after completing treatment. If negative, cytology should be repeated again in six months. If both tests are negative, the woman can return to routine screening intervals, but if either test is positive for ASC-US or greater colposcopy should be completed.
  4. **Immunosuppressed women,** including all women who are HIV positive, with ASC-US should be referred for immediate colposcopy instead of HPV testing or serial cytology.
  5. **Adolescents.** Initial colposcopy or reflex HPV testing may be deferred in adolescents because the risk of invasive cancer is near zero and the prevalence of transient HPV infection is very high . Instead, serial cytology should be completed at six and 12 months or HPV DNA testing at 12 months with referral to colposcopy for positive results (ASC or greater, high risk HPV DNA types).
C. **Management after colposcopy/biopsy.** Colposcopy/biopsy of women with ASC-US will either yield a histologic abnormality (eg, CIN II or III), which should be treated as appropriate, or show no abnormal findings. If no abnormal findings are found and HPV testing was not performed or showed a low-risk type, then follow-up cytological testing in 12 months is recommended.

D. Women who test positive for high risk HPV types, but have CIN I or less on colposcopy/biopsy require a repeat cervical cytology at 6 and 12 months, or perform an HPV test at 12 months, with colposcopy for ASC or higher or a positive HPV test.

II. **Evaluation of atypical squamous cells–cannot exclude high-grade squamous intraepithelial lesion (ASC-H)**

A. Most women with ASC-H on cytological examination should be referred for colposcopy and ECC (ECC is not performed in pregnancy), without HPV testing. Twenty-four to 94% of these women will have CIN II or higher. Biopsy proven CIN II or III is treated, as appropriate.

B. If no lesion or a CIN I lesion is identified, the cytology sample, colposcopy, and any biopsy specimens should be reviewed, if possible, to address any possible cytological-histological discordancy, with further management dependent upon the results. If review of cytology confirms ASC-H, follow-up cytology in six and 12 months or HPV DNA testing in 12 months is acceptable. Colposcopy should be repeated for ASC-US or greater on cytology or a positive test for high risk HPV DNA.

C. In women age 30 or older with ASC-H, an acceptable alternative is to perform HPV testing for initial triaging. If high risk HPV types are present, the patient is referred for colposcopy.

References: See page 294.

Atypical and Malignant Glandular Cells on Cervical Cytology

Cervical Pap smear cytology showing atypical glandular (AGC) or endometrial carcinoma cells indicates the presence of glandular cells that could originate from the endocervical or endometrial region. The Bethesda 2001 system classifies AGC into two subcategories:

AGC (specify endocervical, endometrial, or glandular cells not otherwise specified [NOS])

AGC, favor neoplastic (specify endocervical or NOS)

Additional categories for glandular cell abnormalities are:

Endocervical adenocarcinoma in situ (AIS)

Adenocarcinoma

I. **Atypical glandular cells**

A. A smear with AGC is associated with a premalignant or malignant lesion of the endocervix or endometrium in 10 to 40% of cases.

B. Women over age 50 with AGC are at higher risk of having uterine cancer than younger women (8 and 1%, respectively). Conversely, premenopausal women with AGC are more likely to have CIN II/III or AIS than postmenopausal women.

C. **Evaluation.** Presence of AGC or AIS on cervical cytology is a significant marker for neoplasia of the endometrium, as well as the squamous and glandular epithelium of the cervix. All women with atypical glandular cells or AIS should be referred for colposcopy with directed cervical biopsies and sampling of the endocervical canal. An endometrial biopsy should be performed on all women over age 35 and on younger women with unexplained or anovulatory bleeding, morbid obesity, oligomenorrhea, or an increased risk of endometrial cancer.

D. Women with only atypical endometrial cells on cytology can be initially evaluated with endometrial biopsy only, rather than colposcopy. If endometrial sampling is normal, then colposcopy and endocervical curettage should be performed.

E. Positive findings, such as any grade of CIN on biopsy, should be managed as appropriate.

F. **Negative colposcopy/endocervical curettage.** The management of women with AGC and a negative initial colposcopy/endocervical sampling depends upon AGC subclassification.

1. **AGC NOS.** Women with AGC NOS who have a normal initial colposcopic evaluation and endocervical biopsy can be followed with cervical cytology at four to six month intervals until four consecutive tests are negative for intraepithelial lesions or malignancy. They are then followed with routine surveillance. However, if any abnormality (ASC or greater) is noted on follow-up cytology smears, another colposcopy is required. Women with persistent AGC NOS (two or more cytology results) are at especially high risk of significant glandular disease and need conization if repeat colposcopy and endometrial biopsy are nondiagnostic.
2. In women with AGC NOS and normal colposcopic evaluation and biopsies, HPV studies may be used for further monitoring and, if negative, repeat cytology and endocervical sampling can be done in one year rather than in four visits over two years.
3. AGC favor neoplasia or AIS. A cold-knife conization is the best procedure for subsequent evaluation of AGC lesions at high risk of associated adenocarcinoma, such as AGC favor neoplasia or AIS or persistent AGC NOS.
4. If conization and endometrial biopsies are also negative, the patient should be evaluated for primary or metastatic disease involving the fallopian tube, ovary, and other pelvic and abdominal organs with pelvic ultrasound examination, colonoscopy, and computed tomography of the abdomen.

II. **Endocervical adenocarcinoma**
   A. Endocervical adenocarcinoma in situ (AIS) and adenocarcinoma requires evaluation and will show invasive cancer in a proportion of women with AIS on cytology. An intermediate category: atypical endocervical cells, favor neoplastic suggests some features of AIS but without criteria for a definitive diagnosis.
   B. Colposcopy with directed biopsy is required. A diagnostic excisional procedure is often needed because colposcopy/biopsy can miss small lesions of AIS or adenocarcinoma and lesions high in the canal.

References: See page 294.

Cervical Intraepithelial Neoplasia

Cervical intraepithelial neoplasia (CIN) refers to a preinvasive pathological intermediate of cervical cancer, which progresses slowly and can be easily detected and treated.

I. **Nomenclature**
   A. Histologic definitions of cervical intraepithelial neoplasia (CIN):
   CIN I refers to cellular dysplasia confined to the basal third of the epithelium
   CIN II refers to lesions confined to the basal two-thirds of the epithelium
   CIN III refers to cellular dysplasia encompassing greater than two-thirds of the epithelial thickness, including full-thickness lesions
   B. **Cytologic definitions.** Cytologic Pap smears are classified according to the Bethesda system. In this system, mild dysplasia/CIN I was combined with koilocytic or condylomatous atypia to create the category low-grade squamous intraepithelial lesion (LSIL or LGSIL). Moderate and severe dysplasia/CIS/CIN II/CIN III were merged to form the category of high-grade squamous intraepithelial lesion (HSIL or HGSIL) because of similarities in both the cytologic features and prognosis of these groups.
   C. Other new terms, such as atypical squamous cells of undetermined significance (ASCUS) and atypical glandular cells (AGC), were introduced to express equivocal findings.

II. Risk factors

A. Sexual activity is a key factor in the etiology of cervical neoplasia. The incidence of squamous cell cancer of the cervix in women who have not had any sexual relationships is almost nonexistent. Sexual risk factors for CIN include sexual activity at an early age, history of sexually transmitted infections (chlamydia, herpes simplex virus), multiple sexual partners, or sexual activity with promiscuous men. The major causal factor is infection with the human papillomavirus (HPV).

B. Other risk factors include cigarette smoking, multiparity, and exogenous or endogenous immunodeficiency.

C. Human papillomavirus infection is endemic among sexually experienced individuals. 80% of sexually active women will have acquired a genital HPV infection by age 50. Most HPV infections are transient, resolving spontaneously in six to 18 months.

D. **Diagnosis**

1. **Cervical cytology.** Women are screened for CIN by cervical cytology (eg, conventional Papanicolaou smear or liquid based, such as ThinPrep or SurePath). Abnormal cytology results should be further evaluated.

2. **Colposcopy** is used to evaluate abnormal cervical cytology. Abnormal areas of the epithelium turn white with dilute acetic acid. Capillaries may be identified within the abnormal epithelium. Capillary thickness and the intercapillary distances correlate with the severity of the lesion; high-grade lesions have a coarser vessel pattern and larger intercapillary distance. Abnormal areas can be targeted for biopsy.

III. Management of cervical intraepithelial neoplasia

A. Treatment of cervical intraepithelial abnormalities is undertaken after a histologic abnormality has been proven by tissue biopsy. Treatment is never performed based upon a cytologic diagnosis alone; but is sometimes initiated at the time of colposcopy/biopsy in women who are at high risk of loss to follow-up ("see-and-treat" protocols).

B. Atypical squamous cells (ASC, subcategories ASC-US and ASC-H) is a cytological screening diagnosis that does not justify treatment because it is not diagnostic of a cancerous or precancerous lesion. ASC does require further evaluation to exclude the presence of histologically confirmed high grade disease, which may require treatment.

C. **Low grade lesions: CIN 1**

1. Aggressive intervention in these patients is usually not indicated because a significant number of these lesions spontaneously regress and infrequently progress.

2. LSIL regresses to normal in 47%; progression to a high grade lesion occurs in 21%, and to cancer in 0.15%.

3. **Management.** Since spontaneous regression is observed in most women, expectant management is generally preferred for the reliable patient with biopsy-confirmed CIN 1, in whom the entire lesion and limits of the transformation zone are completely visualized (ie, satisfactory colposcopic examination). If treatment is desired, ablative or excisional modalities are appropriate. An excisional procedure is the preferred diagnostic/therapeutic approach if the transformation zone is not fully visualizedby culposcopy.

4. **Expectant management.** 80 to 85% of women referred for initial colposcopy because of LSIL or HPV DNA positive ASC-US have CIN 1 or less detected on biopsy. 9 to 16% of these women will have histologically confirmed CIN 2 or 3 within two years. Expectant management of women with biopsy confirmed CIN 1 and satisfac-

tory colposcopy consists of repeat cytology at 6 and 12 months or HPV testing at 12 months.

- **a. Colposcopy** should be repeated if repeat cytology shows ASC or greater or HPV DNA testing is positive for a high risk type.
- **b.** After two negative smears or a negative HPV DNA test, annual screening may be resumed.
- **c.** Colposcopy and repeat cytology at 12 months is an acceptable alternative to semiannual cytology or annual HPV testing.

5. **Ablation or excision**
   - **a.** Some women may elect to have ablation or excision of the lesion to relieve their anxiety. Immediate therapy may also be warranted in the patient at high risk for loss to follow-up.
   - **b.** Endocervical sampling is recommended before ablation, and excision is recommended for patients with recurrent disease after ablation. Ablative treatment is unacceptable if colposcopy is not satisfactory. In such cases, a diagnostic and therapeutic excisional procedure should be performed.

6. **Special circumstances**
   - **a. Pregnant and adolescent women**. Expectant management of pregnant or adolescent women with biopsy confirmed CIN 1, even in the setting of an unsatisfactory colposcopic examination, is an acceptable alternative to ablative/excisional therapy because undetected high grade disease is uncommon in this setting.
   - **b. CIN 1.** Expectant management is recommended for the reliable patient in whom the entire lesion and limits of the transformation zone are completely visualized. Repeat cytology should be done at 6 and 12 months or HPV testing at 12 months.

D. **High grade lesions: CIN 2/3**
   1. 43 to 58% of CIN 2 lesions will regress if left untreated, while 22% progress to CIN 3 and 5% progress to invasive cancer.
   2. **Management.** The entire transformation zone should be eliminated. Prior to any therapeutic intervention, an assessment needs to be made as to whether a patient qualifies for ablative therapy or if she requires a more invasive excisional procedure for further diagnostic work-up.
   3. **Ablative therapy.** Prerequisites for ablative treatment are:
      - **a.** Accurate histologic diagnosis/no discrepancy between cytology/colposcopy/histology
      - **b.** No evidence of microinvasion/invasion
      - **c.** No evidence of a glandular lesion (adenocarcinoma in situ or invasive adenocarcinoma)
      - **d.** Satisfactory colposcopy (eg, the transformation zone is fully visualized)
      - **e.** The lesion is limited to the ectocervix and seen in its entirety
      - **f.** There is no evidence of endocervical involvement as determined by colposcopy/endocervical curettage
   4. The most commonly used ablative treatment techniques are cryotherapy and laser ablation.
   5. **Excisional therapy.** Indications for excisional therapy are:
      - **a.** Suspected microinvasion
      - **b.** Unsatisfactory colposcopy (the transformation zone is not fully visualized)
      - **c.** Lesion extending into the endocervical canal
      - **d.** Endocervical curettage revealing dysplasia
      - **e.** Lack of correlation between the cytology and colposcopy/biopsies
      - **f.** Suspected adenocarcinoma in situ
      - **g.** Colposcopist unable to rule out invasive disease
      - **h.** Recurrence after an ablative procedure

6. **Excisional treatment** can be performed by cold knife conization, laser conization, or the loop electrosurgical excision procedure (LEEP). With suspected microinvasion or ACIS, cold knife conization is recommended so that margins can be evaluated without cautery artifact.

7. **Special circumstances**

   a. **Pregnancy.** High-grade lesions discovered during pregnancy have a high rate of regression in the postpartum period. 70% of CIN 3 regress and none progress to invasive carcinoma. Treatment of CIN 2/3 is not indicated during pregnancy. The patient should be monitored with colposcopy (without endocervical curettage) each trimester. Colposcopy and cervical cytology should be performed 6 to 12 weeks postpartum. However, conization during pregnancy is usually required in women with suspected invasive disease.

   b. **Adolescents.** Observation with colposcopy and cytology at six-month intervals for one year is acceptable for reliable adolescents with biopsy-confirmed CIN 2, provided colposcopy is satisfactory, endocervical curettage is negative. In this population, the rate of regression is high and progression to invasive cancer is extremely small.

      (1) Ablation or excision is recommended for adolescents with CIN 3.

      (2) **CIN 2/3.** Ablative and excisional procedures have equally effective cure rates. A loop electrosurgical excisional procedure (LEEP) is recommended over an ablative or other excisional procedures (cold knife cone). LEEP is an office procedure with ease of use, providing a histologic specimen at low cost and morbidity, and high rate of success.

      (3) **Cold knife conization** is recommended for women with suspected microinvasion, unsatisfactory colposcopy (eg, the transformation zone is not fully visualized), lesion extending into the endocervical canal, and suspected adenocarcinoma in situ.

E. **Therapeutic procedures.** The five most common techniques for treatment of CIN are:

   1. Loop electrosurgical excision procedure (LEEP)
   2. Cryotherapy (nitrous oxide or carbon dioxide)
   3. Carbon dioxide (CO2) laser ablation
   4. Conization (cold knife or laser)
   5. These techniques were equally effective, averaging approximately 90% cure.

F. **Loop electrosurgical excision procedure.** The loop electrosurgical excision procedure (LEEP) has become the approach of choice for treating CIN 2 and 3 because of its ease of use, low cost, and high rate of success.

G. **Cryotherapy** refers to the application of a super-cooled probe (nitrous oxide or carbon dioxide) directly to the cervical lesion using one or more cooling and thawing cycles. The probe must be able to cover the entire lesion and the lesion cannot extend into the endocervical canal. Anesthesia is not required.

   1. Blanching extend at least 7 to 8 mm beyond the edge of the cryoprobe to reach the full depth of the cervical crypts. Typically, the cervix is frozen for two to three minutes, followed by a thaw period lasting five minutes. After the cervix has returned to a pink color, an additional two to three minute freeze application is performed.

   2. **Conization** refers to the excision of a cone shaped portion of the cervix. The procedure is usually performed using a scalpel, but laser conization is also possible. Endocervical curettage can be per-

formed after the conization to evaluate the remaining endocervical
canal.

H. **Prognosis and follow-up.** Overall, the rate of recurrent or persistent
disease is 5 to 17% despite therapy with any of the excisional or
ablative techniques.

1. **Negative margins.** There is a high rate of cure in patients who
have their entire lesion excised.
2. **Follow-up.** Cervical cytology or a combination of cytology and
colposcopy with endocervical curettage every six months is suggested for follow-up after treatment of biopsy confirmed CIN 2/3.
Repeat colposcopy is indicated if ASC or greater is detected. After
three results negative for SIL or malignancy have been obtained,
annual follow-up is acceptable and should be continued until at
least three additional consecutive negative results have been
documented.
3. **Positive margins.** In contrast, patients with positive margins after
LEEP or cold knife conization are at increased risk for residual
disease as determined at subsequent hysterectomy or repeat
conization.
4. **Follow-up.** Women who have positive margins on the specimens
excised by cold knife conization or LEEP or in the concomitant
endocervical curettage specimen should receive follow-up with
cytology and colposcopy/biopsy/endocervical curettage (instead of
immediate retreatment) if the patient is likely to be compliant with
frequent monitoring. Alternatively, a repeat excisional procedure
can be offered to women with positive margins who are averse to
the risk of progression. Hysterectomy is an option for women who
have completed childbearing.
5. **Negative histopathology.** A completely negative LEEP/cone
biopsy performed for high grade lesions is also of concern, and
these patients should be followed similarly to those with positive
margins, with cytology and endocervical curettage every six months
for at least the first three visits.

References: See page 294.

Contraception

Approximately 31% of births are unintended; about 22% were "mistimed," while
9% were "unwanted."

I. **Oral contraceptives**
   A. Combined (estrogen-progestin) oral contraceptives are reliable, and they
   have noncontraceptive benefits, which include reduction in dysmenorrhea, iron deficiency, ovarian cancer, endometrial cancer.

Combination Oral Contraceptives		
Drug	Progestin, mg	Estrogen
Monophasic combinations		
Ortho-Novum 1 /35 21, 28	Norethindrone (1)	Ethinyl estradiol (35)
Ovcon 35 21, 28	Norethindrone (0.4)	Ethinyl estradiol (35)
Brevicon 21, 28	Norethindrone (0.5)	Ethinyl estradiol (35)
Modicon 28	Norethindrone (0.5)	Ethinyl estradiol (35)
Necon 0.5/35E 21, 28	Norethindrone (0.5)	Ethinyl estradiol (35)
Nortrel 0.5/35 28	Norethindrone (0.5)	Ethinyl estradiol (35)
Necon 1 /35 21, 28	Norethindrone (1)	Ethinyl estradiol (35)
Norinyl 1 /35 21, 28	Norethindrone (1)	Ethinyl estradiol (35)
Nortrel 1 /35 21, 28	Norethindrone (1)	Ethinyl estradiol (35)
Loestrin 1 /20 21, 28	Norethindrone acetate (1)	Ethinyl estradiol (20)
Microgestin 1 /20 28	Norethindrone acetate (1)	Ethinyl estradiol (20)
Loestrin 1.5/30 21, 28	Norethindrone acetate (1.5)	Ethinyl estradiol (30)
Microgestin 1.5/30 28	Norethindrone acetate (1.5)	Ethinyl estradiol (30)
Alesse 21, 28	Levonorgestrel (0.1)	Ethinyl estradiol (20)
Aviane 21, 28	Levonorgestrel (0.1)	Ethinyl estradiol (20)
Lessina 28	Levonorgestrel (0.1)	Ethinyl estradiol (20)
Levlite 28	Levonorgestrel (0.1)	Ethinyl estradiol (20)
Necon 1/50 21, 28	Norethindrone (1)	Mestranol (50)
Norinyl 1150 21, 28	Norethindrone (1)	Mestranol (50)
Ortho-Novum 1/50 28	Norethindrone (1)	Mestranol (50)
Ovcon 50 28	Norethindrone (1)	Ethinyl estradiol (50)
Cyclessa 28	Desogestrel (0.1)	Ethinyl estradiol (25)
Apri 28	Desogestrel (0.15)	Ethinyl estradiol (30)
Desogen 28	Desogestrel (0.15)	Ethinyl estradiol (30)

Drug	Progestin, mg	Estrogen
Ortho-Cept 21, 28	Desogestrel (0.15)	Ethinyl estradiol (30)
Yasmin 28	Drospirenone (3)	Ethinyl estradiol (30)
Demulen 1 /35 21, 28	Ethynodiol diacetate (1)	Ethinyl estradiol (35)
Zovia 1 /35 21, 28	Ethynodiol diacetate (1)	Ethinyl estradiol (35)
Demulen 1/50 21, 28	Ethynodiol diacetate (1)	Ethinyl estradiol (50)
Zovia 1 /50 21, 28	Ethynodiol diacetate (1)	Ethinyl estradiol (50)
Levlen 21, 28	Levonorgestrel (0.15)	Ethinyl estradiol (30)
Levora 21, 28	Levonorgestrel (0.15)	Ethinyl estradiol (30)
Nordette 21, 28	Levonorgestrel (0.15)	Ethinyl estradiol (30)
Ortho-Cyclen 21, 28	Norgestimate (0.25)	Ethinyl estradiol (35)
Lo/Ovral 21, 28	Norgestrel (0.3)	Ethinyl estradiol (30)
Low-Ogestrel 21, 28	Norgestrel (0.3)	Ethinyl estradiol (30)
Ogestrel 28	Norgestrel (0.5)	Ethinyl estradiol (50)
Ovral 21, 28	Norgestrel (0.5)	Ethinyl estradiol (50)
Seasonale	Levonorgestrel (0.15)	Ethinyl estradiol (0.03)
Multiphasic Combinations		
Kariva 28	Desogestrel (0.15)	Ethinyl estradiol (20, 0, 10)
Mircette 28	Desogestrel (0.15)	Ethinyl estradiol (20, 0, 10)
Tri-Levlen 21, 28	Levonorgestrel (0.05, 0.075, 0.125)	Ethinyl estradiol (30, 40, 30)
Triphasil 21, 28	Levonorgestrel (0.05, 0.075, 0.125)	Ethinyl estradiol (30, 40, 30)
Trivora 28	Levonorgestrel (0.05, 0.075, 0.125)	Ethinyl estradiol (30, 40, 30)
Necon 10/11 21, 28	Norethindrone (0.5, 1)	Ethinyl estradiol (35)
Ortho-Novum 10/11 28	Norethindrone (0.5, 1)	Ethinyl estradiol (35)
Ortho-Novum 7/7/7 21, 28	Norethindrone (0.5, 0.75, 1)	Ethinyl estradiol (35)

Drug	Progestin, mg	Estrogen
Tri-Norinyl 21, 28	Norethindrone (0.5, 1, 0.5)	Ethinyl estradiol (35)
Estrostep 28	Norethindrone acetate (1)	Ethinyl estradiol (20, 30, 35)
Ortho Tri-Cyclen 21, 28	Norgestimate (0.18, 0.215, 0.25)	Ethinyl estradiol (35)

B. Pharmacology
1. Ethinyl estradiol is the estrogen in virtually all OCs.
2. Commonly used progestins include norethindrone, norethindrone acetate, and levonorgestrel. Ethynodiol diacetate is a progestin, which also has significant estrogenic activity. New progestins have been developed with less androgenic activity; however, these agents may be associated with deep vein thrombosis.

C. Mechanisms of action
1. The most important mechanism of action is estrogen-induced inhibition of the midcycle surge of gonadotropin secretion, so that ovulation does not occur.
2. Another potential mechanism of contraceptive action is suppression of gonadotropin secretion during the follicular phase of the cycle, thereby preventing follicular maturation.
3. Progestin-related mechanisms also may contribute to the contraceptive effect. These include rendering the endometrium is less suitable for implantation and making the cervical mucus less permeable to penetration by sperm.

D. Contraindications
1. **Absolute contraindications to OCs:**
   a. Previous thromboembolic event or stroke
   b. History of an estrogen-dependent tumor
   c. Active liver disease
   d. Pregnancy
   e. Undiagnosed abnormal uterine bleeding
   f. Hypertriglyceridemia
   g. Women over age 35 years who smoke heavily (>15 cigarettes per day)
2. **Screening requirements.** Hormonal contraception can be safely provided after a careful medical history and blood pressure measurement. Pap smears are not required before a prescription for OCs.

E. Efficacy.
When taken properly, OCs are a very effective form of contraception. The actual failure rate is 2 to 3% due primarily to missed pills or failure to resume therapy after the seven-day pill-free interval.

Noncontraceptive Benefits of Oral Contraceptive Pills	
Dysmenorrhea	Functional ovarian cysts
Mittelschmerz	Benign breast cysts
Metrorrhagia	Ectopic pregnancy
Premenstrual syndrome	Acne
Hirsutism	Endometriosis
Ovarian and endometrial cancer	

F. Drug interactions.
The metabolism of OCs is accelerated by phenobarbital, phenytoin and rifampin. The contraceptive efficacy of an OC is likely to be decreased in women taking these drugs. Other antibiotics (with the

exception of rifampin) do not affect the pharmacokinetics of ethinyl estradiol.

G. Preparations

1. There are two types of oral contraceptive pills: combination pills that contain both estrogen and progestin, and the progestin-only pill ("mini-pill"). Progestin-only pills, which are associated with more break-through bleeding than combination pills, are rarely prescribed except in lactating women. Combination pills are packaged in 21-day or 28-day cycles. The last seven pills of a 28-day pack are placebo pills.

2. Monophasic combination pills contain the same dose of estrogen and progestin in each of the 21 hormonally active pills. Current pills contain on average 30 to 35 μg. Pills containing less than 50 μg of ethinyl estradiol are "low-dose" pills.

3. **20 μg preparations.** Several preparations containing only 20 μg of ethinyl estradiol are now available (Lo-Estrin 1/20, Mircette, Alesse, Aviane). These are often used for perimenopausal women who want contraception with the lowest estrogen dose possible. These preparations provide enough estrogen to relieve vasomotor flashes. Perimenopausal women often experience hot flashes and premenstrual mood disturbances during the seven-day pill-free interval. Mircette, contains 10 μg of ethinyl estradiol on five of the seven "placebo" days, which reduces flashes and mood symptoms.

4. **Seasonale** is a 91-day oral contraceptive. Tablets containing the active hormones are taken for 12 weeks (84 days), followed by 1 week (7 days) of placebo tablets. Seasonale contains levonorgestrel (0.15 mg) and ethinyl estradiol (0.03 mg). Many women, especially in the first few cycles, have more spotting between menstrual periods. Seasonale is as effective and safe as traditional birth control pills.

5. **Yasmin** contains 30 mcg of ethinyl estradiol and drospirenone. Drospirenone has anti-mineralocorticoid activity. It can help prevent bloating, weight gain, and hypertension, but it can increase serum potassium. Yasmin is contraindicated in patients at risk for hyperkalemia due to renal, hepatic, or adrenal disease. Yasmin should not be combined with other drugs that can increase potassium, such as ACE inhibitors, angiotensin receptor blockers, potassium-sparing diuretics, potassium supplements, NSAIDs, or salt substitutes.

6. **Third-generation progestins**
   a. More selective progestins include norgestimate, desogestrel, and gestodene. They have some structural modifications that lower their androgen activity. Norgestimate (eg, Ortho-Cyclen or Tri-Cyclen) and desogestrel (eg, Desogen or Ortho-Cept) are the least androgenic compounds in this class. The new progestins are not much less androgenic than norethindrone.
   b. The newer OCs are more effective in reducing acne and hirsutism in hyperandrogenic women. They are therefore an option for women who have difficulty tolerating older OCs. There is an increased risk of deep venous thrombosis with the use of these agents, and they should not be routinely used.

H. Recommendations

1. Monophasic OCs containing the second generation progestin, norethindrone (Ovcon 35) are recommended when starting a patient on OCs for the first time. This progestin has very low androgenicity when compared to other second generation progestins, and also compares favorably to the third generation progestins in androgenicity.

2. The pill should be started on the first day of the period to provide the maximum contraceptive effect in the first cycle. However, most women start their pill on the first Sunday after the period starts. Some form of back-up contraception is needed for the first month if one chooses the Sunday start, because the full contraceptive effect might not be provided in the first pill pack.

Factors to Consider in Starting or Switching Oral Contraceptive Pills

Objective	Action	Products that achieve the objective
To minimize high risk of thrombosis	Select a product with a lower dosage of estrogen.	Alesse, Aviane, Loestrin 1/20, Levlite, Mircette
To minimize nausea, breast tenderness or vascular headaches	Select a product with a lower dosage of estrogen.	Alesse, Aviane, Levlite, Loestrin 1/20, Mircette
To minimize spotting or breakthrough bleeding	Select a product with a higher dosage of estrogen or a progestin with greater potency.	Lo/Ovral, Nordette, Ortho-Cept, Ortho-Cyclen, Ortho Tri-Cyclen
To minimize androgenic effects	Select a product containing a low-dose norethindrone or ethynodiol diacetate.	Ovcon 35, Brevicon, Demulen 1/35, Modicon
To avoid dyslipidemia	Select a product containing a low-dose norethindrone or ethynodiol diacetate.	Ovcon 35, Brevicon, Demulen 1/35, Modicon

Instructions on the Use of Oral Contraceptive Pills

Initiation of use (choose one):
The patient begins taking the pills on the first day of menstrual bleeding.
The patient begins taking the pills on the first Sunday after menstrual bleeding begins.
The patient begins taking the pills immediately if she is definitely not pregnant and has not had unprotected sex since her last menstrual period.

Missed pill
If it has been less than 24 hours since the last pill was taken, the patient takes a pill right away and then returns to normal pill-taking routine.
If it has been 24 hours since the last pill was taken, the patient takes both the missed pill and the next scheduled pill at the same time.
If it has been more than 24 hours since the last pill was taken (ie, two or more missed pills), the patient takes the last pill that was missed, throws out the other missed pills and takes the next pill on time. Additional contraception is used for the remainder of the cycle.

Additional contraceptive method
Use an additional contraceptive method for the first 7 days after initially starting oral contraceptive pills.
Use an additional contraceptive method for 7 days if more than 12 hours late in taking an oral contraceptive pill.
Use an additional contraceptive method while taking an interacting drug and for 7 days thereafter.

II. **Hormonal contraceptive methods other than oral contraceptives**
   A. **Contraceptive vaginal ring (NuvaRing)** delivers 15 µg ethinyl estradiol and 120 µg of etonogestrel daily.
      1. **Advantages of the ring** include rapid return to ovulation after discontinuation, lower doses of hormones, ease and convenience, and improved cycle control. Benefits, risks, and contraindications to use

are similar to those with combined oral contraceptive pills, except for the convenience of monthly administration.

2. In women who have not used hormonal contraception in the past month, the ring is inserted on or before day 5 of the menstrual cycle, even if bleeding is not complete, and an additional form of contraception should be used for the following 7 days. New rings should be inserted at approximately the same time of day the ring was removed the previous week.

3. If the ring accidentally falls out, it may be rinsed with cool or warm water and replaced within 3 hours. If it is out of place for more than 3 hours contraceptive effectiveness decreases, so an additional form of contraception should be used until the ring has been inserted for 7 continuous days. If the ring remains in place more than 3 but ≤4 weeks, it is removed and a new one is inserted after a 1-week ring-free interval; if the ring is left in place for >4 weeks, backup contraception is recommended until a new ring has been in place for 7 days.

B. **Transdermal contraceptive patch**

1. **Ortho Evra** is a transdermal contraceptive patch, which is as effective as oral contraceptives. Ortho Evra delivers 20 μg of ethinyl estradiol and 150 μg of norelgestromin daily for 6 to 13 months. Compliance is better with the patch. The patch is applied at the beginning of the menstrual cycle. A new patch is applied each week for 3 weeks; week 4 is patch-free. It is sold in packages of 3 patches. Effectiveness is similar to oral contraceptives.

2. Breakthrough bleeding during the first two cycles, dysmenorrhea, and breast discomfort are more common in women using the patch. A reaction at the site of application of the patch occurs in 1.9% of the women. Contraceptive efficacy may be slightly lower in women weighing more than 90 kg.

C. **Depot medroxyprogesterone acetate** (DMPA, Depo-Provera) is an injectable contraceptive. Deep intramuscular injection of 150 mg results in effective contraception for three to four months. Effectiveness is 99.7%.

D. Women who receive the first injection after the seventh day of the menstrual cycle should use a second method of contraception for seven days. The first injection should be administered within five days after the onset of menses, in which case alternative contraception is not necessary.

E. Ovulation is suppressed for at least 14 weeks after injection of a 150 mg dose of DMPA. Therefore, injections should repeated every three months. A pregnancy test must be administered to women who are more than two weeks late for an injection.

F. Return of fertility can be delayed for up to 18 months after cessation of DMPA. DMPA is not ideal for women who may wish to become pregnant soon after cessation of contraception.

G. Amenorrhea, irregular bleeding, and weight gain (typically 1 to 3 kg) are the most common adverse effects of DMPA. Adverse effects also include acne, headache, and depression. Fifty% of women report amenorrhea by one year. Persistent bleeding may be treated with 50 μg of ethinyl estradiol for 14 days.

H. **Medroxyprogesterone acetate/estradiol cypionate (MPA/E2C, Lunelle)** is a combined (25 mg MPA and 5 mg E2C), injectable contraceptive.

1. Although monthly IM injections are required, MPA/E2C has several desirable features:
   a. It has nearly 100% effectiveness in preventing pregnancy.
   b. Fertility returns within three to four months after it is discontinued.
   c. Irregular bleeding is less common than in women given MPA alone.

2. Weight gain, hypertension, headache, mastalgia, or other nonmenstrual complaints are common.

3. Lunelle should be considered for women who forget to take their birth control pills or those who want a discreet method of contraception. The initial injection should be given during the first 5 days of the menstrual cycle or within 7 days of stopping oral contraceptives. Lunelle injections should be given every 28 to 30 days; 33 days at the most.

III. Barrier methods

A. Barrier methods of contraception, such as the condom, diaphragm, cervical cap, and spermicides, have fewer side effects than hormonal contraception.

B. The diaphragm and cervical cap require fitting by a clinician and are only effective when used with a spermicide. They must be left in the vagina for six to eight hours after intercourse; the diaphragm needs to be removed after this period of time, while the cervical cap can be left in place for up to 24 hours. These considerations have caused them to be less desirable methods of contraception. A major advantage of barrier contraceptives is their efficacy in protecting against sexually transmitted diseases and HIV infection.

IV. Intrauterine devices

A. The currently available intrauterine devices (IUDs) are safe and effective methods of contraception:

1. **Copper T380 IUD** induces a foreign body reaction in the endometrium. It is effective for 8 to 10 years.

2. **Progesterone-releasing IUDs** inhibit sperm survival and implantation. They also decrease menstrual blood loss and relieve dysmenorrhea. **Paragard** is replaced every 10 years. **Progestasert** IUDs must be replaced after one year.

3. **Levonorgestrel IUD (Mirena)** provides effective contraception for five years.

B. Infection

1. Women who are at low risk for sexually transmitted diseases do not have a higher incidence of pelvic inflammatory disease with use of an IUD. An IUD should not be inserted in women at high risk for sexually transmitted infections, and women should be screened for the presence of sexually transmitted diseases before insertion.

2. **Contraindications to IUDs:**
   a. Women at high risk for bacterial endocarditis (eg, rheumatic heart disease, prosthetic valves, or a history of endocarditis).
   b. Women at high risk for infections, including those with AIDS and a history of intravenous drug use.
   c. Women with uterine leiomyomas which alter the size or shape of the uterine cavity.

V. Lactation

A. Women who breast-feed have a delay in resumption of ovulation postpartum. It is probably safest to resume contraceptive use in the third postpartum month for those who breast-feed full time, and in the third postpartum week for those who do not breast-feed.

B. A nonhormonal contraceptive or progesterone-containing hormonal contraceptive can be started at any time; an estrogen-containing oral contraceptive pill should not be started before the third week postpartum because women are still at increased risk of thromboembolism prior to this time. Oral contraceptive pills can decrease breast milk, while progesterone-containing contraceptives may increase breast milk.

VI. Progestin-only agents

A. Progestin-only agents are slightly less effective than combination oral contraceptives. They have failure rates of 0.5% compared with the 0.1% rate with combination oral contraceptives.

B. Progestin-only oral contraceptives (Micronor, Nor-QD, Ovrette) provide a useful alternative in women who cannot take estrogen. Progestin-only contraception is recommended for nursing mothers. Milk production is unaffected by use of progestin-only agents.

C. If the usual time of ingestion is delayed for more than three hours, an alternative form of birth control should be used for the following 48 hours. Because progestin-only agents are taken continuously, without hormone-free periods, menses may be irregular, infrequent or absent.

VII. Postcoital contraception

A. Emergency postcoital contraception consists of administration of drugs within 72 hours to women who have had unprotected intercourse (including sexual assault), or to those who have had a failure of another method of contraception (eg, broken condom).

B. Preparations

1. Menstrual bleeding typically occurs within three days after administration of most forms of hormonal postcoital contraception. A pregnancy test should be performed if bleeding has not occurred within four weeks.

2. **Preven Emergency Contraceptive Kit** includes four combination tablets, each containing 50 µg of ethinyl estradiol and 0.25 mg of levonorgestrel, and a pregnancy test to rule out pregnancy before taking the tablets. Instructions are to take two of the tablets as soon as possible within 72 hours of coitus, and the other two tablets twelve hours later.

3. An oral contraceptive such as Ovral (two tablets twelve hours apart) or Lo/Ovral (4 tablets twelve hours apart) can also be used.

4. Nausea and vomiting are the major side effects. Meclizine 50 mg, taken one hour before the first dose, reduces nausea and vomiting but can cause some sedation.

5. **Plan B** is a pill pack that contains two 0.75 mg tablets of levonorgestrel to be taken twelve hours apart. The cost is comparable to the Preven kit ($20). This regimen may be more effective and better tolerated than an estrogen-progestin regimen.

6. **Copper T380 IUD.** A copper intrauterine device (IUD) placed within 120 hours of unprotected intercourse can also be used as a form of emergency contraception. An advantage of this method is that it provides continuing contraception after the initial event.

Emergency Contraception

1. Consider pretreatment one hour before each oral contraceptive pill dose, using one of the following orally administered antiemetic agents:
   Prochlorperazine (Compazine), 5 to 10 mg
   Promethazine (Phenergan), 12.5 to 25 mg
   Trimethobenzamide (Tigan), 250 mg
   Meclizine (Antivert) 50 mg
2. Administer the first dose of oral contraceptive pill within 72 hours of unprotected coitus, and administer the second dose 12 hours after the first dose. Brand name options for emergency contraception include the following:
   Preven Kit – two pills per dose (0.5 mg of levonorgestrel and 100 µg of ethinyl estradiol per dose)
   Plan B – one pill per dose (0.75 mg of levonorgestrel per dose)
   Ovral – two pills per dose (0.5 mg of levonorgestrel and 100 µg of ethinyl estradiol per dose)
   Nordette – four pills per dose (0.6 mg of levonorgestrel and 120 µg of ethinyl estradiol per dose)
   Triphasil – four pills per dose (0.5 mg of levonorgestrel and 120 µg of ethinyl estradiol per dose)

VIII. **Sterilization**
  A. Sterilization is the most common and effective form of contraception. While tubal ligation and vasectomy may be reversible, these procedures should be considered permanent.
  B. **Essure microinsert sterilization device** is a permanent, hysteroscopic, tubal sterilization device which is 99.9% effective. The coil-like device is inserted in the office under local anesthesia into the fallopian tubes where it is incorporated by tissue. After placement, women use alternative contraception for three months, after which hysterosalpingography is performed to assure correct placement. Postoperative discomfort is minimal.
  C. **Tubal ligation** is usually performed as a laparoscopic procedure in outpatients or in postpartum women in the hospital. The techniques used are unipolar or bipolar coagulation, silicone rubber band or spring clip application, and partial salpingectomy.
  D. **Vasectomy** (ligation of the vas deferens) can be performed in the office under local anesthesia. A semen analysis should be done three to six months after the procedure to confirm azoospermia.

References: See page 294.

Premenstrual Syndrome and Premenstrual Dysphoric Disorder

Premenstrual syndrome (PMS) is characterized by physical and behavioral symptoms that occur repetitively in the second half of the menstrual cycle and interfere with some aspects of the woman's life. Premenstrual dysphoric disorder (PMDD) is the most severe form of PMS, with the prominence anger, irritability, and internal tension. PMS affects up to 75% of women with regular menstrual cycles, while PMDD affects only 3 to 8% of women.

I. **Symptoms**
  A. The most common physical manifestation of PMS is abdominal bloating, which occurs in 90% of women with this disorder; breast tenderness and headaches are also common, occurring in more than 50% of cases.
  B. The most common behavioral symptom of PMS is an extreme sense of fatigue which is seen in more than 90%. Other frequent behavioral complaints include irritability, tension, depressed mood, labile mood (80%), increased appetite (70%), and forgetfulness and difficulty concentrating (50%).

Symptom Clusters Commonly Noted in Patients with PMS

Affective Symptoms	Cognitive or performance
Depression or sadness	Mood instability or mood swings
Irritability	Difficulty in concentrating
Tension	Decreased efficiency
Anxiety	Confusion
Tearfulness or crying easily	Forgetfulness
Restlessness or jitteriness	Accident-prone
Anger	Social avoidance
Loneliness	Temper outbursts
Appetite change	Energetic
Food cravings	**Fluid retention**
Changes in sexual interest	Breast tenderness or swelling
Pain	Weight gain
Headache or migraine	Abdominal bloating or swelling
Back pain	Swelling of extremities
Breast pain	**General somatic**
Abdominal cramps	Fatigue or tiredness
General or muscular pain	Dizziness or vertigo

	Nausea Insomnia

C. Other common findings include acne, oversensitivity to environmental stimuli, anger, easy crying, and gastrointestinal upset. Hot flashes, heart palpitations, and dizziness occur in 15 to 20% of patients. Symptoms should occur in the luteal phase only.

UCSD Criteria for Premenstrual Syndrome

At least one of the following affective and somatic symptoms during the five days before menses in each of the three previous cycles:
Affective symptoms: depression, angry outbursts, irritability, anxiety, confusion, social withdrawal
Somatic symptoms: breast tenderness, abdominal bloating, headache, swelling of extremities Symptoms relieved from days 4 through 13 of the menstrual cycle

DSM-IV Criteria for Premenstrual Dysphoric Disorder

- Five or more symptoms
- At least one of the following four symptoms:
    Markedly depressed mood, feelings of hopelessness, or self-deprecating thoughts
    Marked anxiety, tension, feeling of being "keyed up" or "on edge"
    Marked affective lability
    Persistent and marked anger or irritability or increase in interpersonal conflicts
- Additional symptoms that may be used to fulfill the criteria:
    Decreased interest in usual activities
    Subjective sense of difficulty in concentrating
    Lethargy, easy fatigability, or marked lack of energy
    Marked change in appetite, overeating, or specific food cravings
    Hypersomnia or insomnia
    Subjective sense of being overwhelmed or out of control
- Other physical symptoms such as breast tenderness or swelling, headaches, joint or muscle pain, a sensation of bloating, or weight gain
- Symptoms occurring during last week of luteal phase
- Symptoms are absent postmenstrually
- Disturbances that interfere with work or school or with usual social activities and relationships
- Disturbances that are not an exacerbation of symptoms of another disorder

Differential Diagnosis of Premenstrual Syndrome

Affective disorder (eg, depression, anxiety, dysthymia, panic) Anemia Anorexia or bulimia Chronic medical conditions (eg, diabetes mellitus) Dysmenorrhea	Endometriosis Hypothyroidism Oral contraceptive pill use Perimenopause Personality disorder Substance abuse disorders

D. Differential diagnosis
1. PMDD should be differentiated from premenstrual exacerbation of an underlying major psychiatric disorder, as well as medical conditions such as hyper- or hypothyroidism.
2. About 13% of women with PMS are found to have a psychiatric disorder alone with no evidence of PMS, while 38% had premenstrual exacerbation of underlying depressive and anxiety disorders.

3. 39% of women with PMDD meet criteria for mood or anxiety disorders.

4. The assessment of patients with possible PMS or PMDD should begin with the history, physical examination, chemistry profile, complete blood count, and serum TSH. The history should focus in particular on the regularity of menstrual cycles. Appropriate gynecologic endocrine evaluation should be performed if the cycles are irregular (lengths less than 25 or >36 days).

5. The patient should be asked to record symptoms prospectively for two months. If the patient fails to demonstrate a symptom free interval in the follicular phase, she should be evaluated for a mood or anxiety disorder.

II. Nonpharmacologic therapy

A. Relaxation therapy and cognitive behavioral therapy have shown some benefit. Behavioral measures include keeping a symptom diary, getting adequate rest and exercise, and making dietary changes.

B. Sleep disturbances, ranging from insomnia to excessive sleep, are common. A structured sleep schedule with consistent sleep and wake times is recommended. Sodium restriction may minimize bloating, fluid retention, and breast swelling and tenderness. Caffeine restriction and aerobic exercise often reduce symptoms.

III. Dietary Supplementation

A. Vitamin E supplementation is a treatment for mastalgia. The administration of 400 IU per day of vitamin E during the luteal phase improves affective and somatic symptoms.

B. Calcium carbonate in a dosage of 1200 mg per day for three menstrual cycles results in symptom improvement in 48% of women with PMS.

IV. Pharmacologic Therapy

A. Fluoxetine (Sarafem) and sertraline (Zoloft) have been approved for the treatment of PMDD. SSRIs are recommended as initial drug therapy in women with PMS and PMDD. Common side effects of SSRIs include insomnia, drowsiness, fatigue, nausea, nervousness, headache, mild tremor, and sexual dysfunction.

B. Fluoxetine (Sarafem) 20 mg or sertraline (Zoloft) 50 mg, taken in the morning, is best tolerated and sufficient to improve symptoms. Fluoxetine or sertraline can be given during the 14 days before the menstrual period.

C. Benefit has also been demonstrated for citalopram (Celexa) during the 14 days before the menstrual period.

D. **Diuretics.** Spironolactone (Aldactone) is the only diuretic that has been shown to effectively relieve breast tenderness and fluid retention. Spironolactone is administered only during the luteal phase.

E. **Prostaglandin Inhibitors.** Nonsteroidal anti-inflammatory drugs (NSAIDs) are traditional therapy for primary dysmenorrhea and menorrhagia. These agents include mefenamic acid (Ponstel) and naproxen sodium (Anaprox, Aleve).

References: See page 294.

Prescription Medications Commonly Used in the Treatment of Premenstrual Syndrome (PMS)

Drug class and representative agents	Dosage	Recommendations	Side effects
SSRIs			
Fluoxetine (Sarafem)	10 to 20 mg per day	First-choice agents for the treatment of PMDD. Effective in alleviating behavioral and physical symptoms of PMS and PMDD Administer during luteal phase (14 days before menses).	Insomnia, drowsiness, fatigue, nausea, nervousness, headache, mild tremor, sexual dysfunction
Sertraline (Zoloft)	50 to 150 mg per day		
Paroxetine (Paxil)	10 to 30 mg per day		
Fluvoxamine (Luvox)	25 to 50 mg per day		
Citalopram (Celexa)	20 to 40 mg per day		
Diuretics			
Spironolactone (Aldactone)	25 to 100 mg per day luteal phase	Effective in alleviating breast tenderness and bloating.	Antiestrogenic effects, hyperkalemia
NSAIDs			
Naproxen sodium (Anaprox)	275 to 550 mg twice daily	Effective in alleviating various physical symptoms of PMS. Any NSAID should be effective.	Nausea, gastric ulceration, renal dysfunction. Use with caution in women with pre-existing gastrointestinal or renal disease.
Mefenamic acid (Ponstel)	250 mg tid with meals		
Androgens			
Danazol (Danocrine)	100 to 400 mg twice daily	Somewhat effective in alleviating mastalgia when taken during luteal phase.	Weight gain, decreased breast size, deepening of voice. Monitor lipid profile and liver function.

Drug class and representative agents	Dosage	Recommendations	Side effects
GnRH agonists			
Leuprolide (Lupron)	3.75 mg IM every month or 11.25 mg IM every three months	Somewhat effective in alleviating physical and behavioral symptoms of PMS Side effect profile and cost limit use.	Hot flashes, cardiovascular effects, and osteoporosis
Goserelin (Zoladex)	3.6 mg SC every month or 10.8 mg SC every three months		
Nafarelin (Synarel)	200 to 400 mcg intranasally twice daily		

References: See page 294.

Secondary Amenorrhea

Amenorrhea (absence of menses) can be a transient, intermittent, or permanent condition resulting from dysfunction of the hypothalamus, pituitary, ovaries, uterus, or vagina. Amenorrhea is classified as either primary (absence of menarche by age 16 years) or secondary (absence of menses for more than three cycles or six months in women who previously had menses). Pregnancy is the most common cause of secondary amenorrhea.

I. Diagnosis of secondary amenorrhea
   A. **Step 1: Rule out pregnancy.** A pregnancy test is the first step in evaluating secondary amenorrhea. Measurement of serum beta subunit of hCG is the most sensitive test.
   B. **Step 2: Assess the history**
      1. Recent stress; change in weight, diet or exercise habits; or illnesses that might result in hypothalamic amenorrhea should be sought.
      2. Drugs associated with amenorrhea, systemic illnesses that can cause hypothalamic amenorrhea, recent initiation or discontinuation of an oral contraceptive, androgenic drugs (danazol) or high-dose progestin, and antipsychotic drugs should be evaluated.
      3. Headaches, visual field defects, fatigue, or polyuria and polydipsia may suggest hypothalamic-pituitary disease.
      4. Symptoms of estrogen deficiency include hot flashes, vaginal dryness, poor sleep, or decreased libido.
      5. Galactorrhea is suggestive of hyperprolactinemia. Hirsutism, acne, and a history of irregular menses are suggestive of hyperandrogenism.
      6. A history of obstetrical catastrophe, severe bleeding, dilatation and curettage, or endometritis or other infection that might have caused scarring of the endometrial lining suggests Asherman's syndrome.
   C. **Step 3: Physical examination.** Measurements of height and weight, signs of other illnesses, and evidence of cachexia should be assessed. The skin, breasts, and genital tissues should be evaluated for estrogen deficiency. The breasts should be palpated, including an attempt to express galactorrhea. The skin should be examined for hirsutism, acne,

striae, acanthosis nigricans, vitiligo, thickness or thinness, and easy bruisability.

D. **Step 4: Basic laboratory testing**. In addition to measurement of serum hCG to rule out pregnancy, minimal laboratory testing should include measurements of serum prolactin, thyrotropin, and FSH to rule out hyperprolactinemia, thyroid disease, and ovarian failure (high serum FSH). If there is hirsutism, acne or irregular menses, serum dehydroepiandrosterone sulfate (DHEA-S) and testosterone should be measured.

E. **Step 5: Follow-up laboratory evaluation**
   1. **High serum prolactin concentration**. Prolactin secretion can be transiently increased by stress or eating. Therefore, serum prolactin should be measured at least twice before cranial imaging is obtained, particularly in those women with small elevations (<50 ng/mL). These women should be screened for thyroid disease with a TSH and free T4 because hypothyroidism can cause hyperprolactinemia.
   2. Women with verified high serum prolactin values should have a cranial MRI unless a very clear explanation is found for the elevation (eg, antipsychotics). Imaging should rule out a hypothalamic or pituitary tumor.
   3. **High serum FSH concentration.** A high serum FSH concentration indicates the presence of ovarian failure. This test should be repeated monthly on three occasions to confirm. A karyotype should be considered in most women with secondary amenorrhea age 30 years or younger.

Causes of Primary and Secondary Amenorrhea	
Abnormality	**Causes**
Pregnancy	
Anatomic abnormalities	
Congenital abnormality in Müllerian development	Isolated defect Testicular feminization syndrome 5-Alpha-reductase deficiency Vanishing testes syndrome Defect in testis determining factor
Congenital defect of urogenital sinus development	Agenesis of lower vagina Imperforate hymen
Acquired ablation or scarring of the endometrium	Asherman's syndrome Tuberculosis
Disorders of hypothalamic-pituitary ovarian axis Hypothalamic dysfunction Pituitary dysfunction Ovarian dysfunction	

Causes of Amenorrhea due to Abnormalities in the Hypothalamic-Pituitary-Ovarian Axis

Abnormality	Causes

Hypothalamic dysfunction	Functional hypothalamic amenorrhea
	    Weight loss, eating disorders
	    Exercise
	    Stress
	    Severe or prolonged illness
	Congenital gonadotropin-releasing hormone deficiency
	Inflammatory or infiltrative diseases
	Brain tumors - eg, craniopharyngioma
	Pituitary stalk dissection or compression
	Cranial irradiation
	Brain injury - trauma, hemorrhage, hydrocephalus
	Other syndromes - Prader-Willi, Laurence-Moon-Biedl

Pituitary dysfunction	Hyperprolactinemia Other pituitary tumors- acromegaly, corticotroph adenomas (Cushing's disease) Other tumors - meningioma, germinoma, glioma Empty sella syndrome Pituitary infarct or apoplexy

Ovarian dysfunction	Ovarian failure (menopause)
	    Spontaneous
	    Premature (before age 40 years)
	    Surgical

Other	Hyperthyroidism Hypothyroidism Diabetes mellitus Exogenous androgen use

Drugs Associated with Amenorrhea

Drugs that Increase Prolactin	Antipsychotics Tricyclic antidepressants Calcium channel blockers
Drugs with Estrogenic Activity	Digoxin, marijuana, oral contraceptives
Drugs with Ovarian Toxicity	Chemotherapeutic agents

4. **High serum androgen concentrations**. A high serum androgen value may suggest the diagnosis of polycystic ovary syndrome or may suggest an androgen-secreting tumor of the ovary or adrenal gland. Further testing for a tumor might include a 24-hour urine collection for cortisol and 17-ketosteroids, determination of serum 17-hydroxy-progesterone after intravenous injection of corticotropin (ACTH), and a dexamethasone suppression test. Elevation of 17-ketosteroids, DHEA-S, or 17-hydroxyprogesterone is more consistent with an adrenal, rather than ovarian, source of excess androgen.

5. **Normal or low serum gonadotropin concentrations and all other tests normal**
   a. This result is one of the most common outcomes of laboratory testing in women with amenorrhea. Women with hypothalamic amenorrhea (caused by excessive exercise or weight loss) have normal to low serum FSH values. Cranial MRI is indicated in all women without an a clear explanation for hypogonadotropic hypogonadism or in most women who have visual field defects or headaches. No further testing is required if the onset of amenorrhea is recent or is easily explained (eg, weight loss, excessive exercise) and there are no symptoms suggestive of other disease.
   b. High serum transferrin saturation may indicate hemochromatosis, high serum angiotensin-converting enzyme values suggest sarcoidosis, and high fasting blood glucose or hemoglobin A1c values indicate diabetes mellitus.
6. **Normal serum prolactin and FSH concentrations with history of uterine instrumentation preceding amenorrhea**
   a. Evaluation for Asherman's syndrome should be completed. A progestin challenge should be performed (medroxyprogesterone acetate 10 mg for 10 days). If withdrawal bleeding occurs, an outflow tract disorder has been ruled out. If bleeding does not occur, estrogen and progestin should be administered.
   b. Oral conjugated estrogens (0.625 to 2.5 mg daily for 35 days) with medroxyprogesterone added (10 mg daily for days 26 to 35); failure to bleed upon cessation of this therapy strongly suggests endometrial scarring. In this situation, a hysterosalpingogram or hysteroscopy can confirm the diagnosis of Asherman syndrome.

II. Treatment
   A. **Athletic women** should be counseled on the need for increased caloric intake or reduced exercise. Resumption of menses usually occurs.
   B. **Nonathletic women who are underweight** should receive nutritional counseling and treatment of eating disorders.
   C. **Hyperprolactinemia** is treated with a dopamine agonist. Cabergoline (Dostinex) or bromocriptine (Parlodel) are used for most adenomas. Ovulation, regular menstrual cycles, and pregnancy may usually result.
   D. **Ovarian failure** should be treated with hormone replacement therapy.
   E. **Hyperandrogenism** is treated with measures to reduce hirsutism, resume menses, and fertility and preventing endometrial hyperplasia, obesity, and metabolic defects.
   F. **Asherman's syndrome** is treated with hysteroscopic lysis of adhesions followed by long-term estrogen administration to stimulate regrowth of endometrial tissue.

Benign Breast Disease

Benign breast disease includes breast pain, breast lumps, or nipple discharge. The most common cause of breast nodularity and tenderness is fibrocystic change, which occurs in 60% of premenopausal women.

I. **Benign breast lesions,** which are discovered by breast palpation or mammography, have been subdivided into those that are associated with an increased risk of breast cancer and those that are not.
   A. **No increased risk of breast cancer**
      1. **Fibrocystic changes** consist of an increased number of cysts or fibrous tissue in an otherwise normal breast. Fibrocystic changes do not constitute a disease state.
      2. **Fibrocystic disease** is diagnosed when fibrocystic changes occur in conjunction with pain, nipple discharge, or a degree of lumpiness sufficient to cause suspicion of cancer.

      3. **Duct ectasia** is characterized by distention of subareolar ducts.
      4. **Solitary papillomas** consist of papillary cells that grow from the wall of a cyst into its lumen.
      5. **Simple fibroadenomas** are benign solid tumors, usually presenting as a well-defined, mobile mass.

  B. Increased risk of breast cancer
      1. **Ductal hyperplasia** without atypia is the most common lesion associated with increased risk of breast cancer.
      2. **Sclerosing adenosis** consists of lobular tissue that has undergone hyperplastic change.
      3. **Diffuse papillomatosis** refers to the formation of multiple papillomas.
      4. **Complex fibroadenomas** are tumors that contain cysts >3 mm in diameter, sclerosing adenosis, epithelial calcification, or papillary apocrine changes.
      5. **Atypical hyperplasia** is associated with a four to sixfold increased risk of breast cancer.
      6. **Radial scars** are benign breast lesions of uncertain pathogenesis that are occasionally detected by mammography. Thus, histologic confirmation is required to exclude spiculated carcinoma.

II. Symptoms and signs of benign breast disease

  A. Women with fibrocystic changes can have breast tenderness during the luteal phase of the menstrual cycle. Fibrocystic disease is characterized by more severe or prolonged pain.

  B. Women in their 30s sometimes present with multiple breast nodules 2 to 10 mm in size as a result of proliferation of glandular cells.

  C. Women in their 30s and 40s present with solitary or multiple cysts. Acute enlargement of cysts may cause severe, localized pain of sudden onset. Nipple discharge is common, varying from pale green to brown.

III. Differential diagnosis

  A. Breast pain
      1. Women with mastitis usually complain of the sudden onset of pain, fever, erythema, tenderness, and induration.
      2. Large pendulous breasts may cause pain due to stretching of Cooper's ligaments.
      3. Hidradenitis suppurativa can present as breast nodules and pain.
      4. Chest wall pain induced by trauma or trauma-induced fat necrosis, intercostal neuralgia, costochondritis, underlying pleuritic lesions, or arthritis of the thoracic spine can mimic benign breast disease.

  B. Nipple discharge is uncommon in cancer and, if present, is unilateral. Approximately 3% of cases of unilateral nipple discharge are due to breast cancer; a mass is usually also present.
      1. Nonspontaneous, nonbloody, or bilateral nipple discharge is unlikely to be due to cancer.
         a. Purulent discharge is often caused by mastitis or a breast abscess.
         b. Milky discharge commonly occurs after childbearing and can last several years; it also may be associated with oral contraceptives or tricyclic antidepressants. Serum prolactin should be measured if the discharge is sustained, particularly if it is associated with menstrual abnormalities.
         c. A green, yellow, white, grey, or brown discharge can be caused by duct ectasia.
      2. Evaluation of nipple discharge for suspected cancer may include cytology and galactography. Occult blood can be detected with a guaiac test.

IV. Clinical evaluation

  A. History
      1. The relationship of symptoms to the menstrual cycles, the timing of onset of breast lumps and their subsequent course, the color and location of nipple discharge, and hormone use should be assessed.
      2. Risk factors for breast cancer should be determined, including menarche before age 12 years, first live birth at age $\geq$30 years, and meno-

pause at age ≥55 years; the number of previous breast biopsies, the presence of atypical ductal hyperplasia on biopsy, obesity, nulliparity, increased age, the amount of alcohol consumed, and the number and ages of first-degree family members with breast cancer with two such relatives with breast cancer at any early age should be determined.

B. **Physical examination.** The examination is performed when the breasts are least stimulated, seven to nine days after the onset of menses. The four breast quadrants, subareolar areas, and the axillae should be systematically examined with the woman both lying and sitting with her hands on her hips.

   1. **The specific goals of the examination are to:**
      a. Delineate and document breast masses
      b. Elicit discharge from a nipple
      c. Identify localized areas of tenderness
      d. Detect enlarged axillary or supraclavicular lymph nodes
      e. Detect skin changes, noting the symmetry and contour of the breasts, position of the nipples, scars, dimpling, edema or erythema, ulceration or crusting of the nipple

   2. **"Classic" characteristics of breast cancers:**
      a. Single lesion
      b. Hard
      c. Immovable
      d. Irregular border
      e. Size ≥2 cm

C. **Mammography**

   1. Although 90% or more of palpable breast masses in women in their 20s to early 50s are benign, excluding breast cancer is a crucial step in the evaluation. Mammography is recommended for any woman age 35 years or older who has a breast mass.

   2. Mammography usually is not ordered routinely in women under age 35 years. The breast tissue in younger women is often too dense to evaluate the lump. Ultrasonography is useful in these women to evaluate lumps and to assess for cysts.

   3. Round dense lesions on mammography often represent cystic fluid. Solid and cystic lesions can often be distinguished by ultrasonography and mammography, and needle aspiration under ultrasound guidance further documents the cystic nature of the lesion.

D. **Breast pain.** Women who present with breast pain as their only symptom often undergo mammography. Only 0.4% of women with breast pain have breast cancer. The vast majority of women have normal findings (87%); benign abnormalities are noted in 9%.

E. **Ductal lavage.** The cytologic detection of cellular atypia can identify women with a higher risk of developing breast cancer.

V. Treatment

A. **Fibrocystic disease.** The major aim of therapy in fibrocystic disease is to relieve breast pain or discomfort. Symptomatic relief also may be achieved with a soft brassiere with good support, acetaminophen or a nonsteroidal anti-inflammatory drug, or both.

   1. Breast pain or discomfort may be relieved with a thiazide diuretic.

   2. **Avoidance of caffeine** may provide some patients with relief of pain.

   3. **Vitamin E,** 400 IU twice daily reduces breast pain.

   4. **Evening primrose oil** in doses of 1500-3000 mg daily, relieves breast pain in 30 to 80%.

   5. **Danazol** in doses of 100 to 200 mg daily reduces breast pain. Common side effects include weight gain, acne, hirsutism, bloating, and amenorrhea.

   6. **Tamoxifen** reduces breast pain in about 70% of women. It is safe and well-tolerated as 10 mg twice daily, or bromocriptine 1.25 to 5 mg daily can be tried.

   7. **Oral contraceptives.** The frequency of fibrocystic changes decreases with prolonged oral contraceptive therapy. Oral contracep-

tives containing 19-norprogestins, such as norlutate, have androgenic properties that are beneficial.

References: See page 294.

Menopause

Menopause is defined as the cessation of menstrual periods, menopause occurs at a mean age of 51.4 years in normal women.

I. Definitions
   A. **Menopausal transition** begins with variation in menstrual cycle length and an elevated FSH concentration and ends with the final menstrual period (12 months of amenorrhea). Stage -2 (early) is characterized by variable cycle length (>7 days different from normal menstrual cycle length, which is 21 to 35 days). Stage -1 (late) is characterized by >2 skipped cycles and an interval of amenorrhea >60 days; women at this stage often have hot flashes as well.
   B. **Perimenopause** begins in stage -2 of the menopausal transition and ends 12 months after the last menstrual period.
   C. **Menopause** is defined by 12 months of amenorrhea after the final menstrual period. It results from complete, or near complete, ovarian follicular depletion and absence of ovarian estrogen secretion.
   D. **Postmenopause.** Stage +1 (early) is defined as the first five years after the final menstrual period. It is characterized by further and complete decline in ovarian function and accelerated bone loss; many women in this stage continue to have hot flashes. Stage +2 (late) begins five years after the final menstrual period and ends with death.
II. Epidemiology
   A. The average age at menopause is 51 years; however, for 5% of women it occurs after age 55 (late menopause), and for another 5%, between ages 40 to 45 years (early menopause). Menopause that occurs before age 40 years is premature ovarian failure.
   B. The age of menopause is reduced by about two years in women who smoke. Women who have never had children and who have had regular cycles tend to have an earlier age of menopause.
III. Clinical manifestations
   A. **Bleeding patterns.** Chronic anovulation and progesterone deficiency in this transition period may cause long periods of unopposed estrogen exposure and result in anovulatory bleeding and endometrial hyperplasia.
   B. **Oligomenorrhea** (irregular cycles) for six or more months, or an episode of heavy dysfunctional bleeding is an indication for endometrial surveillance. Endometrial biopsy is the standard to rule out the occurrence of endometrial hyperplasia.
   C. **Irregular or heavy bleeding** during the menopausal transition may be treated with low-dose oral contraceptives or intermittent progestin therapy.
   D. **Hot flashes**
      1. The most common symptom during menopause is the hot flash, occurring in up to 75%. Hot flashes are self-limited, usually resolving without treatment within one to five years, although some women will continue to have hot flashes until after age 70.
      2. Hot flashes begin as the sudden sensation of heat in the upper chest and face that rapidly becomes generalized. The sensation of heat lasts from two to four minutes, is often associated with perspiration and occasionally palpitations, and is often followed by chills and shivering, and sometimes anxiety. Hot flashes usually occur several times per day and are common at night.
   E. **Genitourinary symptoms**
      1. **Vaginal dryness.** The vagina and urethra are very sensitive to estrogen, and estrogen deficiency leads to thinning of the vaginal epithe-

lium. This results in vaginal atrophy (atrophic vaginitis), causing symptoms of vaginal dryness, itching and often, dyspareunia.

2. The vagina typically appears pale, with lack of the normal rugae and often has visible blood vessels or petechial hemorrhages.

3. **Sexual dysfunction.** Estrogen deficiency causes a decrease in blood flow to the vagina and vulva, decreased vaginal lubrication, and sexual dysfunction.

4. Atrophic urethritis results from low estrogen production after the menopause, predisposing to stress and urge urinary incontinence. The prevalence of incontinence increases with age.

IV. **Diagnosis**

A. Menopause is defined as 12 months of amenorrhea in a woman over age 45 in the absence of other causes. Further evaluation is not necessary for women in this group.

B. The best approach to diagnosing the menopausal transition is an assessment of menstrual cycle history and menopausal symptoms (vasomotor flushes, mood changes, sleep disturbances). Measuring serum FSH, estradiol, or inhibin levels is usually not necessary. Serum FSH concentrations increase across the menopausal transition, but at times may be suppressed into the normal premenopausal range (after a recent ovulation).

C. **Differential diagnosis.** Hyperthyroidism should be considered in the differential diagnosis because irregular menses, sweats (although different from typical hot flashes), and mood changes are all potential clinical manifestations of hyperthyroidism. Other etiologies for menstrual cycle changes that should be considered include pregnancy, hyperprolactinemia, and thyroid disease. Atypical hot flashes and night sweats may be caused by medications, carcinoid, pheochromocytoma, or underlying malignancy.

V. **Treatment of menopausal symptoms in women not taking systemic estrogen**

A. Many women cannot or choose not to take estrogen to treat symptoms of estrogen deficiency at menopause because of an increased risk of breast cancer and cardiovascular disease.

B. Therapy prevents bone loss and fracture, but does not confir a protective effect on the heart. Continuous combined therapy with conjugated estrogen (0.625 mg/day) and medroxyprogesterone acetate (2.5 mg/day) is ineffective for either primary or secondary prevention of CHD, and slightly increases risk. Other risks included an increased risk of stroke, venous thromboembolism, and breast cancer.

C. **Patient selection**. Estrogen is a reasonable short-term option for most symptomatic postmenopausal women, with the exception of those with a history of breast cancer, coronary heart disease, a previous venous thromboembolic event or stroke, or those at high risk for these complications. Short-term therapy is six months to five years.

D. **Vasomotor instability**. Hot flashes can result in sleep disturbances, headache, and irritability. Although estrogen is the gold standard for relief of hot flashes, a number of other drugs have been shown to be somewhat better than placebo. Venlafaxine (Effexor, 75 mg daily) reduces hot flashes by 61%. Mouth dryness, anorexia, nausea, and constipation are common. Gabapentin (Neurontin) has been used for hot flashes at a dose of 200mg orally once daily to 400mg orally four times daily.

E. **Urogenital atrophy**

1. Both systemic and vaginal estrogen are effective for genitourinary atrophy; however, vaginal estrogen has lesser systemic levels than estrogen tablets.

2. **Moisturizers and lubricants.** The long-acting vaginal moisturizer, Replens, produces a moist film over the vaginal tissue. A water soluble lubricant, such as Astroglide and K-Y Personal Lubricant, should be used at the time of intercourse.

3. Low-dose vaginal estrogen

a. **Estrogen Cream (Premarin)** 0.5 g of cream, or one-eighth of an applicatorful daily into the vagina for three weeks followed by twice weekly administration thereafter. Estrace, which is crystalline estradiol, can also by given by vaginal applicator at a dose of one-eighth of an applicator or 0.5 g (which contains 50 microgram of estradiol).

b. **Vaginal ring** is a silastic ring impregnated with estradiol (Estring, Phadia) involves insertion of a silastic ring that delivers 6 to 9 mcg of estradiol to the vagina daily for a period of three months.

c. With low-dose vaginal estrogen, a progestin is not necessary.

F. Osteoporosis. Estrogen is no longer a primary therapy for osteoporosis. Exercise, and daily intake of calcium (1500 mg/day) and vitamin D (400 to 800 IU/day) are recommended for prevention of bone loss in perimenopausal and postmenopausal women.

VI. Treatment of menopausal symptoms with hormone therapy

A. Estrogen prevents bone loss and fracture, but is not cardioprotective, and slightly increases risk. Other risks seen with combined therapy included an increased risk of stroke, venous thromboembolism, and breast cancer.

B. Menopausal symptoms

1. **Hot flashes.** Estrogen therapy remains the gold standard for relief of menopausal symptoms, in particular, hot flashes, and therefore is a reasonable option for most postmenopausal women, with the exception of those with a history of breast cancer, CHD, a previous venous thromboembolic event or stroke, or those at high risk for these complications. In otherwise healthy women, the absolute risk of an adverse event is extremely low.

2. Short-term therapy (with a goal of symptom management) is less than five years.

3. **Adding a progestin.** Endometrial hyperplasia and cancer can occur after as little as six months of unopposed estrogen therapy; as a result, a progestin should be added in women who have not had a hysterectomy. Women who have undergone hysterectomy should not receive a progestin.

4. Hormone preparations: Combined, continuous conjugated estrogens (0.625 mg) and medroxyprogesterone acetate (MPA 2.5 mg) is commonly used. However, low dose estrogen is a better option (eg, 0.3 mg conjugated estrogens or 0.5 mg estradiol).

5. **A low-estrogen oral contraceptive** (20 mcg of ethinyl estradiol) remains an appropriate treatment for perimenopausal women who seek relief of menopausal symptoms, and who also desire contraception, and in some instances need bleeding control (in cases of dysfunctional uterine bleeding). Most of these women are between the ages of 40 and 50 years and are still candidates for oral contraception.

6. When women taking a low-dose oral contraceptive during menopause reach age 50 or 51 years, options include stopping the pill altogether, or changing to an estrogen replacement regimen if necessary for symptoms. Tapering the oral contraceptive by one pill per week is recommended.

References: See page 294.

Osteoporosis

Over 1.3 million osteoporotic fractures occur each year in the United States. The risk of all fractures increases with age; among persons who survive until age 90, 33% of women will have a hip fracture. The lifetime risk of hip fracture for white women at age 50 is 16%. Osteoporosis is characterized by low bone mass, microarchitectural disruption, and increased skeletal fragility.

Risk Factors for Osteoporotic Fractures	
Personal history of fracture as an adult History of fracture in a first-degree relative Current cigarette smoking Low body weight (less than 58 kg [127 lb]) Female sex Estrogen deficiency (menopause before age 45 years or bilateral ovariectomy, prolonged premenopausal amenorrhea [>one year])	White race Advanced age Lifelong low calcium intake Alcoholism Inadequate physical activity Recurrent falls Dementia Impaired eyesight despite adequate correction Poor health/frailty

I. **Screening for osteoporosis and osteopenia**
   A. **Normal bone density** is defined as a bone mineral density (BMD) value within one standard deviation of the mean value in young adults of the same sex and race.
   B. **Osteopenia** is defined as a BMD between 1 and 2.5 standard deviations below the mean.
   C. **Osteoporosis** is defined as a value more than 2.5 standard deviations below the mean; this level is the fracture threshold. These values are referred to as T-scores (number of standard deviations above or below the mean value).
   D. **Dual x-ray absorptiometry.** In dual x-ray absorptiometry (DXA), two photons emitted from an x-ray tube. DXA is the most commonly used method for measuring bone density because it gives very precise measurements with minimal radiation. DXA measurements of the spine and hip are recommended.
II. **Recommendations for screening for osteoporosis of the National Osteoporosis Foundation**
   A. All women should be counseled about the risk factors for osteoporosis, especially smoking cessation and limiting alcohol. All women should be encouraged to participate in regular weight-bearing and exercise.
   B. Measurement of BMD is recommended for all women 65 years and older regardless of risk factors. BMD should also be measured in all women under the age of 65 years who have one or more risk factors for osteoporosis (in addition to menopause). The hip is the recommended site of measurement.
   C. All adults should be advised to consume at least 1,200 mg of calcium per day and 400 to 800 IU of vitamin D per day. A daily multivitamin (which provides 400 IU) is recommended. In patients with documented vitamin D deficiency, osteoporosis, or previous fracture, two multivitamins may be reasonable, particularly if dietary intake is inadequate and access to sunlight is poor.
   D. Treatment is recommended for women without risk factors who have a BMD that is 2 SD below the mean for young women, and in women with risk factors who have a BMD that is 1.5 SD below the mean.
III. **Nonpharmacologic therapy of osteoporosis in women**
   A. **Diet.** An optimal diet for treatment (or prevention) of osteoporosis includes an adequate intake of calories (to avoid malnutrition), calcium, and vitamin D.
   B. **Calcium.** Postmenopausal women should be advised to take 1000 to 1500 mg/day of elemental calcium, in divided doses, with meals.
   C. **Vitamin D** total of 800 IU daily should be taken.
   D. **Exercise.** Women should exercise for at least 30 minutes three times per week. Any weight-bearing exercise regimen, including walking, is acceptable.
   E. **Cessation of smoking** is recommended for all women because smoking cigarettes accelerates bone loss.

IV. Drug therapy of osteoporosis in women

A. Selected postmenopausal women with osteoporosis or at high risk for the disease should be considered for drug therapy. Particular attention should be paid to treating women with a recent fragility fracture, including hip fracture, because they are at high risk for a second fracture.

B. Candidates for drug therapy are women who already have postmenopausal osteoporosis (less than -2.5) and women with osteopenia (T score -1 to -2.5) soon after menopause.

C. **Bisphosphonates**

1. **Alendronate (Fosamax)** (10 mg/day or 70 mg once weekly) or **risedronate (Actonel)** (5 mg/day or 35 mg once weekly) are good choices for the treatment of osteoporosis. Bisphosphonate therapy increases bone mass and reduces the incidence of vertebral and nonvertebral fractures.

2. Alendronate (5 mg/day or 35 mg once weekly) and risedronate (5 mg/day of 35 mg once weekly) have been approved for prevention of osteoporosis.

3. Alendronate or risedronate should be taken with a full glass of water 30 minutes before the first meal or beverage of the day. Patients should not lie down for at least 30 minutes after taking the dose to avoid the unusual complication of pill-induced esophagitis.

4. Alendronate is well tolerated and effective for at least seven years.

5. The bisphosphonates (alendronate or risedronate) and raloxifene are first-line treatments for *prevention* of osteoporosis. The bisphosphonates are first-line therapy for *treatment* of osteoporosis. Bisphosphonates are preferred for prevention and treatment of osteoporosis because they increase bone mineral density more than raloxifene.

D. **Selective estrogen receptor modulators**

1. **Raloxifene (Evista)** (5 mg daily or a once-a-week preparation) is a selective estrogen receptor modulator (SERM) for prevention and treatment of osteoporosis. It increases bone mineral density and reduces serum total and low-density-lipoprotein (LDL) cholesterol. It also appears to reduce the incidence of vertebral fractures and is one of the first-line drugs for prevention of osteoporosis.

2. Raloxifene is somewhat less effective than the bisphosphonates for the prevention and treatment of osteoporosis. Venous thromboembolism is a risk.

Treatment Guidelines for Osteoporosis

Calcium supplements with or without vitamin D supplements or calcium-rich diet
Weight-bearing exercise
Avoidance of alcohol tobacco products
Alendronate (Fosamax)
Risedronate (Actonel)
Raloxifene (Evista)

Agents for Treating Osteoporosis

Medication	Dosage	Route
Calcium	1,000 to 1,500 mg per day	Oral
Vitamin D	400 IU per day (800 IU per day in winter in northern latitudes)	Oral

Medication	Dosage	Route
Alendronate (Fosamax)	**Prevention:** 5 mg per day or 35 mg once-a-week **Treatment:** 10 mg per day or 70 mg once-a-week	Oral
Risedronate (Actonel)	5 mg daily or 35 mg once weekly	Oral
Raloxifene (Evista)	60 mg per day	Oral

- **E. Monitoring the response to therapy**
    1. Bone mineral density and a marker of bone turnover should be measured at baseline, followed by a repeat measurement of the marker in three months.
    2. If the marker falls appropriately, the drug is having the desired effect, and therapy should be continued for two years, at which time bone mineral density can be measured again. The anticipated three-month decline in markers is 50% with alendronate.
- **F. Estrogen/progestin therapy**
    1. Estrogen-progestin therapy is no longer a first-line approach for the treatment of osteoporosis in postmenopausal women because of increases in the risk of breast cancer, stroke, venous thromboembolism, and coronary disease.
    2. Indications for estrogen-progestin in postmenopausal women include persistent menopausal symptoms and patients with an indication for antiresorptive therapy who cannot tolerate the other drugs.

References: See page 294.

Abnormal Vaginal Bleeding

Menorrhagia (excessive bleeding) is most commonly caused by anovulatory menstrual cycles. Occasionally it is caused by thyroid dysfunction, infections or cancer.

- **I. Pathophysiology of normal menstruation**
    - **A.** In response to gonadotropin-releasing hormone from the hypothalamus, the pituitary gland synthesizes follicle-stimulating hormone (FSH) and luteinizing hormone (LH), which induce the ovaries to produce estrogen and progesterone.
    - **B.** During the follicular phase, estrogen stimulation causes an increase in endometrial thickness. After ovulation, progesterone causes endometrial maturation. Menstruation is caused by estrogen and progesterone withdrawal.
    - **C.** **Abnormal bleeding** is defined as bleeding that occurs at intervals of less than 21 days, more than 36 days, lasting longer than 7 days, or blood loss >80 mL.
- **II. Clinical evaluation of abnormal vaginal bleeding**
    - **A.** A menstrual and reproductive history should include last menstrual period, regularity, duration, frequency; the number of pads used per day, and intermenstrual bleeding.
    - **B.** Stress, exercise, weight changes and systemic diseases, particularly thyroid, renal or hepatic diseases or coagulopathies, should be sought. The method of birth control should be determined.
    - **C.** Pregnancy complications, such as spontaneous abortion, ectopic pregnancy, placenta previa and abruptio placentae, can cause heavy bleeding. Pregnancy should always be considered as a possible cause of abnormal vaginal bleeding.

III. Puberty and adolescence – menarche to age 16

A. Irregularity is normal during the first few months of menstruation; however, soaking more than 25 pads or 30 tampons during a menstrual period is abnormal.

B. Absence of premenstrual symptoms (breast tenderness, bloating, cramping) is associated with anovulatory cycles.

C. Fever, particularly in association with pelvic or abdominal pain may, indicate pelvic inflammatory disease. A history of easy bruising suggests a coagulation defect. Headaches and visual changes suggest a pituitary tumor.

D. Physical findings
1. Pallor not associated with tachycardia or signs of hypovolemia suggests chronic excessive blood loss secondary to anovulatory bleeding, adenomyosis, uterine myomas, or blood dyscrasia.
2. Fever, leukocytosis, and pelvic tenderness suggests PID.
3. Signs of impending shock indicate that the blood loss is related to pregnancy (including ectopic), trauma, sepsis, or neoplasia.
4. Pelvic masses may represent pregnancy, uterine or ovarian neoplasia, or a pelvic abscess or hematoma.
5. Fine, thinning hair, and hypoactive reflexes suggest hypothyroidism.
6. Ecchymoses or multiple bruises may indicate trauma, coagulation defects, medication use, or dietary extremes.

E. Laboratory tests
1. CBC and platelet count and a urine or serum pregnancy test should be obtained.
2. Screening for sexually transmitted diseases, thyroid function, and coagulation disorders (partial thromboplastin time, INR, bleeding time) should be completed.
3. **Endometrial sampling** is rarely necessary for those under age 20.

F. Treatment of infrequent bleeding
1. Therapy should be directed at the underlying cause when possible. If the CBC and other initial laboratory tests are normal and the history and physical examination are normal, reassurance is usually all that is necessary.
2. Ferrous gluconate, 325 mg bid-tid, should be prescribed.

G. Treatment of frequent or heavy bleeding
1. Treatment with nonsteroidal anti-inflammatory drugs (NSAIDs) improves platelet aggregation and increases uterine vasoconstriction. NSAIDs are the first choice in the treatment of menorrhagia because they are well tolerated and do not have the hormonal effects of oral contraceptives.
   a. **Mefenamic acid (Ponstel)** 500 mg tid during the menstrual period.
   b. **Naproxen (Anaprox, Naprosyn)** 500 mg loading dose, then 250 mg tid during the menstrual period.
   c. **Ibuprofen (Motrin, Nuprin)** 400 mg tid during the menstrual period.
   d. Gastrointestinal distress is common. NSAIDs are contraindicated in renal failure and peptic ulcer disease.
2. Iron should also be added as ferrous gluconate 325 mg tid.

H. Patients with hypovolemia and a hemoglobin level below 7 g/dL should be hospitalized for hormonal therapy and iron replacement.
1. Hormonal therapy consists of estrogen (Premarin) 25 mg IV q6h until bleeding stops. Thereafter, oral contraceptive pills should be administered q6h x 7 days, then taper slowly to one pill qd.
2. If bleeding continues, IV vasopressin (DDAVP) should be administered. Hysteroscopy may be necessary, and dilation and curettage is a last resort. Transfusion may be indicated in severe hemorrhage.
3. Iron should also be added as ferrous gluconate 325 mg tid.

IV. Primary childbearing years – ages 16 to early 40s

A. Contraceptive complications and pregnancy are the most common causes of abnormal bleeding in this age group. Anovulation accounts for 20% of cases.

B. Adenomyosis, endometriosis, and fibroids increase in frequency as a woman ages, as do endometrial hyperplasia and endometrial polyps. Pelvic inflammatory disease and endocrine dysfunction may also occur.

C. **Laboratory tests**
   1. CBC and platelet count, Pap smear, and pregnancy test.
   2. Screening for sexually transmitted diseases, thyroid-stimulating hormone, and coagulation disorders (partial thromboplastin time, INR, bleeding time).
   3. If a non-pregnant woman has a pelvic mass, ultrasonography or hysterosonography (with uterine saline infusion) is required.

D. **Endometrial sampling**
   1. Long-term unopposed estrogen stimulation in anovulatory patients can result in endometrial hyperplasia, which can progress to adenocarcinoma; therefore, in perimenopausal patients who have been anovulatory for an extended interval, the endometrium should be biopsied.
   2. Biopsy is also recommended before initiation of hormonal therapy for women over age 30 and for those over age 20 who have had prolonged bleeding.
   3. Hysteroscopy and endometrial biopsy with a Pipelle aspirator should be done on the first day of menstruation (to avoid an unexpected pregnancy) or anytime if bleeding is continuous.

E. **Treatment**
   1. Medical protocols for anovulatory bleeding (dysfunctional uterine bleeding) are similar to those described above for adolescents.
   2. **Hormonal therapy**
      a. In women who do not desire immediate fertility, hormonal therapy may be used to treat menorrhagia.
      b. A 21-day package of oral contraceptives is used. The patient should take one pill three times a day for 7 days. During the 7 days of therapy, bleeding should subside, and, following treatment, heavy flow will occur. After 7 days off the hormones, another 21-day package is initiated, taking one pill each day for 21 days, then no pills for 7 days.
      c. Alternatively, medroxyprogesterone (Provera), 10-20 mg per day for days 16 through 25 of each month, will result in a reduction of menstrual blood loss. Pregnancy will not be prevented.
      d. Patients with severe bleeding may have hypotension and tachycardia. These patients require hospitalization, and estrogen (Premarin) should be administered IV as 25 mg q4-6h until bleeding slows (up to a maximum of four doses). Oral contraceptives should be initiated concurrently as described above.
   3. Iron should also be added as ferrous gluconate 325 mg tid.
   4. Surgical treatment can be considered if childbearing is completed and medical management fails to provide relief.

V. **Premenopausal, perimenopausal, and postmenopausal years--age 40 and over**

   A. Anovulatory bleeding accounts for about 90% of abnormal vaginal bleeding in this age group. However, bleeding should be considered to be from cancer until proven otherwise.

   B. History, physical examination and laboratory testing are indicated as described above. Menopausal symptoms, personal or family history of malignancy and use of estrogen should be sought. A pelvic mass requires an evaluation with ultrasonography.

   C. **Endometrial carcinoma**
      1. In a perimenopausal or postmenopausal woman, amenorrhea preceding abnormal bleeding suggests endometrial cancer. Endometrial evaluation is necessary before treatment of abnormal vaginal bleeding.

2. Before endometrial sampling, determination of endometrial thickness by transvaginal ultrasonography is useful because biopsy is often not required when the endometrium is less than 5 mm thick.

D. **Treatment**
   1. Cystic hyperplasia or endometrial hyperplasia without cytologic atypia is treated with depo-medroxyprogesterone, 200 mg IM, then 100 to 200 mg IM every 3 to 4 weeks for 6 to 12 months. Endometrial hyperplasia requires repeat endometrial biopsy every 3 to 6 months.
   2. Atypical hyperplasia requires fractional dilation and curettage, followed by progestin therapy or hysterectomy.
   3. If the patient's endometrium is normal (or atrophic) and contraception is a concern, a low-dose oral contraceptive may be used. If contraception is not needed, estrogen and progesterone therapy should be prescribed.
   4. **Surgical management**
      a. **Vaginal or abdominal hysterectomy** is the most absolute curative treatment.
      b. **Dilatation and curettage** can be used as a temporizing measure to stop bleeding.
      c. **Endometrial ablation and resection** by laser, electrodiathermy "rollerball," or excisional resection are alternatives to hysterectomy.

References: See page 294.

Pelvic Inflammatory Disease

Pelvic inflammatory disease (PID) is an acute infection of the upper genital tract structures in women, involving the uterus, oviducts, and ovaries. PID usually is a community-acquired infection initiated by a sexually transmitted agent. The estimated number of cases of PID in women 15 to 44 years of age in the United States was 168,837 in 2003.

I. **Clinical features**
   A. **Lower abdominal pain** is the cardinal presenting symptom in women with PID. The recent onset of pain that worsens during coitus or with jarring movement may be the only presenting symptom of PID; the onset of pain during or shortly after menses is particularly suggestive. The abdominal pain is usually bilateral and rarely of more than two weeks' duration.
   B. **Abnormal uterine bleeding** occurs in one-third or more of patients with PID. New vaginal discharge, urethritis, proctitis, fever, and chills can be associated signs. The presence of PID is less likely if symptoms referable to the bowel or urinary tract predominate.
   C. **Risk factors for sexually transmitted diseases:**
      1. Age less than 25 years
      2. Young age at first sex
      3. Nonbarrier contraception
      4. New, multiple, or symptomatic sexual partners
      5. Oral contraception
      6. Cervical ectopy
   D. **Factors that facilitate pelvic inflammatory disease:**
      1. Previous episode of PID
      2. Sex during menses
      3. Vaginal douching
      4. Bacterial vaginosis
      5. Intrauterine device
   E. **Physical examination.** Only one-half of patients with PID have fever. Abdominal examination reveals diffuse tenderness greatest in the lower quadrants, which may or may not be symmetrical. Rebound tenderness and decreased bowel sounds are common. Marked tenderness in the

right upper quadrant does not exclude PID, since 10% of these patients have perihepatitis (Fitz-Hugh Curtis syndrome).

F. **Pelvic examination.** Purulent endocervical discharge and/or acute cervical motion and adnexal tenderness with bimanual examination is strongly suggestive of PID. Significant lateralization of adnexal tenderness is uncommon in PID.

G. **Subclinical pelvic inflammatory disease.** Lower genital tract infection with gonorrhea, chlamydia, or bacterial vaginosis is a risk factor for subclinical PID, defined by the presence of neutrophils and plasma cells in endometrial tissue.

II. Diagnostic considerations

A. Laparoscopy is recommended for the following:
1. A sick patient with high suspicion of a competing diagnosis (appendicitis)
2. An acutely ill patient who has failed outpatient treatment for PID
3. Any patient not clearly improving after 72 hours of inpatient treatment for PID. Consent for laparotomy at the same procedure should be obtained in advance for these patients.

B. **Diagnostic criteria.** The index of suspicion for the clinical diagnosis of PID should be high, especially in adolescent women, even if they deny sexual activity. Empiric treatment is recommended for women with abdominal pain who have at least one of the following:
1. Cervical motion tenderness or uterine/adnexal tenderness
2. Oral temperature >101 F (>38.3 C)
3. Peripheral leukocytosis/left shift
4. Abnormal cervical or vaginal mucopurulent discharge
5. Presence of white blood cells (WBCs) on saline microscopy of vaginal secretions
6. Elevated erythrocyte sedimentation rate
7. Elevated C-reactive protein

III. Differential diagnosis.
In addition to PID, the differential diagnosis of lower abdominal pain in a young woman includes the following conditions:

A. Gastrointestinal: Appendicitis, cholecystitis, constipation, gastroenteritis, inflammatory bowel disease

B. Renal: Cystitis, pyelonephritis, nephrolithiasis, urethritis

C. Obstetric/Gynecologic: Dysmenorrhea, ectopic pregnancy, intrauterine pregnancy complication, ovarian cyst, ovarian torsion, ovarian tumor.

Differential Diagnosis of Pelvic Inflammatory Disease	
Appendicitis Ectopic pregnancy Hemorrhagic ovarian cyst Ovarian torsion Endometriosis Urinary tract Infection	Irritable bowel syndrome Somatization Gastroenteritis Cholecystitis Nephrolithiasis

IV. Diagnostic testing

A. **Laboratory testing** for patients suspected of PID always begins with a pregnancy test to rule out ectopic pregnancy and complications of an intrauterine pregnancy. A urinalysis (preferably on a catheterized specimen) and a stool for occult blood should be obtained since abnormalities in either lessen the probability of PID. Although PID is usually an acute process, fewer than one-half of PID patients exhibit leukocytosis. A hematocrit of less than 0.30 makes PID less likely.

B. **Gram stain and microscopic examination** of vaginal discharge. If a cervical Gram stain is positive for Gram negative intracellular diplococci, the probability of PID greatly increases; if negative, it is of little use.

    C. Increased white blood cells (WBC) in vaginal fluid is the most sensitive single laboratory test for PID (78% for $\geq$3 WBC per high power field. However, the specificity is only 39%.

    D. **Recommended laboratory tests:**
1. Pregnancy test
2. Microscopic exam of vaginal discharge in saline
3. Complete blood counts
4. Nucleic acid amplification tests for chlamydia and gonococcus
5. Urinalysis
6. Fecal occult blood test
7. C-reactive protein (optional)
8. Ultrasounds are reserved for acutely ill patients with PID in whom a pelvic abscess is a consideration.

V. Treatment and sequelae of pelvic inflammatory disease

    A. **Outpatient therapy.** The CDC recommends either oral ofloxacin (Floxin, 400 mg twice daily) or levofloxacin (Levaquin, 500 mg once daily) with or without metronidazole (Flagyl) 500 mg twice daily) for 14 days. Metronidazole is added when anaerobic coverage is of concern. Beyond 48 hours of symptoms, the most frequent isolates are anaerobes.

    B. An alternative is an initial single dose of ceftriaxone (Rocephin, 250 mg IM), cefoxitin (Mefoxin, 2 g IM plus probenecid 1 g orally), or another parenteral third-generation cephalosporin, followed by doxycycline (100 mg orally twice daily) with or without metronidazole for 14 days. The combination of amoxicillin-clavulanate and doxycycline is also an alternative that has achieved short-term clinical response. For patients younger than 18 years of age, one of the alternative regimens should be used since neither ofloxacin nor levofloxacin is approved for systemic use in this age group.

    C. **For women younger than 18 years** treatment consists of an initial single dose of ceftriaxone (Rocephin, 250 mg IM) or cefoxitin (Mefoxin, 2 g IM plus probenecid 1 g orally), or another parenteral third-generation cephalosporin, followed by doxycycline (100 mg orally twice daily) with or without metronidazole for 14 days. For those who are unlikely to complete at least seven days of doxycycline, some providers suggest administration of azithromycin 1 g PO should be given at the time of parenteral adminstration of cephalosporin to ensure eradication of chlamydia.

    D. **For women >18 years azithromycin (Zithromax)** 1 g PO should be given for Chlamydia coverage, and either cefixime (Suprax) 400 mg PO or ceftriaxone (Rocephin) 125 mg IM (for gonococcus coverage) given for one dose by directly observed therapy, followed by amoxicillin-clavulanate 875 mg PO twice daily for 7 to 10 days. For penicillin-allergic patients, a fluoroquinolone or spectinomycin may be used for initial single-dose gonococcus coverage, followed by doxycycline and metronidazole for 14 days.

    E. Reevaluation two to three days after the initiation of therapy to assure accuracy of diagnosis and response to therapy is an extremely important aspect of outpatient treatment of PID.

    F. **Inpatient therapy.** The CDC suggest either of the following regimens:
1. Cefotetan (Cefotan, 2 g IV every12h) or cefoxitin (Mefoxin, 2 g IV every 6h) plus doxycycline (100 mg IV or PO every 12h), or
2. Clindamycin (900 mg IV every 8h) plus gentamicin loading dose (2 mg/kg of body weight) followed by a maintenance dose (1.5 mg/kg) every 8 hours. Single daily dosing of gentamicin may be substituted.
3. **Alternative regimens:**
    a. Ofloxacin (Floxin, 400 mg IV every12h) or levofloxacin (Levoquin, 500 mg IV daily) with or without metronidazole (Flagyl, 500 mg IV every 8h), or
    b. Ampicillin-sulbactam (Unasyn, 3 g IV every 6h) plus doxycycline (100 mg IV or PO every12h).

       c. Ofloxacin has been studied as monotherapy for the treatment of PID; however, due to concerns regarding its lack of activity against anaerobic flora, some clinicians prefer to also add metronidazole. Ampicillin-sulbactam plus oral doxycycline is effective coverage against Chlamydia trachomatis, Neisseria gonorrhoeae, and anaerobes.

   4. Parenteral administration of antibiotics should be continued for 24 hours after a clear clinical response, followed by doxycycline (100 mg PO BID) or clindamycin (450 mg PO QID) for a total of 14 days.

G. Recommended regimens:

   1. Levofloxacin (Levoquin, 500 mg IV Q24h) plus metronidazole (500 mg IV Q8h)

   2. A broad spectrum cephalosporin plus doxycycline with or without metronidazole

   3. Ertapenem (Invanz, 1 g IV Q24h)

H. For patients younger than 18 years of age, the second regimen should be used since levofloxacin is not approved for use in this age group when other effective alternatives are available.

I. Some providers prescribe azithromycin (Zithromax, 1 g PO once) as soon as the patient is tolerating oral intake if the patient is unlikely to comply with doxycycline administration. Parenteral therapy should continue until the pelvic tenderness is absent (two to five days).

J. Treatment for PID must be accompanied by a discussion of sexually transmitted infections, partner treatment, and future safe sex practices. Male sex partners of women with PID should be examined and empiri-cally treated if they had sexual contact during the preceding 60 days. Other important components of the evaluation include:

   1. Serology for human immunodeficiency virus (HIV)

   2. Papanicolaou smear

   3. Hepatitis B surface antigen determination and initiation of the vaccine series for patients who are antigen negative and unvaccinated

   4. Hepatitis C virus serology

   5. Serologic tests for syphilis

References: See page 294.

Genital Chlamydia Trachomatis Infections

Chlamydia trachomatis is the most common sexually transmitted genital infection. Infants born to mothers through an infected birth canal can develop conjunctivitis and pneumonia. These syndromes are caused by the C. trachomatis serovars B and D through K. The L serovars cause lymphogranuloma venereum (LGV), a genital ulcer syndrome. Chlamydia trachomatis serovars A to C cause endemic trachoma, a common ocular infection in the developing world.

I. Microbiology and epidemiology

   A. C. trachomatis is a small gram-negative bacterium and an obligate intracellular parasite.

   B. Chlamydia cannot be cultured on artificial media; tissue culture has been required. Rapid screening tests are now available.

   C. 4,000,000 cases of C. trachomatis infection occur annually. C. trachomatis and Neisseria gonorrhoeae cause similar clinical syndromes, but chlamydia infections tend to have fewer acute symptoms and more significant long-term complications.

   D. Prevalence. The rates of chlamydia are highest in adolescent women. Between 18 and 26 years of age, the prevalence of chlamydial infection is 4.2%. The highest rates are in African American women (14%) and are higher in women than men.

   E. Risk factors for Chlamydia trachomatis infection:

     1. Adolescents and young adults

      2. Multiple sex partners or a partner with other partners during the last three months or a recent new sex partner
      3. Inconsistent use of barrier contraceptives
      4. Clinical evidence of mucopurulent cervicitis
      5. Cervical ectopy
      6. Unmarried status
      7. History of prior sexually transmitted disease
      8. Lower socioeconomic class or education not beyond high school.

II. Clinical manifestations

  A. The majority of women with C. trachomatis infection are asymptomatic; however, cervicitis or pelvic inflammatory disease may occur.

  B. Cervicitis. Cervical infection is the most common chlamydial syndrome in women. More than 50% of these women are asymptomatic. Vaginal discharge, poorly differentiated abdominal pain, or lower abdominal pain are the most frequent symptoms.

  C. Physical examination is often unremarkable, mucopurulent cervical discharge, cervical friability, cervical edema, and endocervical ulcers may be seen.

  D. Perihepatitis (Fitzhugh-Curtis syndrome). Patients with chlamydia infection occasionally develop perihepatitis, an inflammation of the liver capsule and adjacent peritoneal surfaces. Perihepatitis is more commonly seen in PID, occurring in 5% of cases.

  E. Pelvic inflammatory disease. 30% of women with chlamydia infection will develop PID if left untreated. While PID caused by N. gonorrhoeae infection may be more acutely symptomatic, PID due to C. trachomatis tends to cause higher rates of infertility.

  F. Pregnancy. Untreated chlamydia infection can increase the risk for premature rupture of the membranes and low birth weight. If the mother is untreated, 20 to 50% of newborns will develop conjunctivitis, and 10 to 20% will develop pneumonia.

III. Diagnosis

  A. Nucleic acid amplification (NAAT) uses polymerase chain reaction (PCR). These sensitive and specific tests have replaced poorly standardized cell culture methods as the "gold standard."
      1. Another advantage of NAATs is the ability to perform testing on urine as well as urethral specimens. Since urine collection is noninvasive, it is a preferred method.
      2. The PCR assay has a sensitivity and specificity of 83 and 99.5% for urine samples and 86 and 99.6% for cervical samples.

  B. Antigen detection requires a swab from the cervix or urethra. The sensitivity of this method is 80 to 95% compared to culture.

IV. Chlamydia screening

  A. Clinical practice guidelines strongly recommend routine chlamydia screening for sexually-active women below the age of 25.

V. Treatment.

Chlamydiae are susceptible to the tetracyclines and the macrolides. Treatment efficacy with recommended regimens is >95%.

  A. Azithromycin (Zithromax, 1 g PO as a single dose) or doxycycline (100 mg PO BID for 7 days) are the two recommended regimens.

  B. Alternative regimens include seven days of erythromycin base (500 mg PO QID), erythromycin ethylsuccinate (800 mg PO), ofloxacin (300 mg PO BID), or levofloxacin (500 mg PO QD). Erythromycin is associated with significant gastrointestinal side effects; ofloxacin and levofloxacin are expensive alternatives.

Treatment of chlamydia trachomatis infection and related syndromes

Urethritis, cervicitis, conjunctivitis, or proctitis

Azithromycin (Zithromax) 1 g oral once **OR**
Doxycycline 100 mg oral twice daily for seven days
Alternatives
Ofloxacin (Floxin) 300 mg oral twice daily for seven days
Levofloxacin (Levaquin) 500 mg oral daily for seven days
Erythromycin 500 mg oral four times daily for seven days

Infection in pregnancy

Azithromycin (Zithromax) 1 g oral once **OR**
Amoxicillin 500 mg oral three times daily for seven days
Alternatives
Erythromycin 500 mg oral four times daily for seven days

Neonatal ophthalmia or pneumonia

Azithromycin 20 mg/kg oral once daily for three days
Alternatives
Erythromycin 12.5 mg/kg oral four times daily for 14 days§

Lymphogranuloma venereum

Doxycycline 100 mg oral twice daily for 21 days
Alternatives
Erythromycin 500 mg oral four times daily for 21 days

C. **Adjunctive measures:**
   1. Presumptive treatment of partners
   2. Evaluation for other STDs (syphilis serology, gonococcal testing)
   3. HIV counseling and testing
   4. Safer-sex counseling and condom provision
   5. Contraception provision or referral
   6. Test of cure. Testing for C. trachomatis following treatment with azithromycin or doxycycline is not recommended. Exceptions include:
      a. Patients with persisting symptoms or
      b. Those in whom compliance with the treatment regimen is suspected.
      c. Pregnant females
   7. If a test for cure is performed, this should be done more than three weeks after the completion of therapy.
   8. Repeat screening should be considered within the first three to four months after therapy is completed or at least when the patient has her next encounter with the healthcare system within the first 12 months because patients who have the disease once are at a higher risk for acquiring it again.
References: See page 294.

Vaginitis

Approximately 8-18% of women report an episode of vaginal symptoms each year. The etiology of vaginal complaints includes infection of the vagina, cervix, and upper genital tract, chemicals or irritants (eg, spermicides or douching), hormone deficiency, and rarely systemic diseases.

I. Clinical evaluation
A. Symptoms of vaginitis include vaginal discharge, pruritus, irritation, soreness, odor, dyspareunia and dysuria. Dyspareunia is a common feature of atrophic vaginitis. Abdominal pain is suggestive of pelvic inflammatory disease and suprapubic pain is suggestive of cystitis.

B. A new sexual partner increases the risk of acquiring sexually transmitted diseases, such as trichomonas, chlamydia, or Neisseria gonorrheae. Trichomoniasis often occurs during or immediately after the menstrual period; candida vulvovaginitis often occurs during the premenstrual period.

C. Antibiotics and high-estrogen oral contraceptive pills may predispose to candida vulvovaginitis; increased physiologic discharge can occur with oral contraceptives; pruritus unresponsive to antifungal agents suggests vulvar dermatitis.

II. Physical examination
A. The vulva usually appears normal in bacterial vaginosis. Erythema, edema, or fissure formation suggest candidiasis, trichomoniasis, or dermatitis.

B. Trichomonas is associated with a purulent discharge; candidiasis is associated with a thick, adherent, "cottage cheese-like" discharge; and bacterial vaginosis is associated with a thin, homogeneous, "fishy smelling" discharge. The cervix in women with cervicitis is usually erythematous and friable, with a mucopurulent discharge.

C. Abdominal or cervical motion tenderness is suggestive of PID.

III. Diagnostic studies
A. **Vaginal pH.** The pH of the normal vaginal secretions is 4.0 to 4.5. A pH above 4.5 suggests bacterial vaginosis or trichomoniasis (pH 5 to 6), and helps to exclude candida vulvovaginitis (pH 4 to 4.5).

B. **Saline microscopy** should look for candidal buds or hyphae, motile trichomonads, epithelial cells studded with adherent coccobacilli (clue cells), and polymorphonuclear cells (PMNs). The addition of 10% potassium hydroxide to the wet mount is helpful in diagnosing candida vaginitis. Culture for candida and trichomonas may be useful if microscopy is negative.

C. **Cervical culture.** A diagnosis of cervicitis, typically due to Neisseria gonorrhoeae or Chlamydia trachomatis, must always be considered in women with purulent vaginal discharge. The presence of high-risk behavior or any sexually transmitted disease requires screening for HIV, hepatitis B, and other STDs.

Clinical Manifestations of Vaginitis	
Candidal Vaginitis	Nonmalodorous, thick, white, "cottage cheese-like" discharge that adheres to vaginal walls Hyphal forms or budding yeast cells on wet-mount Pruritus Normal pH (<4.5)
Bacterial Vaginosis	Thin, dark or dull grey, homogeneous, malodorous discharge that adheres to the vaginal walls Elevated pH level (>4.5) Positive KOH (whiff test) Clue cells on wet-mount microscopic evaluation

Trichomonas Vaginalis	Copious, yellow-gray or green, homogeneous or frothy, malodorous discharge Elevated pH level (>4.5) Mobile, flagellated organisms and leukocytes on wet-mount microscopic evaluation Vulvovaginal irritation, dysuria
Atrophic Vaginitis	Vaginal dryness or burning

IV. **Bacterial vaginosis**
   A. **Incidence.** Bacterial vaginosis is the most common cause of vaginitis in women of childbearing age, with prevalence of 5-60%.
   B. **Microbiology and risk factors.** Bacterial vaginosis represents a change in vaginal flora characterized by a reduction of lactobacilli and an increase of Gardnerella vaginalis, Mobiluncus species, Mycoplasma hominis, anaerobic gram-negative rods, and Peptostreptococcus species. Risk factors for bacterial vaginosis include multiple or new sexual partners, early age of first coitus, douching, cigarette smoking, and use of an intrauterine contraceptive device.
   C. **Clinical features.** Symptoms include a "fishy smelling" discharge that is more noticeable after unprotected intercourse. The discharge is off-white, thin, and homogeneous. Pruritus and inflammation are absent.
   D. **Complications**
      1. Pregnant women appear to be at higher risk of preterm delivery.
      2. Bacterial vaginosis may cause plasma-cell endometritis, postpartum fever, post-hysterectomy vaginal-cuff cellulitis, and postabortal infection.
      3. Bacterial vaginosis is a risk factor for HIV acquisition and transmission.
   E. **Diagnosis.** Three of the four criteria listed below are necessary for diagnosis.
      1. Homogeneous, grayish-white discharge
      2. Vaginal pH >4.5
      3. Positive whiff-amine test, defined as the presence of a fishy odor when 10% KOH is added to vaginal discharge samples
      4. Clue cells on saline wet mount (epithelial cells studded with coccobacilli)
   F. **Therapy.** Treatment is indicated in women with symptomatic infection and those with asymptomatic infection prior to abortion or hysterectomy.
      1. Metronidazole or clindamycin administered either orally or intravaginally will result in a high rate of clinical cure (70-80%). Oral medication is more convenient.
      2. The oral regimen is 500 mg twice daily for 7 days. Topical vaginal therapy with 0.75% metronidazole gel (MetroGel, 5 g once daily for 5 days) is as effective as oral metronidazole.
      3. Single-dose therapy with 2 g of metronidazole achieves a similar immediate rate of clinical response.
      4. Side effects of metronidazole include a metallic taste, nausea, a disulfiram-like effect with alcohol, interaction with warfarin, and peripheral neuropathy.
   G. **Relapse**
      1. Approximately 30% of patients have a recurrence within three months. Recurrence usually reflects a failure to eradicate the offending organisms. Management of symptomatic relapse includes prolonged therapy for 10 to 14 days.
      2. Most women with a history of recurrent infection benefit from suppressive therapy with metronidazole gel 0.75% for 10 days, followed by twice-weekly applications for three to six months.
V. **Candida vulvovaginitis**
   A. **Incidence.** Candida vulvovaginitis accounts for one-third of vaginitis. Up to 75% of women report having had at least one episode of candidiasis. The

condition is rare before menarche. It is less common in postmenopausal women, unless they are taking estrogen replacement therapy.

B. Microbiology and risk factors. Candida albicans is responsible for 80-92% of vulvovaginal candidiasis.

1. **Antibiotics.** A minority of women are prone to vulvovaginal candidiasis while taking antibiotics.

2. **Intrauterine devices** have been associated with vulvovaginal candidiasis.

3. **Pregnancy.** Symptomatic infection is more common in pregnancy.

C. Clinical features. Vulvar pruritus is the dominant feature. Women may also complain of dysuria (external rather than urethral), soreness, irritation, and dyspareunia. There is often little or no discharge. Physical examination often reveals erythema of the vulva and vaginal mucosa. The discharge is thick, adherent, and "cottage cheese-like."

D. Diagnosis

1. The vaginal pH is typically 4 to 4.5, which distinguishes candidiasis from Trichomonas or bacterial vaginosis. The diagnosis is confirmed by finding the organism on a wet mount; adding 10% potassium hydroxide facilitates recognition of budding yeast and hyphae. Microscopy is negative in 50% of patients with vulvovaginal candidiasis.

2. Empiric therapy is often considered in women with typical clinical features, a normal vaginal pH, and no other pathogens visible on microscopy. Culture should be performed in patients with persistent or recurrent symptoms.

E. Therapy

1. Women with mild infection usually respond to treatment within a couple of days. More severe infections require a longer course of therapy and may take up to 14 days to fully resolve.

2. **Uncomplicated infection.** Both oral and topical antimycotic drugs achieve comparable clinical cure rates that are in excess of 80%.

3. Oral azole agents are more convenient. Side effects of single-dose fluconazole (150 mg) tend to be mild and infrequent, including gastrointestinal intolerance, headache, and rash.

Treatment regimens for yeast vaginitis*

1-day regimens
Clotrimazole vaginal tablets (Mycelex G), 500 mg hs**
Fluconazole tablets (Diflucan), 150 mg PO
Itraconazole capsules (Sporanox), 200 mg PO bid
Tioconazole 6.5% vaginal ointment (Vagistat-1), 4.6 g hs** [5 g]

3-day regimens
Butoconazole nitrate 2% vaginal cream (Femstat 3), 5 g hs [28 g]
Clotrimazole vaginal inserts (Gyne-Lotrimin 3), 200 mg hs**
Miconazole vaginal suppositories (Monistat 3), 200 mg hs**
Terconazole 0.8% vaginal cream (Terazol 3), 5 g hs
Terconazole vaginal suppositories (Terazol 3), 80 mg hs
Itraconazole capsules (Sporanox), 200 mg PO qd

5-day regimen
Ketoconazole tablets (Nizoral), 400 mg PO bid

7-day regimens
Clotrimazole 1% cream (Gyne-Lotrimin, Mycelex-7, Sweet'n Fresh Clotrimazole-7), 5 g hs**
Clotrimazole vaginal tablets (Gyne-Lotrimin, Mycelex-7, Sweet'n Fresh Clotrimazole-7), 100 mg hs**
Miconazole 2% vaginal cream (Femizol-M, Monistat 7), 5 g hs**
Miconazole vaginal suppositories (Monistat 7), 100 mg hs**
Terconazole 0.4% vaginal cream (Terazol 7), 5 g hs

14-day regimens
Nystatin vaginal tablets (Mycostatin), 100,000 U hs

*Suppositories can be used if inflammation is predominantly vaginal; creams if vulvar; a combination if both. Cream-suppository combination packs available: clotrimazole (Gyne-Lotrimin, Mycelex); miconazole (Monistat, M-Zole). Use 1-day or 3-day regimen if compliance is an issue. Miconazole nitrate may be used during pregnancy.

**Nonprescription formulation. If nonprescription therapies fail, use terconazole 0.4% cream or 80-mg suppositories at bedtime for 7 days.

4. **Complicated infections.** Factors that predispose to complicated infection include uncontrolled diabetes, immunosuppression, and a history of recurrent vulvovaginal candidiasis. Women with severe inflammation or complicated infection require seven to 14 days of topical therapy or two doses of oral therapy 72 hours apart.

Management options for complicated or recurrent yeast vaginitis

Extend any 7-day regimen to 10 to 14 days
Eliminate use of nylon or tight-fitting clothing
Consider discontinuing oral contraceptives
Consider eating 8 oz yogurt (with Lactobacillus acidophilus culture) per day
Improve glycemic control in diabetic patients
For long-term suppression of recurrent vaginitis, use ketoconazole, 100 mg (½ of 200-mg tablet) qd for 6 months

5. **Partner treatment** is not necessary since this is not a primary route of transmission.
6. **Pregnancy.** Topical azoles applied for seven days are recommended for treatment during pregnancy.

VI. **Trichomoniasis**
A. Trichomoniasis, the third most common cause of vaginitis, is caused by the flagellated protozoan, Trichomonas vaginalis. The disorder is virtually always sexually transmitted.
B. **Clinical features.** Trichomoniasis in women ranges from an asymptomatic state to a severe, acute, inflammatory disease. Signs and symptoms include a purulent, malodorous, thin discharge (70%) with associated burning, pruritus, dysuria, and dyspareunia. Physical examination reveals erythema of the vulva and vaginal mucosa; the classic green-yellow frothy discharge is observed in 10-30%. Punctate hemorrhages may be visible on the vagina and cervix in 2%.
C. **Complications.** Infection is associated with premature rupture of the membranes and prematurity; however, treatment of asymptomatic infection has not been shown to reduce these complications. Trichomoniasis is a risk factor for development of post-hysterectomy cellulitis. The infection facilitates transmission of the human immunodeficiency virus.
D. **Diagnosis**
1. The presence of motile trichomonads on wet mount is diagnostic of infection, but this occurs in only 50-70% of cases. Other findings include an elevated vaginal pH (>4.5) and an increase in polymorphonuclear leukocytes on saline microscopy.
E. **Culture on Diamond's medium** has a high sensitivity (95%) and specificity (>95%) and should be considered in patients with elevated vaginal pH, increased numbers of polymorphonuclear leukocytes and an absence of motile trichomonads and clue cells on wet mount.
F. **The OSOM Trichomonas Rapid Test for Trichomonas** antigens has a sensitivity of 88.3% and specificity of 98.8%. Results can be read in 10 minutes. The Affirm VP III Microbial Identification System (Becton Dickinson) test uses a nucleic acid probe and is read in 45 minutes.

G. **Cervical cytology.** Trichomonads are sometimes reported on conventional Papanicolaou (Pap) smears. Conventional Pap smears are inadequate for diagnosis of trichomoniasis because this technique has a sensitivity of only 60 to 70% and false positive results are common (at least 8%). Asymptomatic women with trichomonads identified on conventional Pap smear should be evaluated by wet mount and should not be treated until the diagnosis is confirmed.

H. Treatment of asymptomatic women with trichomonads noted on liquid-based cervical cytology is appropriate.

VII. **Treatment of Trichomonas vaginitis**

A. **Nonpregnant women**

1. The 5-nitroimidazole drugs (metronidazole or tinidazole) are the only class of drugs that provide curative therapy of trichomoniasis. Cure rates are 90 to 95%.

2. Treatment consists of a single oral dose of 2 grams (four 500 mg tablets) of either tinidazole (Fasigyn) or metronidazole (Flagyl). Cure rates with tinidazole are comparable to those of metronidazole, but better tolerated.

3. Similar cure rates are obtained with single and multiple dose regimens (82 to 88%). Side effects (eg, nausea, vomiting, headache, metallic taste, dizziness) appear to be dose related and occur less frequently with the lower doses of multiple dose, prolonged therapy (eg, metronidazole 500 mg twice daily for seven days. There is no multiple dose regimen for tinidazole).

4. Oral is preferred to vaginal therapy since systemic administration achieves therapeutic drug levels in the urethra and periurethral glands.

5. Patients should be advised to not consume alcohol for 24 hours after metronidazole treatment and 72 hours after tinidazole treatment because of the possibility of a disulfiram-like (Antabuse effect) reaction.

6. Follow-up is unnecessary for women who become asymptomatic after treatment.

B. **Male partners.** T vaginalis infection in men is often asymptomatic and transient (spontaneous resolution within 10 days). Symptoms, when present, consist of a clear or mucopurulent urethral discharge and/or dysuria. Complications include prostatitis, balanoposthitis, epididymitis, and infertility. Maximal cure rates are achieved when sexual partners are treated simultaneously with the affected woman. Neither partner should resume intercourse until both partners have completed treatment, otherwise reinfection can occur.

C. **Pregnancy**

1. Metronidazole is the drug of choice for treatment of symptomatic trichomoniasis in pregnancy. Meta-analysis has not found any relationship between metronidazole exposure during the first trimester of pregnancy and birth defects. The Centers for Disease Control and Prevention no longer discourage the use of metronidazole in the first trimester.

2. In pregnant women, some clinicians prefer metronidazole 500 mg twice daily for five to seven days to the 2 g single dose regimen because of the lower frequency of side effects.

3. Asymptomatic infections during pregnancy should not be treated because treatment does not prevent, and may even increase, the risk of preterm delivery.

Treatment options for trichomoniasis

Initial measures
Tinidazole (Fasigyn) 2 g PO in a single dose. Cure rates with tinidazole are compara-
ble to those of metronidazole, but better tolerated.
Metronidazole (Flagyl, Protostat), 2 g PO in a single dose, or metronidazole, 500 mg
PO bid X 7 days, or metronidazole, 375 mg PO bid X 7 days
Treat male sexual partners

Measures for treatment failure
Treatment sexual contacts
Re-treat with tinazole 2 gm PO or metronidazole, 500 mg PO bid X 7 days
If infection persists, confirm with culture and re-treat with metronidazole,
2-4 g PO qd X 3-10 days

VIII. **Other causes of vaginitis and vaginal discharge**
  A. **Atrophic vaginitis**
    1. Reduced endogenous estrogen causes thinning of the vaginal epithe-
       lium. Symptoms include vaginal soreness, postcoital burning, dyspare-
       unia, and spotting. The vaginal mucosa is thin with diffuse erythema,
       occasional petechiae or ecchymoses, and few or no vaginal folds.
       There may be a serosanguineous or watery discharge with a pH of 5.0-
       7.0.
    2. Treatment consists of topical vaginal estrogen. **Vaginal ring estradiol
       (Estring)**, a silastic ring impregnated with estradiol, is the preferred
       means of delivering estrogen to the vagina. The silastic ring delivers 6
       to 9 µg of estradiol to the vagina daily. The rings are changed once
       every three months. Concomitant progestin therapy is not necessary.
    3. **Conjugated estrogens (Premarin)**, 0.5 gm of cream, or one-eighth of
       an applicatorful daily into the vagina for three weeks, followed by twice
       weekly thereafter is also effective. Concomitant progestin therapy is
       not necessary.
    4. **Estrace cream (estradiol)** can also by given by vaginal applicator at a
       dose of one-eighth of an applicator or 0.5 g (which contains 50 µg of
       estradiol) daily into the vagina for three weeks, followed by twice
       weekly thereafter. Concomitant progestin therapy is not necessary.
    5. **Oral estrogen (Premarin)** 0.3 mg qd should also provide relief.
  B. **Desquamative inflammatory vaginitis**
    1. Chronic purulent vaginitis usually occurs perimenopausally, with
       diffuse exudative vaginitis, massive vaginal-cell exfoliation, purulent
       vaginal discharge, and occasional vaginal and cervical spotted rash.
    2. Laboratory findings included an elevated pH, increased numbers of
       parabasal cells, the absence of gram-positive bacilli and their replace-
       ment by gram-positive cocci on Gram staining. Clindamycin 2% cream
       is usually effective.
  C. **Noninfectious vaginitis and vulvitis**
    1. Noninfectious causes of vaginitis include irritants (eg, minipads,
       spermicides, povidone-iodine, topical antimycotic drugs, soaps and
       perfumes) and contact dermatitis (eg, latex condoms and antimycotic
       creams).
    2. Typical symptoms include pruritus, irritation, burning, soreness, and
       variable discharge. The diagnosis should be suspected in symptomatic
       women who do not have an otherwise apparent infectious cause.
    3. Management of noninfectious vaginitis includes identifying and elimi-
       nating the offending agent. Sodium bicarbonate sitz baths and topical
       vegetable oils. Topical corticosteroids are not recommended.
References: See page 294.

Urinary Incontinence

I. **Terminology**
   A. **Urinary incontinence** is involuntary leakage of urine.
   B. **Urgency** is the complaint of a sudden and compelling desire to pass urine, that is difficult to defer.
   C. **Urge incontinence** is the complaint of involuntary leakage accompanied by urgency. Common precipitants include running water, hand washing, and exposure to cold.
   D. **Stress incontinence** is involuntary leakage with effort, exertion, sneezing, or coughing.
   E. Mixed incontinence is the complaint of involuntary leakage associated with urgency and also with exertion, effort, sneezing, or coughing.
   F. **Overactive bladder** is a symptom syndrome consisting of urgency, frequency, and nocturia, with or without urge incontinence.
   G. **Hesitancy** describes difficulty in initiating voiding.
   H. **Straining to void** is the muscular effort used either to initiate, maintain, or improve the urinary stream.

II. **Types of urinary incontinence**
   A. **Incontinence related to reversible conditions.** Incontinence affects up to one-third of community-dwelling older persons and is often caused by medical and functional factors. Medications often precipitate or worsen urinary incontinence in older individuals.
   B. **Urge incontinence.** The etiology of the overactive bladder syndrome is uninhibited bladder contractions (called detrusor overactivity).
   C. **Most common causes of detrusor overactivity:**
      1. Age-related changes
      2. Interruption of central nervous system (CNS) inhibitory pathways (eg, by stroke, cervical stenosis)
      3. Bladder irritation caused by infection, bladder stones, inflammation, or neoplasms
      4. Detrusor overactivity in many cases may be idiopathic.
      5. Urge urinary incontinence in younger women may be due to interstitial cystitis, characterized by urgency and frequent voiding of small amounts of urine, often with dysuria or pain.
   D. **Urge urinary incontinence** in frail older persons frequently coexists with impaired detrusor contractile function, a condition termed detrusor hyperactivity with impaired contractility (DHIC). DHIC is characterized by urgency and an elevated postvoid residual in the absence of outlet obstruction.
   E. **Stress incontinence** occurs when increases in intraabdominal pressure overcome sphincter closure mechanisms. Stress urinary incontinence is the most common cause of urinary incontinence in younger women, second most common cause in older women, and may occur in older men after transurethral or radical prostatectomy.
      1. **Causes of stress incontinence:**
         a. Stress urinary incontinence in women most often results from impaired urethral support from pelvic endofascia and muscles.
         b. Stress urinary incontinence is less frequently caused failure of urethral closure, called intrinsic sphincter deficiency (ISD). This usually results from operative trauma and scarring, but it can also occur with postmenopausal mucosal atrophy. Unlike the episodic, stress-maneuver-related leakage of stress urinary incontinence, ISD leakage typically is continual.
   F. **Mixed incontinence** is the most common type of urinary incontinence in women, caused by detrusor overactivity and impaired urethral sphincter function.
   G. **Overflow incontinence** is dribbling and/or continuous leakage associated with incomplete bladder emptying caused by impaired detrusor contractility and/or bladder outlet obstruction. The postvoid residual is

elevated, and there may be a weak urinary stream, dribbling, intermittency, hesitancy, frequency, and nocturia. Stress-related leakage may occur.

1. Outlet obstruction is the second most common cause of urinary incontinence in older men (after detrusor overactivity), resulting from benign prostatic hyperplasia, prostate cancer, or urethral stricture.

III. **Diagnostic evaluation**
   A. **History.** The onset and course of incontinence and associated lower urinary tract symptoms.
   B. Leakage frequency, volume, timing, and associated symptoms (eg, urgency, effort maneuvers, urinary frequency, nocturia, hesitancy, interrupted voiding, incomplete emptying, straining to empty, sense of warning).
   C. Precipitants: medications, caffeinated beverages, alcohol, physical activity, cough, laughing, sound of water.
   D. Bowel and sexual function (impaction can cause overflow urinary incontinence; bowel control and sexual function share sacral cord innervation with voiding).
   E. Status of other medical conditions, parity, and medications, along with their temporal relationship to urinary incontinence onset.

Key Questions in Evaluating Patients for Urinary Incontinence

Do you leak urine when you cough, laugh, lift something or sneeze? How often?
Do you ever leak urine when you have a strong urge on the way to the bathroom? How often?
How frequently do you empty your bladder during the day?
How many times do you get up to urinate after going to sleep? Is it the urge to urinate that wakes you?
Do you ever leak urine during sex?
Do you wear pads that protect you from leaking urine? How often do you have to change them?
Do you ever find urine on your pads or clothes and were unaware of when the leakage occurred?
Does it hurt when you urinate?
Do you ever feel that you are unable to completely empty your bladder?

Drugs That Can Influence Bladder Function

Drug	Side effect
Antidepressants, antipsychotics, sedatives/hypnotics	Sedation, retention (overflow)
Diuretics	Frequency, urgency (OAB)
Caffeine	Frequency, urgency (OAB)
Anticholinergics	Retention (overflow)
Alcohol	Sedation, frequency (OAB)
Narcotics	Retention, constipation, sedation (OAB and overflow)
Alpha-adrenergic blockers	Decreased urethral tone (stress incontinence)

Drug	Side effect
Alpha-adrenergic agonists	Increased urethral tone, retention (over-flow)
Beta-adrenergic agonists	Inhibited detrusor function, retention (overflow)

IV. Physical examination

   A. General examination should include the level of alertness and functional status. Vital signs should include orthostatic vital signs.

   B. Neck examination should investigate limitations in cervical lateral rotation and lateral flexion, interosseous muscle wasting, and an abnormal Babinski reflex. These changes suggest cervical spondylosis or stenosis, with secondary interruption of inhibitory tracts to the detrusor, thus causing detrusor overactivity.

   C. Back examination may reveal dimpling or a hair tuft at the spinal cord base, suggestive of occult dysraphism (incomplete spina bifida). Evidence of prior laminectomy should be sought.

   D. Cardiovascular examination should look for evidence of volume overload (eg, rales, pedal edema).

   E. Abdomen should be palpated for masses, tenderness, and bladder distention.

   F. Extremities should be examined for joint mobility and function.

   G. Genital examination in women should include inspection of the vaginal mucosa for atrophy (thinning, pallor, loss of rugae), narrowing of the introitus by posterior synechia, vault stenosis, and inflammation (erythema, petechiae, telangiectasia, friability). A bimanual examination should be done to evaluate for masses or tenderness.

   1. The adequacy of pelvic support may be assessed by a split-speculum exam, removing the top blade of the speculum and holding the bottom blade firmly against the posterior vaginal wall. While the woman to coughs, assess whether the urethra remains firmly fixed or swings quickly forward (urethral hypermobility) and for bulging of the anterior vaginal wall (cystocoele).

   2. Check for rectocele by turning the single blade of the speculum to support the anterior vaginal wall and having the patient cough again.

   3. Uncircumcised men should be checked for phimosis, paraphimosis, and balanitis.

   H. Rectal examination should check for masses and fecal impaction, and for prostate consistency and symmetry in men (estimation of prostate size by digital examination is unreliable).

   I. Neurologic examination assess sacral root integrity, including perineal sensation, resting and volitional tone of the anal sphincter, anal wink (anal contraction in response to a light scratch of the perineal skin lateral to the anus), and the bulbocavernosus reflex (anal contraction in response to a light squeeze of the clitoris or glans penis). Cognitive status and affect should be assessed, as well as motor strength and tone (especially with regard to mobility), and vibration and peripheral sensation for peripheral neuropathy.

   J. Clinical testing

   1. Stress test is best done when the patient has not recently voided and is in a standing position with a relaxed perineum. The patient should give a single vigorous cough. A pad is held underneath the perineum, and the physician or nurse observes directly whether there is leakage from the urethra.

   a. Leakage instantaneous with cough suggests impaired sphincter function, while a several-second delay before leakage suggests an effort-induced uninhibited detrusor contraction.

2. **Postvoid residual volume (PVR)** by catheterization or ultrasound. Elevated PVR is found most commonly in:
   a. Frail elderly men with symptoms of bladder outlet obstruction
   b. Patients with symptoms of decreased bladder emptying or abdominal distention
   c. Women with previous anti-incontinence surgery
   d. Persons with suprasacral and sacral spinal cord injury
   e. Patients who have failed empiric antimuscarinic drug therapy
   f. A PVR of less than 50 mL is considered adequate emptying, and a PVR >200 mL is suggestive of either detrusor weakness or obstruction.

K. **Laboratory tests.** Renal function tests, glucose, calcium, and, in older people, a vitamin B12 level should be obtained. A urinalysis should be performed. Urine cytology and cystoscopy are indicated only if there is hematuria or pelvic pain.

L. **Urodynamic testing** is not usually necessary in the evaluation of urinary incontinence.

V. **Treatment of urinary incontinence**

A. **Lifestyle.** Adequate fluid intake (up to two liters per day); avoidance of caffeinated beverages and alcohol; minimizing evening intake; management of constipation; smoking cessation; and treatment of pulmonary disease if cough is exacerbating incontinence.

B. **Behavioral therapy**
   1. **Cognitively intact patients**
      a. **Bladder training** involves timed voiding every two hours while awake. Bladder relaxation techniques involve having the patients sit down when an urge occurs and concentrate on making the urge decrease and pass by taking a deep breath, contracting their pelvic muscles. Once in control of the urge, they walk to a bathroom and void.
      b. **Supplemental biofeedback** may be helpful for some patients in addition to bladder training.
   2. **Cognitively impaired patients**. Prompted voiding involves regular monitoring of continence; prompting to toilet on a scheduled basis; and praise when individuals are continent and attempt to toilet.

C. **Pelvic muscle (Kegel) exercises** (PME) strengthen the urethral closure mechanism with small numbers of isometric repetitions at maximal exertion. The basic recommended regimen is three sets of 8 to 12 slow velocity contractions sustained for six to eight seconds each, performed three or four times a week and continued for at least 15 to 20 weeks.

VI. **Pharmacological therapy.** Medications are not useful in the treatment of with stress incontinence.

A. **Antimuscarinics.** Anticholinergics with antimuscarinic effects are frequently prescribed for urge incontinence. These agents result in a 40% higher rate of cure or improvement; dry mouth is common.
   1. **Oxybutynin (Ditropan)** has direct antispasmodic effects and inhibits the action of acetylcholine on smooth muscle. Oxybutynin is available in both immediate release (IR), extended release (ER), and transdermal formulations. Efficacy is similar.
      a. The initial dosage for IR is 2.5 mg two to three times daily, followed by titration as needed up to 20 mg/day in divided doses. The ER formulation is started at 5 mg once daily and titrated up to 20 to 30 mg once daily. The transdermal patch is available at 3.8 mg and should be changed twice a week.
      b. **Anticholinergic side effects**, especially dry mouth, can limit therapy; dry mouth is less frequent with extended release and transdermal preparations. The postvoid residual should be monitored in older patients. Worsening of urinary incontinence can result from subclinical retention.

2. **Tolterodine (Detrol LA**, 1 to 2 mg twice a day immediate release, 2 to 4 mg per day extended release) has similar efficacy to oxybutynin. It causes dry mouth less frequently than oxybutynin IR 5 mg three times daily, but has similar side effects to ER oxybutynin 10 mg/day. Tolterodine is more expensive than generic oxybutynin IR. Oxybutynin and tolterodine have similar clinical efficacy, but tolterodine causes less dry mouth.

3. **Trospium (Sanctura**, 20 mg twice daily) is approved for the treatment of overactive bladder. Dose should be reduced to 20 mg once a day in the elderly and renal impairment. Trospium must be taken on an empty stomach. Dry mouth occurs in 22% and constipation in 10%.

4. **Solifenacin (Vesicare**, 5 to 10 mg daily) and darifenacin **(Enablex**, 7.5 to 15 mg daily) are approved for overactive bladder. Solifenacin and darifenacin are more selective for the M-3 muscarinic receptor in the bladder. Incontinence episodes decrease with solifenacin, similar to tolterodine (58%). The rate of dry mouth is 14% and the rate of constipation is 7%.

5. **Duloxetine (Cymbalta)** is a serotonin and norepinephrine reuptake inhibitor that is only approved for major depression and neuropathic pain. It stimulates pudendal motor neuron alpha adrenergic and 5-hydroxytryptamine-2 receptors. 40 mg twice daily results in significant decreases in the frequency of incontinence compared with placebo (50 to 54%). Nausea is common. Duloxetine is contraindicated in chronic liver disease.

B. **Stress incontinence may be treated** with topical estrogen. Up to 2 g of vaginal cream daily, intravaginal estrogen rings, or dissolving tablets (Vagifem) are effective for urinary incontinence. Topical estrogen is applied as 0.3 mg of conjugated estrogens or 0.5 mg of estradiol daily for three weeks, and then twice a week thereafter.

Medications Used to Treat Urinary Incontinence

Drug	Dosage
Stress Incontinence	
Estrogen dissolving tablets (Vagifem)	One tablet inserted vaginally once daily for the first two weeks. Then one tablet twice weekly
Vaginal estrogen ring (Estring)	Insert into vagina every three months
Vaginal estrogen cream	0.5 g, apply in vagina every night
Overactive bladder	
Oxybutynin transdermal (Oxytrol)	39 cm^2 patch 2 times/week
Oxybutynin ER (Ditropan XL)	5 to 15 mg, every morning
Tolterodine LA (Detrol LA)	2-4 mg qd
Generic oxybutynin	2.5 to 10 mg, two to four times daily
Tolterodine (Detrol)	1 to 2 mg, two times daily

Drug	Dosage
Trospium (Sanctura)	20 mg twice daily
Solifenacin (Vesicare)	5 to 10 mg daily
Darifenacin (Enablex)	7.5 to 15 mg daily
Duloxetine (Cymbalta)	20 mg twice daily, and increasing to 40 mg twice daily after two weeks

VII. Surgery
- **A. Urge incontinence.** Potential surgical treatments for severe cases of intractable urge urinary incontinence are sacral nerve modulation and augmentation cystoplasty; however, these are not first-line treatments.
- **B. Stress incontinence.** Surgery offers the highest cure rates for stress urinary incontinence. However, it is invasive and potentially morbid.
  1. **Bladder neck suspension procedures** such as the transvaginal Burch colposuspension are used to treat urethral hypermobility and stress urinary incontinence.
  2. **Sling procedures** (using material to support the urethra or bladder neck) including tension-free vaginal tape (TVT) are increasingly being used for stress incontinence in women.
  3. **Periurethral bulking injections** with collagen are preferable for intrinsic sphincter deficiency.

VIII. Continence pessaries may benefit women with stress urinary incontinence related to pelvic floor prolapse or laxity. The use of these devices may be very appealing to women, who wish to avoid surgery.

References: See page 294.

Genital Warts

Genital warts or condyloma acuminata are caused by infection with human papillomavirus (HPV). Types 16, 18, 31, and 45 have been associated strongly with premalignant and malignant cervical carcinoma. About 18% to 33% of sexually active female adolescents test positive for HPV DNA. Common warts are associated with different HPV types than those that cause genital warts.

I. Symptoms and Signs
- **A.** The lesions of condylomata acuminata are usually flesh- to gray-colored papillomatous growths. They range in size from less than 1 millimeter in diameter to several square centimeters. The presence of koilocytotic cells on Papanicolaou smears from the cervix suggest condyloma.
- **B.** Among adolescent and adult males, venereal warts usually are localized to the penis. Lesions present as brown to slate blue pigmented macules and papules.

II. Treatment
- **A.** Cryotherapy with liquid nitrogen or a cryoprobe is the most effective method of treating single or multiple small lesions. Cryosurgery is more effective than topical therapies. Lesions should be frozen until a 2 mm margin of freeze appears, then allowed to thaw, then refrozen. Repeat freeze several times. Side effects include burning, which resolves within a few hours, and ulceration, which heals in 7 to 10 days with little or no scarring.
- **B.** Repeated weekly application of podophyllin as a 10% solution in benzoin has been the principal mode of therapy for many years. Podophyllin can cause chemical burns and neurologic, hematologic, and febrile complica-

tions. Podophyllotoxin (podofilox) is more efficacious and less toxic than podophyllin.

C. Other treatment modalities include 5-fluorouracil as a 5% cream and a solution of trichloroacetic acid, both of which are painful and can cause ulcers.

D. **Imiquimod (Aldara)** induces interferon. A cream formulation containing 5% imiquimod has resulted in good total clearance rates and tolerable side effects (erythema). The cream is applied three times a week prior to normal sleeping hours and is washed off after 6 to 10 hours with mild soap and water.

E. Surgical techniques include conventional surgery, electrocautery, and laser therapy. Intralesional or systemic administration of interferon is effective for recalcitrant disease.

F. Sexual transmission of HPV can be decreased by using condoms. Examination of sex partners is unnecessary; most probably are infected with HPV already, and no test for asymptomatic infection is available.

III. **Prevention of HPV infection**
   A. Quadrivalent HPV 6/11/16/18 L1 virus-live particle vaccine (Gardasil) provides protection against persistent HPV 16/18 infection in 89 percent of women who received vaccination. The vaccine should be administered in girls and women 9 to 26 years of age.

References: See page 294.

Pubic Infections

I. **Molluscum contagiosum**
   A. This disease is produced by a virus of the pox virus family and is spread by sexual or close personal contact. Lesions are usually asymptomatic and multiple, with a central umbilication. Lesions can be spread by autoinoculation and last from 6 months to many years.
   B. **Diagnosis.** The characteristic appearance is adequate for diagnosis, but biopsy may be used to confirm the diagnosis.
   C. **Treatment.** Lesions are removed by sharp dermal curette, liquid nitrogen cryosurgery, or electrodesiccation.

II. **Pediculosis pubis (crabs)**
   A. Phthirus pubis is a blood sucking louse that is unable to survive more than 24 hours off the body. It is often transmitted sexually and is principally found on the pubic hairs. Diagnosis is confirmed by locating nits or adult lice on the hair shafts.
   B. **Treatment**
      1. **Permethrin cream (Elimite),** 5% is the most effective treatment; it is applied for 10 minutes and washed off.
      2. **Kwell shampoo,** lathered for at least 4 minutes, can also be used, but it is contraindicated in pregnancy or lactation.
      3. All contaminated clothing and linen should be laundered.

III. **Pubic scabies**
   A. This highly contagious infestation is caused by the Sarcoptes scabiei (0.2-0.4 mm in length). The infestation is transmitted by intimate contact or by contact with infested clothing. The female mite burrows into the skin, and after 1 month, severe pruritus develops. A multiform eruption may develop, characterized by papules, vesicles, pustules, urticarial wheals, and secondary infections on the hands, wrists, elbows, belt line, buttocks, genitalia, and outer feet.
   B. **Diagnosis** is confirmed by visualization of burrows and observation of parasites, eggs, larvae, or red fecal compactions under microscopy.
   C. **Treatment.** Permethrin 5% cream (Elimite) is massaged in from the neck down and remove by washing after 8 hours.

References: See page 294.

Urologic Disorders

Benign Prostatic Hyperplasia

Benign prostatic hyperplasia (BPH) is a common disorder that increases in frequency with age in men older than 50 years. Symptoms or BPH include increased frequency of urination, nocturia, hesitancy, urgency, and weak urinary stream. The correlation between symptoms and the presence of prostatic enlargement on rectal examination or by transrectal ultrasonographic assessment of prostate size is poor.

I. **Clinical evaluation of obstructive urinary symptoms**
   A. History of type 2 diabetes, which can cause nocturia
   B. Symptoms of neurologic disease that would suggest a neurogenic bladder
   C. Sexual dysfunction
   D. Gross hematuria or pain in the bladder region suggestive of a bladder tumor or calculi
   E. History of urethral trauma, urethritis, or urethral instrumentation that could lead to urethral stricture
   F. Family history of BPH and prostate cancer
   G. Treatment with drugs that can impair bladder function (anticholinergic drugs) or increase outflow resistance (sympathomimetic drugs)
   H. A 24-hour voiding chart of frequency and volume should be obtained.
   I. Symptoms are classified as mild (total score 0 to 7), moderate (total score 8 to 19) and severe (total score 20 to 35).
   J. **Other disorders that can cause difficulty urinating:**
      1. Urethral stricture
      2. Bladder neck contracture
      3. Carcinoma of the prostate
      4. Carcinoma of the bladder
      5. Bladder calculi
      6. Urinary tract infection and prostatitis
      7. Neurogenic bladder

Benign Prostatic Hyperplasia Symptom Score

For each question, circle the answer that best describes your situation. Add the circled number together to get your total score. See the key at the bottom of this form to determine the overall rating of your symptoms.

	Not at all	Less than one in five times	Less than half of the time	About half of the time	More than half of the time	Almost always
In the past month, how often have you had a sensation of not emptying your bladder completely after you finished voiding?	0	1	2	3	4	5
In the past month, how often have you had to urinate again less than 2 hours after you finished urinating before?	0	1	2	3	4	5

	Not at all	Less than one in five times	Less than half of the time	About half of the time	More than half of the time	Almost always
In the past month, how often have you found you stopped and started again several times when you urinated?	0	1	2	3	4	5
In the past month, how often have you found it difficult to postpone urination?	0	1	2	3	4	5
In the past month, how often have you had a weak urinary stream?	0	1	2	3	4	5
In the past month, how often have you had to push or strain to begin urination?	0	1	2	3	4	5
In the past month, how many times did you typically get up to urinate from the time you went to bed until you arose in the morning?	0	1	2	3	4	5

K. **Physical examination.** A digital rectal examination should be done to assess prostate size and consistency, nodules, induration, and asymmetry, which raise suspicion for malignancy. Rectal sphincter tone should be determined, and a neurological examination performed.

L. **Urinalysis** should be done to detect urinary infection and blood, which could indicate bladder cancer or calculi.

M. **Optional tests**

1. **Serum prostate specific antigen.** Prostate cancer can cause obstructive symptoms. Measurements of serum PSA may be used as a screening test for prostate cancer in men with BPH, preferably in men between the ages of 50 to 69 years. Blood should not be obtained for PSA assay within 24 hours after vigorous digital rectal examination or ejaculation.

   a. The results should be interpreted according to age- and race-based norms. High values occur in men with prostatic diseases other than cancer, including BPH. Some men with prostatic cancer have serum PSA concentrations of 4.0 ng/mL or less.

   b. A combination of digital rectal examination and serum PSA determination provides the most acceptable means for excluding prostate cancer.

2. **Maximal urinary flow rates** greater than 15 mL/sec are thought to exclude bladder outlet obstruction. Maximal flow rates below 15 mL/sec are compatible with obstruction due to prostatic or urethral disease.

3. **Post-void residual urine volume** can be determined by in-out catheterization, radiographic methods, or ultrasonography. Normal men have less than 12 mL of residual urine. A large residual volume is a possible indicator of BPH.

4. Ultrasonography is useful in men who have a high serum creatinine concentration or a urinary tract infection. Total prostate volume can be measured by ultrasonography to assess disease progression, and it is

useful when considering medical treatment with a 5-alpha-reductase inhibitor or when considering surgery.

II. Medical treatment of benign prostatic hyperplasia

A. Indications for therapy

1. Obstructive symptoms only require therapy if they have a significant impact on a patient's quality of life. Benign prostatic hypertrophy may require therapy if obstruction is creating a risk for upper tract injury such as hydronephrosis or renal insufficiency, or lower tract injury such as urinary retention, recurrent infection, or bladder decompensation (eg, low pressure detrusor contractions; >25 percent post-void residuals). Patients who develop these symptoms will require invasive therapy.

B. Alpha-1-adrenergic antagonists are more effective for short-term treatment of BPH; however, only 5-alpha-reductase inhibitors have demonstrated the potential for long-term reduction in prostate volume. The efficacy of these classes are similar with long-term therapy, but 5-alpha-reductase inhibitors have been found to reduce the need for surgery. The use of agents from both classes in combination may be superior to using either class alone.

C. Alpha-1-adrenergic antagonists. Four long-acting alpha-1-antagonists, terazosin, doxazosin, tamsulosin, and alfuzosin have been approved for treatment of the symptoms of BPH.

1. **Mechanism.** Prostatic tissue contains alpha-1 and alpha-2 adrenergic receptors. Alpha-1-adrenergic antagonists target alpha-1A receptors.
2. The alpha-1-antagonists appear to have similar efficacy.
3. Alfuzosin (Uroxatral), terazosin (Hytrin), doxazosin (Cardura), and tamsulosin (Flomax) decrease symptom scores by 30 to 40 percent, and urinary flow rates increase by 16 to 25 percent.
4. **Side effects.** The frequency of side effects with alfuzosin (Uroxatral) and tamsulosin (Flomax) is similar to placebo, but terazosin and doxazosin cause significant side effects in 10 percent.
   a. Side effects include orthostatic hypotension and dizziness. Terazosin and doxazosin need to be initiated at bedtime (to reduce postural lightheadedness) and the dose should be titrated up over several weeks.
   b. The hypotensive action can be useful in older men who have hypertension. Alpha-1-adrenergic antagonists may increase the incidence of heart failure when used for hypertension.

D. Tamsulosin (Flomax) and alfuzosin (Uroxatral) have less effect on blood pressure than either terazosin (Hytrin) or doxazosin (Cardura), and tamsulosin (Flomax) may further have slightly less effect on blood pressure than alfuzosin.

   a. The hypotensive effects of terazosin and doxazosin can be potentiated by sildenafil (Viagra), vardenafil (Levitra), or tadalafil (Cialis).
   b. Other common side effects of alpha-1-antagonists include asthenia and nasal congestion.

Starting dosages of alpha-blocking agents for managing benign prostatic hypertrophy	
Drug	**Starting dosage**
Afuzosin (Uroxatral)	10 mg qd
Tamsulosin (Flomax)	0.4 mg qd
Terazosin (Hytrin)	1 mg qd, adjusted up to 5 mg qd
Doxazosin mesylate (Cardura)	1 mg qd, adjusted up to 4 mg qd

E. **5-Alpha-reductase inhibitors** include finasteride and dutasteride. Treatment for 6 to 12 months is required before prostate size is reduced enough to improve symptoms. The type 2 form of 5-alpha-reductase catalyzes the conversion of testosterone to dihydrotestosterone in prostatic tissue.

1. Efficacy. Finasteride (Proscar) for 12 months reduces obstructive and non-obstructive symptoms by 23-18 percent and increases maximal urinary flow rate by 1.6 mL/sec. The mean prostatic volume is reduced by 19-18 percent.

2. Dutasteride (Avodart) is an inhibitor of both 5-alpha reductase enzymes, and may be more potent than finasteride.

3. Dutasteride and finasteride are similar in effectiveness and the side effect profiles of these agents are similar. The side effect on hair growth for men with dutasteride has not yet been established.

4. Side effects of these drugs are decreased libido and ejaculatory or erectile dysfunction, occurring in 4 to 6 percent of men.

5. Serum prostate-specific antigen (PSA) concentrations decrease by about 50 percent with finasteride. PSA values should be corrected by a factor of 2 for the first 24 months of finasteride use, and by a factor of 2.5 for longer term use.

6. **Combination therapy.** Long-term therapy with combined alpha adrenergic antagonist and 5-alpha-reductase inhibitor therapy appears to be superior to either agent alone.

III. **Recommendations**

A. Men who develop upper tract injury (eg, hydronephrosis, renal dysfunction), or lower tract injury (eg, urinary retention, recurrent infection, bladder decompensation) require invasive therapy.

B. Alpha-adrenergic antagonists provide immediate therapeutic benefits, while 5-alpha-reductase inhibitors require long-term treatment for efficacy. In most men with mild to moderate symptoms of BPH. Initial treatment consists of an alpha-adrenergic antagonist alone. For severe symptoms (large prostate (>40 g), inadequate response to monotherapy), combination treatment with an alpha-adrenergic antagonist and a 5-alpha-reductase inhibitor is recommended.

C. The choice of alpha-adrenergic antagonist and 5-alpha-reductase inhibitor may be made on the basis of cost and side-effect profile. Tamsulosin (Flomax) and alfuzosin (Uroxatral) have less effect on blood pressure than either terazosin (Hytrin) or doxazosin (Cardura), and tamsulosin may further have slightly less effect on blood pressure than alfuzosin.

References: See page 294.

Prostatitis and Prostatodynia

Prostatitis is a common condition, with a 5 percent lifetime prevalence to 9 percent. Prostatitis is divided into three subtypes: acute, chronic bacterial prostatitis and chronic nonbacterial prostatitis/chronic pelvic pain syndrome (CNP/CPPS).

I. **Acute Bacterial Prostatitis**

A. Acute bacterial prostatitis (ABP) should be considered a urinary tract infection. The most common cause is Escherichia coli. Other species frequently found include Klebsiella, Proteus, Enterococci and Pseudomonas. On occasion, cultures grow Staphylococcus aureus, Streptococcus faecalis, Chlamydia or Bacteroides species.

B. Patients may present with fever, chills, low back pain, perineal or ejaculatory pain, dysuria, urinary frequency, urgency, myalgias and obstruction. The prostate gland is tender and may be warm, swollen, firm and irregular. Vigorous digital examination of the prostate should be avoided because it may induce bacteremia.

C. The infecting organism can often be identified by urine culturing.
D. Treatment consists of trimethoprim-sulfamethoxazole (TMP-SMX [Bactrim, Septra]), a quinolone or tetracycline. Men at increased risk for sexually transmitted disease require antibiotic coverage for Chlamydia.

Common Antibiotic Regimens for Acute Bacterial Prostatitis	
Medication	**Standard dosage**
Trimethoprim-sulfamethoxazole (Bactrim, Septra)	1 DS tablet (160/800 mg) twice a day
Doxycycline (Vibramycin)	100 mg twice a day
Ciprofloxacin (Cipro)	500 mg twice a day
Norfloxacin (Noroxin)	400 mg twice a day
Ofloxacin (Floxin)	400 mg twice a day

E. Antibiotic therapy should be continued for three to four weeks. Extremely ill patients should be hospitalized to receive a parenteral broad-spectrum cephalosporin and an aminoglycoside.

II. **Chronic Bacterial Prostatitis**
   A. Chronic bacterial prostatitis (CBP) is a common cause of recurrent urinary tract infections in men. Men experience irritative voiding symptoms, pain in the back, testes, epididymis or penis, low-grade fever, arthralgias and myalgias. Signs may include urethral discharge, hemospermia and secondary epididymo-orchitis. Often the prostate is normal on rectal examination.
   B. CBP presents with negative premassage urine culture results, and greater than 10 to 20 white blood cells per high-power field in the pre- and the postmassage urine specimen. Significant bacteriuria in the postmassage urine specimen suggests chronic bacterial prostatitis.
   C. TMP-SMX is the first-line antibiotic for CBP. Norfloxacin (Noroxin) taken twice a day for 28 days achieves a cure rate in 64 percent. Ofloxacin (Floxin) is also highly effective. Some men require long-term antibiotic suppression with TMP-SMX or nitrofurantoin.

III. **Chronic Nonbacterial Prostatitis/Chronic Pelvic Pain Syndrome (prostatodynia)**
   A. Patients with CNP/CPPS have painful ejaculation pain in the penis, testicles or scrotum, low back pain, rectal or perineal pain, and/or inner thigh pain. They often have irritative or obstructive urinary symptoms and decreased libido or impotence. The physical examination is usually unremarkable, but patients may have a tender prostate.
   B. No bacteria will grow on culture, but leukocytosis may be found in the prostatic secretions.
   C. Treatment begins with 100 mg of doxycycline (Vibramycin) or minocycline (Minocin) twice daily for 14 days. Other therapies may include Allopurinol (Zyloprim), thrice-weekly prostate massage or transurethral microwave thermotherapy.
   D. Hot sitz baths and nonsteroidal anti-inflammatory drugs (NSAIDs) may provide some relief. Some men may notice aggravation of symptoms with alcohol or spicy foods and should avoid them. Anticholinergic agents

(oxybutynin [Ditropan]) or alpha-blocking agents (doxazosin [Cardura], tamsulosin [Flomax] or terazosin [Hytrin]) may be beneficial.

References: See page 294.

Acute Epididymoorchitis

I. **Clinical evaluation of testicular pain**
   A. Epididymoorchitis is indicated by a unilateral painful testicle and a history of unprotected intercourse, new sexual partner, urinary tract infection, dysuria, or discharge. Symptoms may occur following acute lifting or straining.
   B. The epididymis and testicle are painful, swollen, and tender. The scrotum may be erythematosus and warm, with associated spermatic cord thickening or penile discharge.
   C. **Differential diagnosis of painful scrotal swelling**
      1. Epididymitis, testicular torsion, testicular tumor, hernia.
      2. Torsion is characterized by sudden onset, age <20, an elevated testicle, and previous episodes of scrotal pain. The epididymis is usually located anteriorly on either side, and there is an absence of evidence of urethritis and UTI.
      3. Epididymitis is characterized by fever, laboratory evidence of urethritis or cystitis, and increased scrotal warmth.

II. **Laboratory evaluation of epididymoorchitis**
   A. Epididymoorchitis is indicated by leukocytosis with a left shift; UA shows pyuria and bacteriuria. Midstream urine culture will reveal gram negative bacilli. Chlamydia and Neisseria cultures should be obtained.
   B. **Common pathogens**
      1. **Younger men.** Epididymoorchitis is usually associated with sexually transmitted organisms such as Chlamydia and gonorrhea.
      2. **Older men.** Epididymoorchitis is usually associated with a concomitant urinary tract infection or prostatitis caused by E. coli, proteus, Klebsiella, Enterobacter, or Pseudomonas.

III. **Treatment of epididymoorchitis**
   A. Bed rest, scrotal elevation with athletic supporter, an ice pack, analgesics, and antipyretics are prescribed. Sexual and physical activity should be avoided.
   B. **Sexually transmitted epididymitis in sexually active males**
      1. Ceftriaxone (Rocephin) 250 mg IM x 1 dose **AND** doxycycline 100 mg PO bid x 10 days **OR**
      2. Ofloxacin (Floxin) 300 mg bid x 10 days.
      3. Treat sexual partners
   C. **Epididymitis secondary to urinary tract infection**
      1. TMP/SMX DS bid for 10 days **OR**
      2. Ofloxacin (Floxin) 300 mg PO bid for 10 days.

References: See page 294.

Male Sexual Dysfunction

Impotence is defined as the inability to develop or sustain erection 75 percent of the time. It is a common abnormality and may be due to psychological causes, medications, hormonal abnormalities, neurologic, or vascular problems.

I. **Causes of sexual dysfunction in men**
   A. Libido declines with androgen deficiency, depression, and with the use of prescription and recreational drugs. Erectile dysfunction may reflect either inadequate arterial blood flow into (failure to fill) or accelerated venous drainage out of (failure to store) the corpora cavernosae.

II. Sexual history

A. Rapidity of onset. Sexually competent men who have sudden onset of impotence invariably have psychogenic impotence. Psychologic counseling is the preferred therapy in this setting. Only radical prostatectomy or other overt genital tract trauma causes a sudden loss of male sexual function. In comparison, men suffering from impotence of any other cause complain that sexual function failed sporadically at first, then more consistently.

B. Erectile reserve. Most men experience spontaneous erections during REM sleep, and often wake up with an erection, attesting to the integrity of neurogenic reflexes and corpora cavernosae blood flow. Complete loss of nocturnal erections is present in men with neurologic or vascular disease.

C. Nonsustained erection with detumescence after penetration is most commonly due to anxiety or the vascular steal syndrome. In the vascular steal syndrome, blood is diverted from the engorged corpora cavernosae to accommodate the oxygen requirements of the thrusting pelvis. Vascular surgery to ensure equitable genital and pelvic arterial inflow is useful.

D. Assessment of interpersonal conflict. Unexpressed interpersonal conflict is one of the more common causes of male sexual dysfunction. Couples counseling can restore harmony and sexual function in 25 percent of cases.

Agents That May Cause Erectile Dysfunction

Antidepressants
  Monoamine oxidase inhibitors
  Selective serotonin reuptake inhibitors
  Tricyclic antidepressants
Antihypertensives
  Beta blockers
  Centrally acting alpha agonists
  Diuretics
Antipsychotics
Anxiolytics

Miscellaneous
  Cimetidine (Tagamet)
  Corticosteroids
  Finasteride (Proscar)
  Gemfibrozil (Lopid)
Drugs of abuse
  Alcohol
  Anabolic steroids
  Heroin
  Marijuana

Clinical clues to causes of male sexual dysfunction

Finding	Cause
Rapid onset	Psychogenic Genitourinary trauma (eg, radical prostatectomy)
Nonsustained erection	Anxiety Vascular steal
Depression or use of certain drugs	Depression Drug induced
Complete loss of nocturnal erections	Vascular disease Neurologic disease

III. Physical examination

A. Weak or absent femoral and peripheral pulses suggest the presence of vasculogenic impotence. If pulses are normal, the presence of femoral bruits suggests pelvic blood occlusion.

B. Visual field defects in hypogonadal men suggests a pituitary tumor.

    C. **Gynecomastia** suggests Klinefelter's syndrome.
    D. **Penile plaques** suggest Peyronie's disease.
    E.**Testicular atrophy** asymmetry or masses should be sought.
    F.**Cremasteric reflex** is an index of the integrity of the thoracolumbar erection center. This is elicited by stroking the inner thighs and observing ipsilateral contraction of the scrotum.

IV. Laboratory studies and diagnostic tests

    A. **Hormonal testing** should include serum testosterone, prolactin and thyroid function tests.
    B. **Nocturnal penile tumescence testing.** The Rigi-Scan monitor provides quantifies the number, tumescence and rigidity of erectile episodes. Impotent men with normal NPT are considered to have psychogenic impotence whereas those with impaired NPT are considered to have "organic" impotence usually due to vascular or neurologic disease.
    C. **Duplex Doppler ultrasonography or angiography** of the penile deep arteries, are indicated in men with impaired NPT to identify areas of arterial obstruction or venous leak.

V. Treatment of male sexual dysfunction

    A. **First-line therapy** consists of the **phosphodiesterase inhibitors** because of their efficacy, ease of use. **Sildenafil (Viagra), vardenafil (Levitra), and tadalafil (Cialis)** appear to be equally effective, but tadalafil has a longer duration of action. Phosphodiesterase inhibitors are contraindicated in men taking nitrates.
    B. **Second-line therapy** consists of penile self-injectable drugs, intraurethral alprostadil, and vacuum devices.
    C. **Surgical implantation of a penile prosthesis** is reserved for men who have not responded to first- and second-line therapies.
    D. For men with sexual dysfunction and low serum testosterone levels, testosterone replacement therapy should be the initial treatment.
    E. **Phosphodiesterase-5 inhibitors**
        1. **Sildenafil, vardenafil and tadalafil** All act to increase intracavernosal cyclic GMP levels, and each one has been proven to be effective in restoring erectile function.
        2. **Sildenafil (Viagra)** is taken one hour before planned sexual intercourse, it is effective for a wide range of disorders causing erectile dysfunction.
            a. Detumescence is associated with catabolism of cyclic GMP by type 5 phosphodiesterase. PDE-5 inhibitors act by blocking the latter enzyme.
            b. **Efficacy.** 69 percent of all attempts at sexual intercourse are successful. Headache, flushing, and dyspepsia occur in 6 to 18 percent of the men.
            c. **Testosterone** therapy with sildenafil therapy may be useful in men with serum total testosterone concentrations <400 ng/dL who do not respond to sildenafil alone.
            d. **Dose.** Sildenafil should be taken orally one hour before a planned sexual encounter. The initial dose should be 50 mg, and it should be reduced to 25 mg if side effects occur. The dose can be increased to 100 mg if necessary. Each sildenafil pill costs about $10.00 retail.
            e. **Cardiovascular effects**
                (1) Sildenafil is a vasodilator that lowers the blood pressure by about 8 mmHg; this change typically produces no symptoms.
                (2) The combination of sildenafil and nitrates can lead to severe hypotension (eg, more than 50/25 mmHg) and syncope. Sildenafil is contraindicated in patients taking nitrates. Nitrates should not be prescribed within 24 hours (or longer in patients with renal or hepatic dysfunction) of takeing sildinafil.
                (3) Sildenafil has been associated with myocardial infarction and sudden death. Case reports of MI in association with sildenafil may have been unrelated to the drug. PDE-5 inhibitors are safe

for men with stable coronary artery disease who are not taking nitrates.

   (4) The vasodilator properties of sildenafil may have an adverse effect in some patients with a hypertrophic cardiomyopathy; the decrease in preload and afterload can increase the outflow obstruction.

f. Sildenafil is clearly contraindicated in men taking nitrates. Other men in whom it is potentially hazardous include those who have:

   (1) Active coronary ischemia (eg, positive exercise test) who are not taking nitrates
   (2) Heart failure and borderline low blood pressure or low volume status
   (3) A complicated, multidrug, antihypertensive drug regimen

g. Men who are considering sildenafil therapy should be questioned regarding exercise tolerance; resumption of sexual activity after a prolonged period of inactivity is analogous to beginning a new exercise regimen. Sildenafil can be considered in men who are participating in aerobic activities that are roughly equivalent in energy expenditure to sex. If such activity cannot be documented, exercise treadmill testing should be considered.

h. **Alpha adrenergic antagonists**, used for the treatment of benign prostatic hyperplasia, may cause symptomatic hypotension when taken in combination with PDE-5 inhibitors. Sildenafil doses above 25 mg should not be taken within four hours of an alpha-blocker. Tamsulosin (Flomax) is the only alpha adrenergic antagonist which is approved for use with PDE-5 inhibitors, but only with tadalafil.

i. Side effects associated with sildenafil include headache, lightheadedness, dizziness, flushing, distorted vision, and, in some cases, syncope. Flushing, headaches, dyspepsia, and visual disturbances occur in 12,11, 5, and 3 percent, respectively. Sildenafil causes blue vision in approximately 3 percent of men. This effect lasts two to three hours.

j. Interactions. Sildenafil should be avoided in patients taking drugs that can prolong the half-life of sildenafil by blocking CYP3A4 (erythromycin, ketoconazole, protease inhibitors, and grapefruit juice); drugs that induce CYP3A4 (rifampin and phenytoin) reduce the effectiveness of sildenafil.

F. Vardenafil (Levitra) and tadalafil (Cialis) are PDE-5 inhibitors. Vardenafil shares a similar structure, onset and duration of action and side-effect profile with sildenafil, whereas tadalafil (Cialis) differs in chemical structure, has an equally rapid onset but longer duration of action and does not cause blue vision but otherwise shares a similar side-effect profile with the other two phosphodiesterase inhibitors.

G. **Vardenafil (Levitra)** is available as a 10 and 20 mg dose. Vardenafil appears to be as effective as sildenafil.

1. High-fat, but not moderate-fat meals, may lower the peak serum concentration of vardenafil by 18 percent, and delay absorption by one hour.

2. A slight prolongation of the QT interval may occur, but this is not clinically important. However, vardenafil should not be used in men with congenital QT prolongation or in those taking antiarrhythmics drugs, such as quinidine, procainamide, amiodarone, or sotalol.

3. Side effects are similar to those seen with sildenafil, and include headache, flushing, and rhinitis, in 13, 10, 10 and 5 percent, respectively. Changes in color vision (blue vision) have not been reported.

4. Vardenafil appears to be as effective as sildenafil with no evidence of a more rapid onset of action. Vardenafil is contraindicated in men taking nitrates.

5. Patients on alpha-blocker therapy should be stable prior to initiating vardenafil (which should be started at the lowest recommended dose).

H. **Tadalafil (Cialis)** has a different chemical structure than sildenafil and vardenafil. Tadalafil also appears to be as effective as sildenafil but has a longer duration of action. The recommended starting dose is 10 mg, with 5 and 20 mg options available. Food does not interfere with its absorption.

1. With tadalafil, 75 percent of intercourse attempts are successful compared with 32 percent with placebo.

2. **Side effects** are similar to those seen with sildenafil and vardenafil, with headache, dyspepsia, flushing, and rhinitis occurring in 8 to 14, 5 to 10, 4 to 6, and 5 percent, respectively. Mild back pain occurs in six percent. Visual side effects have not been described.

3. **Drug interactions**
   a. Tadalafil is contraindicated in men taking concurrent nitrates. Nitrates should be avoided for at least 48 hours after the last tadalafil dose. Other issues related to sexual activity in men with coronary heart disease are similar to those with sildenafil.
   b. Alpha adrenergic antagonists, used for the treatment of benign prostatic hyperplasia, may cause symptomatic hypotension when taken in combination with PDE-5 inhibitors. Tamulosin is the only alpha adrenergic antagonist which is approved for use with PDE-5 inhibitors, but only with tadalafil.
   c. Excessive alcohol intake (5 or more drinks) in combination with tadalafil may potentiate the hypotensive effect of tadalafil.
   d. Potent CYP3A4 inhibitors (erythromycin, ketoconazole, protease inhibitors, grapefruit juice) should be avoided because these drugs that can prolong the half-life of tadalafil; drugs that induce CYP3A4 (rifampin, phenytoin) reduce the effectiveness of tadalafil. Blue vision has not been reported with this medication.

I. **Comparisons**

1. All PDE-5 inhibitors allow men to have erections after appropriate sexual stimulation but differ in the onset of action as well as duration of effectiveness. Tadalafil differs in two ways. Its absorption is less affected by high fat meals and alcohol and it has a longer duration of action.

2. With sildenafil and vardenafil men are advised that maximum effectiveness is achieved by taking the tablet on an empty stomach (high fat meals and alcohol delay absorption) and then wait at least an hour before attempting sexual intercourse. Tadalafil can be taken without regard to meals.

3. Duration of action that separates one PDE-5 inhibitor from another. Sildenafil and vardenafil are effective as early as 30 minutes and up to 4 hours after dosing whereas tadalafil is effective as early as 16 minutes after and up to 36 hours after dosing.

4. Concomitant treatment with alpha adrenergic antagonists (used for benign prostatic hyperplasia) is contraindicated (due to potential hypotension with combination therapy), with the exception of tamulosin, which may be used safely with tadalafil.

5. Sildenafil and vardenafil must be taken on an empty stomach, while tadalafil can be taken without regard to food.

Oral Treatments for Male Sexual Dysfunction

Medication	Mechanism	Pros and cons	Dosing
Vardenafil (Levitra)	Inhibits phosphodiesterase 5, allowing cyclic GMP to accumulate within penis	No visual side effects Side effects: headaches, dyspepsia, vasodilation, diarrhea. Contraindicated if using nitrates	Taken one hour before sex and effective up to four hours. Stimulation needed for erection. **Dose:** 2.5 to 20 mg
Sildenafil (Viagra)	Same as vardenafil	Similar efficacy/side effects to vardenafil but blue tinge to vision. 100 mg effective in 75 percent of men.	Similar onset and duration as vardenafil **Dose:** 25 to 100 mg
Tadalafil (Cialis)	Same as vardenafil	Similar efficacy/side effects to vardenafil but no visual side effects	Similar onset of action as vardenafil. Duration of action is up to 36 hours. **Dose:** 2.5 to 20 mg
SSRIs	Inhibits serotonin reuptake by neurons	May help patients with premature ejaculation, depression	Sertraline (Zoloft) 50 mg/day. Paroxetine (Paxil) 20 mg as needed 3 hours before intercourse.

Pharmacokinetic Characteristics of PDE-5 Inhibitors

Parameter	Vardenafil (Levitra)	Sildenafil (Viagra)	Tadalafil (Cialis)
Oral dose	20 mg	100 mg	20 mg
Onset of action	30 min	30 min	16 min
Duration of action	4 hours	4 hours	36 hours
Food interaction	Minimal with low-fat foods; delay in time to peak concentration with high-fat foods	With high-fat foods; possible with low-fat foods	None
Alcohol interaction	None	None	Maybe

Parameter	Vardenafil (Levitra)	Sildenafil (Viagra)	Tadalafil (Cialis)
Age >65 yr	Increased half-life dose adjustment not needed	Increased half-life, dose adjustment may be needed	Increased half-life dose adjustment may not be needed

VI. Penile self-injection

A. Intrapenile injection therapy with alprostadil (prostaglandin E1, Caverject), papaverine, or alprostadil with papaverine and phentolamine (Tri-Mix) have all been used for purposes of inducing erection.

B. The technique consists of inserting an insulin syringe with a 26 gauge needle through the shaft of the penis and injecting the vasoactive agent into one corporeal body. A full, firm erection can be expected within a few minutes.

C. **Alprostadil**

   1. Intrapenile alprostadil injections are satisfactory in 87 percent of the men. There is a very high attrition rate with self-injection, suggesting that it may not be a satisfactory long-term solution.

   2. The major side effect of intrapenile alprostadil therapy is penile pain, occurring in 50 percent.

   3. Priapism, or a prolonged erection lasting more than four to six hours, is a medical emergency. Prolonged erections occur in 6 percent of men who use intrapenile alprostadil and about 11 percent of those who use intrapenile papaverine.

VII. Intraurethral alprostadil (MUSE) provides an erection sufficient for intercourse in two-thirds of men. After insertion of the alprostadil into the urethra, the penis should be massaged for up to one minute.

   1. Systemic effects are uncommon, and complications such as priapism and penile fibrosis are less common than after alprostadil given by penile injection.

Suppositories, Injections, and Devices for Sexual Dysfunction			
Treatment	**Effect**	**Pros and cons**	**Usage pattern**
Suppository			
MUSE (alprostadil)	Alprostadil (prostaglandin E1) in gel form delivered by applicator into meatus of penis	Can be used twice daily. Not recommended with pregnant partners	Inserted 5-10 minutes before sex. Effects last one hour
Penile injection			
Alprostadil (Caverject and Edex)	Prostaglandin E1 injected into base of penis.	Effective in 50-85 percent of cases. May be painful and not recommended for daily use. Priapism occurs uncommonly	Inject 10-20 minutes before sex. Erections may last hours

Treatment	Effect	Pros and cons	Usage pattern
Invicorp (VIP and phentolamine)	VIP and alpha-blocker, phentolamine.	Possibly more effective than alprostadil. Causes less pain. Priapism rare	Inject 10-20 minutes before sex. Requires stimulation to have erection
Device			
Vacuum pump	Creates a vacuum, drawing blood into cavernosae. Elastic tourniquet at base.	Safe if erection not maintained more than one hour. May interfere with ejaculation	Inflated just before sexual activity. Erection lasts until elastic ring removed

VIII. **Vacuum-assisted erection devices** have been developed to encourage increased arterial inflow and create an erection sufficient for sexual intercourse. Men cannot ejaculate externally because the occlusive rings compress the penile urethra.

A. Vacuum devices successfully create erections in 67 percent. Satisfaction with vacuum-assisted erections has varied between 25 and 49 percent.

IX. **Penile prostheses** remain a viable option for those men who do not respond to sildenafil and find penile injection or vacuum erection therapy distasteful. There are two general types of prostheses: malleable rods and inflatable prostheses.

X. **Premature ejaculation** is defined as an inability to control ejaculation so that both partners enjoy sexual intercourse. Approximately 20 percent of men complain of premature ejaculation.

A. The selective serotonin reuptake inhibitor (SSRI) sertraline (Zoloft, 50 mg/day) increases the mean ejaculatory latency time to 3.2 minutes. Other SSRIs also appear to be effective.

B. Intermittent use of SSRIs may be as effective as continuous use. Paroxetine (Paxil, 20 mg) as needed three to four hours before planned intercourse increases the mean ejaculatory latency time to 3.2 minutes.

C. Serotonin reuptake inhibitors (SSRIs) are first-line therapy, and clomipramine is second-line therapy for premature ejaculation.

References: See page 294.

Psychiatric Disorders

Depression

The lifetime prevalence of major depression in the United States is 17 percent. In primary care, depression has a prevalence rate of 4.8 to 8.6 percent.

I. Diagnosis
  A. The Diagnostic and Statistical Manual of Mental Disorders (DSM-IV) includes nine symptoms in the diagnosis of major depression.
  B. These nine symptoms can be divided into two clusters: (1) physical or neurovegetative symptoms and (2) psychologic or psychosocial symptoms. The nine symptoms are: depressed mood plus sleep disturbance; interest/pleasure reduction; guilt feelings or thoughts of worthlessness; energy changes/fatigue; concentration/attention impairment; appetite/weight changes; psychomotor disturbances, and suicidal thoughts.

Diagnostic Criteria for Major Depression, DSM IV

Cluster 1: Physical or neurovegetative symptoms
Sleep disturbance
Appetite/weight changes
Attention/concentration problem
Energy-level change/fatigue
Psychomotor disturbance

Cluster 2: Psychologic or psychosocial symptoms
Depressed mood and/or
Interest/pleasure reduction
Guilt feelings
Suicidal thoughts

Note: Diagnosis of major depression requires at least one of the first two symptoms under cluster 2 and four of the remaining symptoms to be present for at least two weeks. Symptoms should not be accounted for by bereavement.

II. Drug Therapy

Characteristics of Common Antidepressants		
Drug	**Recommended Dosage**	**Comments**
Selective Serotonin Reuptake Inhibitors (SSRIs)		
Escitalopram (Lexapro)	10 mg qd	Minimal sedation, activation, or inhibition of hepatic enzymes, nausea, anorgasmia, headache
Citalopram (Celexa)	Initially 20 mg qd; maximum 40 mg/d	
Fluoxetine (Prozac)	10-20 mg qd initially, taken in AM	Anxiety, insomnia, agitation, nausea, anorgasmia, erectile dysfunction, headache, anorexia.

Drug	Recommended Dosage	Comments
Fluvoxamine (LuVox)	50-100 mg qhs; max 300 mg/d [50, 100 mg]	Headache, nausea, sedation, diarrhea
Paroxetine (Paxil)	20 mg/d initially, given in AM; increase in 10-mg/d increments as needed to max of 50 mg/d. [10, 20, 30, 40 mg]	Headache, nausea, somnolence, dizziness, insomnia, abnormal ejaculation, anxiety, diarrhea, dry mouth.
Sertraline (Zoloft)	50 mg/d, increasing as needed to max of 200 mg/d [50, 100 mg]	Insomnia, agitation, dry mouth, headache, nausea, anorexia, sexual dysfunction.
Secondary Amine Tricyclic Antidepressants		
Desipramine (Norpramin, generics)	100-200 mg/d, gradually increasing to 300 mg/d as tolerated.[10, 25, 50, 75, 100, 150 mg]	No sedation; may have stimulant effect; best taken in morning to avoid insomnia.
Nortriptyline (Pamelor)	25 mg tid-qid, max 150 mg/d. [10, 25, 50, 75 mg]	Sedating
Tertiary Amine Tricyclics		
Amitriptyline (Elavil, generics)	75 mg qhs-bid, increasing to 150-200 mg/d. [25, 50, 75, 100, 150 mg]	Sedative effect precedes antidepressant effect. High anticholinergic activity.
Clomipramine (Anafranil)	25 mg/d, increasing gradually to 100 mg/d; max 250 mg/d; may be given once qhs [25, 50, 75 mg].	Relatively high sedation, anticholinergic activity, and seizure risk.
Protriptyline (Vivactil)	5-10 mg PO tid-qid; 15-60 mg/d [5, 10 mg]	Useful in anxious depression; nonsedating
Doxepin (Sinequan, generics)	50-75 mg/d, increasing up to 150-300 mg/d as needed [10, 25, 50, 75, 100, 150 mg]	Sedating. Also indicated for anxiety. Contraindicated in patients with glaucoma or urinary retention.
Imipramine (Tofranil, generics)	75 mg/d in a single dose qhs, increasing to 150 mg/d; 300 mg/d. [10, 25, 50 mg]	High sedation and anticholinergic activity. Use caution in cardiovascular disease.

Drug	Recommended Dosage	Comments
Miscellaneous		
Bupropion (Wellbutrin, Wellbutrin SR)	100 mg bid; increase to 100 mg tid [75, 100 mg] Sustained release: 100-200 mg bid [100, 150 mg]	Agitation, dry mouth, insomnia, headache, nausea, constipation, tremor. Good choice for patients with sexual side effects from other agents; contraindicated in seizure disorders.
Venlafaxine (Effexor)	75 mg/d in 2-3 divided doses with food; increase to 225 mg/d as needed. [25, 37.5, 50, 75, 100 mg]. Extended-release: initially 37.5 mg qAM. The dosage can be increased by 75 mg every four days to a max of 225 mg qd [37.5, 75, 100, 150 mg].	Inhibits norepinephrine and serotonin reuptake. Hypertension, nausea, insomnia, dizziness, abnormal ejaculation, headache, dry mouth, anxiety.
Duloxetine (Cymbalta)	20 mg bid or 60 mg qd or 30 mg bid. Start at a dose of 30 mg and increase the dose to 60 mg daily; up to 120 mg daily [30, 60 mg].	Inhibits norepinephrine and serotonin reuptake. Contraindicated in hepatic or renal insufficiency. Food delays absorption. Nausea, dry mouth, constipation. Diarrhea and vomiting less often. Insomnia, dizziness, somnolence, and sweating also seen. Sexual side effects may be less common than with the SSRIs. Marketed for physical pain associated with depression.
Maprotiline (Ludiomil)	75 to 225 in single or divided doses [25, 50, 75 mg].	Delays cardiac conduction; high anticholinergic activity; contraindicated in seizure disorders.
Mirtazapine (Remeron)	15 to 45 PO qd [15, 30 mg].	High anticholinergic activity; contraindicated in seizure disorders.
Nefazodone (Serzone)	Start at 100 mg PO bid, increase to 150-300 mg PO bid as needed [100, 150, 200, 250 mg].	Headache, somnolence, dry mouth, blurred vision. Postural hypotension, impotence.
Reboxetine (Vestra)	5 mg bid	Selective norepinephrine reuptake inhibitor. Dry mouth, insomnia, constipation, increased sweating
Trazodone (Desyrel, generics)	150 mg/d, increasing by 50 mg/d every 3-4 d 400 mg/d in divided doses [50, 100, 150, 300 mg]	Rarely associated with priapism. Orthostatic hypotension in elderly. Sedating.

A. **Psychotherapy**
   1. The efficacy of cognitive therapy, behavioral therapy, and interpersonal therapy are 46, 55, and 52 percent, respectively, in psychiatric patients with major depression.
   2. Cognitive behavioral therapy is as effective as medication use for maintenance therapy (over two years) in patients with major depression.

B. Selective serotonin reuptake inhibitors
1. Abnormalities in brain serotonergic activity have been implicated in mood disorders. Medications causing increased serotonergic activity are often effective in ameliorating symptoms of depression, anxiety, and obsessive ruminations.
2. The selective-serotonin reuptake inhibitors (SSRIs) block the action of the presynaptic serotonin reuptake pump, thereby increasing the amount of serotonin available in the synapse and increasing postsynaptic serotonin receptor occupancy.
3. **The SSRIs all share several other characteristics:**
   a. They are all hepatically metabolized.
   b. They have relatively little affinity for histaminic, dopaminergic, alpha-adrenergic, and cholinergic receptors.
   c. They tend to have relatively mild side-effect profiles, although they can be associated with sexual dysfunction.
   d. They are relatively safe in overdose.
   e. They all produce changes in sleep architecture (decreased REM latency and decreased total REM sleep).
4. The SSRIs differ in potency, receptor selectivity, and pharmacokinetic properties. The overall efficacy of the different SSRIs appears to be similar. Coadministration of any SSRI with a monoamine oxidase inhibitor (MAOI) is contraindicated due to the potential for producing a sometimes fatal "serotonin syndrome," characterized by agitation, hyperthermia, diaphoresis, tachycardia, and rigidity.
5. **Fluoxetine (Prozac)** has a relatively mild side-effect profile, and a once-daily-dosing schedule. Fluoxetine is indicated for the treatment of major depressive disorder, obsessive-compulsive disorder, and bulimia.
   a. Fluoxetine is 95 percent protein bound. It undergoes oxidative metabolism in the liver by the cytochrome P-450 (CYP) enzyme system. The principal CYP enzymes responsible for its metabolism are CYP2D6 and CYP3A/34. The half-life (t 1/2) of fluoxetine is four to six days. Its active metabolite, norfluoxetine, is formed through demethylation of fluoxetine, is a potent and selective inhibitor of the serotonin reuptake pump, and has a t 1/2 of 7 to 15 days. Fluoxetine is a potent inhibitor of CYP2D6; norfluoxetine is also a mild inhibitor of CYP 3A/34. Drugs metabolized by CYP2D6 (tricyclic antidepressants, antiarrhythmics, beta-blockers) must be used cautiously when coadministered with fluoxetine.
   b. The clinical antidepressant effect may be delayed three to six weeks from the start of treatment.
   c. The usual effective dose of fluoxetine is 20 mg daily. Patients who do not respond to this dosage after several weeks can have their dose increased by 10 to 20 mg as tolerated up to 80 mg daily.
   d. **Fluoxetine (Prozac Weekly)** can be administered once weekly to patients who have responded to daily fluoxetine. Fluoxetine is given as 90 mg per week. Seven days should elapse after the last 20 mg daily dose of fluoxetine before beginning the once weekly regimen.
   e. The most common initial side effects of fluoxetine are nausea, insomnia, and anxiety. These effects usually present at the start of treatment and tend to resolve over one to two weeks. Fluoxetine, like all of the SSRIs, is relatively safe in overdose.
6. **Sertraline (Zoloft)** is approved for the treatment of depressive illness. Sertraline is 98 percent protein bound. Absorption is increased when taken with food. It is metabolized by the hepatic p450 enzyme system and has an active metabolite that is significantly less potent than the active compound. The t 1/2 of sertraline is 26 hours. As opposed to fluoxetine, which is a potent inhibitor of CYP2D6, sertraline has only mild inhibition of this enzyme. Sertraline has a low likelihood of interactions with coadministered medications.

    a. Sertraline is usually started at 50 mg daily; the effective mainte-
nance dose is typically 50 to 100 mg daily, although doses up to
200 mg daily may be necessary. Clinical effect is usually evident by
three to six weeks.

    b. Common initial side effects of sertraline include nausea, diarrhea,
insomnia, and sexual dysfunction. It may be more likely than the
other SSRIs to cause nausea. As with fluoxetine, sexual dysfunction
can persist. Addition of bupropion (Wellbutrin, 75 to 150 mg/day in
divided doses) or buspirone (BuSpar, 10 to 20 mg twice daily) may
alleviate decreased libido, diminished sexual arousal, or impaired
orgasm. Sertraline is relatively safe in overdose.

7. Paroxetine (Paxil) is indicated for the treatment of depression, panic
disorder, generalized anxiety disorder, and social phobia.

    a. Paroxetine is 95 percent protein bound. It inhibits the liver enzyme
CYP2D6 and must be used cautiously when coadministered with
other drugs metabolized by this enzyme (tricyclic antidepressants,
antiarrhythmics, beta-blockers). The t 1/2 is 24 hours. It has a mild
affinity for muscarinic receptors and can cause more anticholinergic
side effects than the other SSRIs (although much less than the
tricyclic antidepressants).

    b. The starting and maintenance dose of paroxetine is 20 mg daily but
can be raised to 40 mg daily if necessary. In contrast to fluoxetine
and sertraline, which can be activating, paroxetine is mildly sedating. Other side effects include nausea, dry mouth, and sexual
dysfunction. Sexual dysfunction may be slightly higher with
paroxetine than with the other SSRIs.

    c. An enteric-coated, controlled-release formulation of paroxetine may
cause less nausea than the immediate-release formulation. The
recommended starting dose of Paxil CR is 12.5 mg/day for panic
disorder and 25 mg/day for depression; the maximum dose is 75
mg/day.

8. Citalopram (Celexa) has mild p450 2D6 inhibition, but it has significantly less p450 interactions than the other SSRIs, making it an
appealing choice in patients who are on other medications where drug-
drug interactions are a concern. Citalopram is touted as causing less
sexual dysfunction than the other SSRIs. Anxiety symptoms are
improved with citalopram compared with sertraline or placebo.

    a. The usual starting dose of citalopram is 20 mg daily. The therapeu-
tic dose range tends to be 20 to 40 mg daily in a single morning
dose.

9. Escitalopram (Lexapro) is a single isomer formulation of citalopram.
Escitalopram is reported to be a more potent serotonin reuptake
inhibitor, and a daily dose of 10 mg is at least comparable to 40 mg of
citalopram. There are no clear advantages of escitalopram compared
with other SSRIs in terms of efficacy or adverse effects, although, like
citalopram, it has little effect on CYP isoenzymes and therefore may
prove to have fewer drug interactions than other SSRIs such as
fluoxetine or paroxetine.

C. Heterocyclic antidepressants

    1. The cyclic antidepressants are less commonly used as first-line
antidepressants with the development of the SSRIs. This is mainly due
to the less benign side-effect profile of the cyclic antidepressants. In
contrast to the SSRIs, the cyclic antidepressants can be fatal in doses
as little as five times the therapeutic dose. The toxicity is usually due to
prolongation of the QT interval, leading to arrhythmias. Overdose of
cyclic antidepressants can also cause anticholinergic toxicity and
seizures.

    2. The cyclic antidepressants tend to have anticholinergic and orthostatic
effects, as well as sedation, weight gain, and sexual dysfunction. In
addition, tricyclic antidepressant users have a higher risk of myocardial
infarction compared with SSRI users.

3. As with all antidepressants, the cyclic antidepressants can take up to three to six weeks before reaching full clinical effect.

4. **Tertiary amines** are not frequently used as primary antidepressant agents because of their tendency to cause significant sedative and anticholinergic side effects.

   a. **Imipramine (Tofranil).** The usual starting dose of imipramine is 25 mg daily. The dose can be increased by 25 to 50 mg every three to four days to a typical therapeutic dose range of 150 to 300 mg daily. Patients with combined blood levels of imipramine and desipramine greater than 225 ng/mL have a superior response. Imipramine is moderately sedating and anticholinergic compared with other cyclic antidepressants.

   b. **Amitriptyline (Elavil).** Amitriptyline is demethylated to nortriptyline, which has antidepressant effects. The usual starting dose of is 25 mg, given at bedtime. Therapeutic doses are generally in the range of 100 to 300 mg daily, but many patients find it difficult to reach these doses due to sedation. Blood levels of amitriptyline plus nortriptyline are 95 to 160 ng/mL.

5. **Secondary amines**

   a. **Desipramine (Norpramin)** is an active metabolite of imipramine. Desipramine differs from the tertiary amines in that it is much more selective in its properties of norepinephrine blockade than in its properties of serotonin reuptake blockade. It tends to have much less sedative and anticholinergic side effects. It does, however, share the side effect of orthostatic hypotension. The usual starting dose of desipramine is 25 mg daily.

   b. **Nortriptyline (Aventyl)** is an active metabolite of amitriptyline. Like desipramine, nortriptyline has significantly more effects on norepinephrine than on serotonin receptors. Although nortriptyline has fewer sedative and anticholinergic side effects than the tertiary amines, it has slightly more than desipramine. It is distinctly different from desipramine in that it has very little orthostatic hypotensive effects. Nortriptyline is twice as potent as the other cyclic antidepressants. The starting dose is 25 mg daily.

6. **Cardiac testing.** Before initiating treatment with any of the cyclic antidepressants, patients must be screened for cardiac conduction system disease, which precludes the use of these medications. Patients over age 40 years should have a baseline electrocardiogram (ECG).

D. **Venlafaxine (Effexor XR)** is a phenylethylamine inhibitor of serotonin reuptake and an inhibitor of norepinephrine reuptake. The t 1/2 of the parent compound plus the active metabolite is 11 hours. There is a slow-release form that allows for once-daily dosing. Venlafaxine is excreted by the kidney, and food does not affect its absorption. Venlafaxine is a weak inhibitor of the p450 2D6 enzyme, but it tends to not interact with most coadministered medications (except MAOIs).

1. Dosing for the immediate-release form of venlafaxine begins at 37.5 mg twice daily. The medication can be increased by 75 mg every four days to a maximum dose of 375 mg daily in three divided doses. The extended-release form of venlafaxine is given as a single-morning dose of 37.5 mg. If this is well tolerated, the dose is increased to 75 mg in a single daily dose. The medication can be increased by 75 mg every four days to a recommended maximum of 225 mg daily in a single-daily dose.

2. The most common side effects of venlafaxine are nausea, dizziness, insomnia, sedation, and constipation. It can also induce sweating. Venlafaxine may cause blood pressure increases. Three to 7 percent of patients have mild blood pressure elevations (average 1 to 2 mm Hg).

3. Medications that inhibit CYP2D6 can increase the plasma level of venlafaxine. This is sometimes encountered when switching a patient

from an SSRI with CYP2D6 inhibiting properties (eg, fluoxetine, paroxetine) to venlafaxine.

4. Venlafaxine overdose is more serious than overdose with SSRIs. Venlafaxine is more likely to cause seizures than tricyclic antidepressants. Rates of serotonin toxicity are also higher with venlafaxine than with tricyclic antidepressants. Venlafaxine should be avoided in patients who are at high risk for deliberate overdose.

5. Patients who do not respond to other antidepressants may respond better to venlafaxine, and venlafaxine may be less likely to lose efficacy over time. Venlafaxine may be more likely to lead to a remission of depression.

E. **Duloxetine (Cymbalta)** is an inhibitor of both serotonin reuptake and norepinephrine reuptake.

1. Duloxetine is metabolized in the liver and should not be administered with hepatic insufficiency. Metabolites are excreted in the urine, and the use of duloxetine is not recommended in end-stage renal disease. Food delays the absorption of duloxetine, and the t 1/2 is 12 hours. Duloxetine is a moderate inhibitor of CYP2D6.

2. Dosage is 20 mg twice daily or 60 mg daily either as a single dose or as 30 mg twice daily. Start at 30 mg daily and increase to 60 mg daily; there may be added benefit to using up to 120 mg daily.

3. Nausea, dry mouth and constipation are common. Diarrhea and vomiting are seen less often. Insomnia, dizziness, somnolence, and sweating occur. Sexual side effects occur, but may be less common than with the SSRIs. Duloxetine is marketed as a treatment for physical pain associated with depression. Duloxetine has shown efficacy in diabetic neuropathy.

4. Medications that inhibit CYP2D6 (paroxetine and fluoxetine) and medications that inhibit CYP1A2 (fluvoxamine) can increase levels of duloxetine.

F. **Mirtazapine (Remeron)** is a tetracyclic compound (a piperazinoazepine), but it is unrelated to TCAs. It has a unique mechanism of action in that it blocks pre- and postsynaptic alpha-2 receptors, as well as the serotonin receptors 5HT2 and 5HT3.

1. Mirtazapine can be particularly helpful in depressed patients with insomnia because of its sedative properties.

2. Mirtazapine is metabolized in the liver primarily by oxidation and demethylation. It is metabolized by several p450 enzymes including 2D6, 1A2, 3A4, and 2C9. Mirtazapine's t 1/2 is 20 to 40 hours, and it is 85 percent protein bound.

3. Some side effects may be greater at lower doses. Sedation appears more pronounced at doses of 15 mg daily than at 30 mg daily. Dosing is most frequently started at 15 mg daily and can be increased to 30 mg or 45 mg daily as needed in one- to two-week intervals. Dosing may be initiated at 30 mg or more in order to reduce sedation.

4. **Side effects** of mirtazapine are sedation, weight gain, and dry mouth. Many patients report a significant increase in appetite. Mirtazapine may have less propensity to cause sexual dysfunction than the SSRIs, TCAs, and MAOIs. Two out of 2796 patients developed agranulocytosis, and a third developed neutropenia. All recovered after the medication was discontinued. There are no FDA recommendations to monitor white blood cell counts. Mild transaminase elevations have been noted in some patients.

G. **Electroconvulsive therapy.** Electroconvulsive therapy (ECT) is highly effective in patients with psychotic depression. Patients who continue to have severe melancholic depression on maximum medical therapy also do well with ETC. The quick response and low side-effect profile make ECT one of the most effective ways to alleviate the symptoms of major depression. The relapse rate after ECT is high, and drug therapy should continue following cessation of ETC.

References: See page 294.

Generalized Anxiety Disorder

Generalized anxiety disorder (GAD) is characterized by excessive worry and anxiety that are difficult to control and cause significant distress and impairment. Commonly patients develop symptoms of GAD secondary to other DSM-IV diagnoses such as panic disorder, major depression, alcohol abuse, or an axis II personality disorder.

I. **Epidemiology.** GAD is a common anxiety disorder. The prevalence is estimated to be 5 percent in the primary care setting. Twice as many women as men have the disorder. GAD may also be associated with substance abuse, post-traumatic stress disorder, and obsessive compulsive disorder. Between 35 and 50 percent of individuals with major depression meet criteria for GAD.

II. **Clinical manifestations and diagnosis**
   A. **The diagnostic criteria for GAD** suggest that patients experience excessive anxiety and worry about a number of events or activities, occurring more days than not for at least six months, that are out of proportion to the likelihood or impact of feared events. Affected patients also present with somatic symptoms, including fatigue, muscle tension, memory loss, and insomnia, and other psychiatric disorders.

DSM-IV-PC Diagnostic Criteria for Generalized Anxiety Disorder

1. Excessive anxiety and worry about a number of events or activities, occurring more days than not for at least six months, that are out of proportion to the likelihood or impact of feared events.
2. The worry is pervasive and difficult to control.
3. The anxiety and worry are associated with three (or more) of the following six symptoms (with at least some symptoms present for more days than not for the past six months):
   Restlessness or feeling keyed up or on edge
   Being easily fatigued
   Difficulty concentrating or mind going blank
   Irritability
   Muscle tension
   Sleep disturbance (difficulty falling or staying asleep, or restless unsatisfying sleep)
4. The anxiety, worry, or physical symptoms cause clinically significant distress or impairment in social, occupational, or other important areas of functioning.

   B. **Comorbid psychiatric disorders** and an organic etiology for anxiety must be excluded by careful history taking, a complete physical examination, and appropriate laboratory studies. The medical history should focus upon current medical disorders, medication side effects, or substance abuse to anxiety (or panic) symptoms.
   C. **Psychosocial history** should screen for major depression and agoraphobia, stressful life events, family psychiatric history, current social history, substance abuse history (including caffeine, nicotine, and alcohol), and past sexual, physical and emotional abuse, or emotional neglect.
   D. **Laboratory studies** include a complete blood count, chemistry panel, serum thyrotropin (TSH) and urinalysis. Urine or serum toxicology measurements or drug levels can be obtained for drugs or medications suspected in the etiology of anxiety.

III. **Treatment**
   A. **Drug therapy.** While benzodiazepines have been the most traditionally used drug treatments for GAD, selective serotonin reuptake inhibitors (SSRIs), selective serotonin and norepinephrine reuptake inhibitors (SNRIs, eg venlafaxine), and buspirone are also effective, and because of their lower side effect profiles and lower risk for tolerance are becoming first-line treatment.

B. Antidepressants

1. **Venlafaxine SR (Effexor)** may be a particularly good choice for patients with coexisting psychiatric illness, such as panic disorder, major depression, or social phobia, or when it is not clear if the patient has GAD, depression, or both. Venlafaxine can be started as venlafaxine XR 37.5 mg daily, with dose increases in increments of 37.5 mg every one to two weeks until a dose of 150 mg to 300 mg is attained.

C. Tricyclic antidepressants, SSRIs, or SNRIs may be associated with side effects such as restlessness and insomnia. These adverse effects can be minimized by starting at lower doses and gradually titrating to full doses as tolerated.

1. **Selective serotonin reuptake inhibitors**
   a. **Paroxetine (Paxil)** 5 to 10 mg qd, increasing to 20 to 40 mg.
   b. **Sertraline (Zoloft)** 12.5 to 25 mg qd, increasing to 50 to 200 mg.
   c. **Fluvoxamine (Luvox)** 25 mg qd, increasing to 100 to 300 mg.
   d. **Fluoxetine (Prozac)** 5 mg qd, increasing to 20 to 40 mg.
   e. **Citalopram (Celexa)** 10 mg qd, increasing to 20 to 40 mg.
   f. Side effects of SSRIs include agitation, headache, gastrointestinal symptoms (diarrhea and nausea), and insomnia. About 20 to 35 percent of patients develop sexual side effects after several weeks or months of SSRI therapy, especially a decreased ability to have an orgasm. Addition of bupropion (75 to 150 mg/day in divided doses) or buspirone (10 to 20 mg twice daily) may alleviate decreased libido, diminished sexual arousal, or impaired orgasm.

Physical Causes of Anxiety-Like Symptoms

Cardiovascular
Angina pectoris, arrhythmias, congestive heart failure, hypertension, hypovolemia, myocardial infarction, syncope (multiple causes), valvular disease, vascular collapse (shock)

Dietary
Caffeine, monosodium glutamate (Chinese restaurant syndrome), vitamin-deficiency diseases

Drug-related
Akathesia (secondary to antipsychotic drugs), anticholinergic toxicity, digitalis toxicity, hallucinogens, hypotensive agents, stimulants (amphetamines, cocaine, related drugs), withdrawal syndromes (alcohol, sedative-hypnotics), bronchodilators (theophylline, sympathomimetics)

Hematologic
Anemias

Immunologic
Anaphylaxis, systemic lupus erythematosus

Metabolic
Hyperadrenalism (Cushing's disease), hyperkalemia, hyperthermia, hyperthyroidism, hypocalcemia, hypoglycemia, hyponatremia, hypothyroidism, menopause, porphyria (acute intermittent)

Neurologic
Encephalopathies (infectious, metabolic, toxic), essential tremor, intracranial mass lesions, postconcussive syndrome, seizure disorders (especially of the temporal lobe), vertigo

Respiratory
Asthma, chronic obstructive pulmonary disease, pneumonia, pneumothorax, pulmonary edema, pulmonary embolism

Secreting tumors
Carcinoid, insulinoma, pheochromocytoma

---

2. **Imipramine (Tofranil)**, a starting dose of 10 to 20 mg po at night can be gradually titrated up to 75 to 300 mg each night. Imipramine has anticholinergic and antiadrenergic side effects. Desipramine

(Norpramin), 25-200 mg qhs, and nortriptyline (Pamelor), 25 mg tid-qid, can be used as alternatives.

3. **Trazodone (Desyrel)** is a serotonergic agent, but because of its side effects (sedation and priapism), it is not an ideal first-line agent. Daily dosages of 200 to 400 mg are helpful in patients who have not responded to other agents.

4. **Nefazodone (Serzone)** has a similar pharmacologic profile to trazodone, but it is better tolerated and is a good alternative; 100 mg bid; increase to 200-300 mg bid.

D. **Buspirone (BuSpar)** appears to be as effective as the benzodiazepines for the treatment of GAD. However, the onset of action can be several weeks, and there are occasional gastrointestinal side effects. Advantages of using buspirone instead of benzodiazepines include the lack of abuse potential, physical dependence, or withdrawal, and lack of potentiation of alcohol or other sedative-hypnotics. Most patients need to be titrated to doses of 30 to 60 mg per day given in two or three divided doses.

E. **Benzodiazepines.** Several controlled studies have demonstrated the efficacy of benzodiazepines (eg, chlordiazepoxide, diazepam, alprazolam) in the treatment of GAD.

1. Many anxious patients who start on benzodiazepines have difficulty stopping them, particularly since rebound anxiety and withdrawal symptoms can be moderate to severe. Methods of facilitating withdrawal and decreasing rebound symptoms include tapering the medication slowly, converting short-acting benzodiazepines to a long-acting preparation (eg, clonazepam) prior to tapering, and treating the patient with an antidepressant before attempting to taper.

2. Symptoms of anxiety can be alleviated in most cases of GAD with clonazepam (Klonopin) 0.25 to 0.5 mg po bid titrated up to 1 mg bid or tid, or lorazepam (Ativan) 0.5 to 1.0 mg po tid titrated up to 1 mg po tid or qid. Often an antidepressant is prescribed concomitantly. After six to eight weeks, when the antidepressant begins to have its optimal effects, the benzodiazepine usually should be tapered over months, achieving roughly a 10 percent dose reduction per week.

Benzodiazepines Commonly Prescribed for Anxiety Disorders			
Name	Half-life (hours)	Dosage range (per day)	Initial dosage
Alprazolam (Xanax)	14	1 to 4 mg	0.25 to 0.5 mg four times daily
Chlordiazepoxide (Librium)	20	15 to 40 mg	5 to 10 mg three times daily
Clonazepam (Klonopin)	50	0.5 to 4.0 mg	0.5 to 1.0 mg twice daily
Clorazepate (Tranxene)	60	15 to 60 mg	7.5 to 15.0 mg twice daily
Diazepam (Valium)	40	6 to 40 mg	2 to 5 mg three times daily
Lorazepam (Ativan)	14	1 to 6 mg	0.5 to 1.0 mg three times daily
Oxazepam (Serax)	9	30 to 90 mg	15 to 30 mg three times daily

F. Agents with short half-lives, such as oxazepam (Serax), do not cause excessive sedation. These agents should be used in the elderly and in patients with liver disease. They are also suitable for use on an "as-needed" basis. Agents with long half-lives, such as clonazepam (Klonopin), should be used in younger patients who do not have concomitant medical problems. The longer-acting agents can be taken less frequently during the day, patients are less likely to experience anxiety between doses and withdrawal symptoms are less severe.

References: See page 294.

Panic Disorder

Panic disorder is characterized by the occurrence of panic attacks--sudden, unexpected periods of intense fear or discomfort. About 15% of the general population experiences panic attacks; 1.6-3.2% of women and 0.4%-1.7% of men have panic disorder.

I. Clinical evaluation
  A. Panic attacks are manifested by the sudden onset of an overwhelming fear, accompanied by feelings of impending doom, for no apparent reason.

DSM-IV Criteria for panic attack

A discrete period of intense fear or discomfort in which four or more of the following symptoms developed abruptly and reached a peak within 10 minutes.
  Chest pain or discomfort
  Choking
  Depersonalization or derealization
  Dizziness, faintness, or unsteadiness
  Fear of "going crazy" or being out of control
  Fear of dying
  Flushes or chills
  Nausea or gastrointestinal distress
  Palpitations or tachycardia
  Paresthesias
  Shortness of breath (or feelings of smothering)
  Sweating
  Trembling or shaking

  B. The essential criterion for panic attack is the presence of 4 of 13 cardiac, neurologic, gastrointestinal, or respiratory symptoms that develop abruptly and reach a peak within 10 minutes. The physical symptoms include shortness of breath, dizziness or faintness, palpitations, accelerated heart rate, and sweating. Trembling, choking, nausea, numbness, flushes, chills, or chest discomfort are also common, as are cognitive symptoms such as fear of dying or losing control.
  C. One third of patients develop agoraphobia, or a fear of places where escape may be difficult, such as bridges, trains, buses, or crowded areas. Medications, substance abuse, and general medical conditions such as hyperthyroidism must be ruled out as a cause of the patient's symptoms.
  D. The history should include details of the panic attack, its onset and course, history of panic, and any treatment. Questioning about a family history of panic disorder, agoraphobia, hypochondriasis, or depression is important. Because panic disorder may be triggered by marijuana or stimulants such as cocaine, a history of substance abuse must be identified. A medication history, including prescription, over-the-counter, and herbal preparations, is essential.
  E. The patient should be asked about stressful life events or problems in daily life that may have preceded onset of the disorder. The extent of any

avoidance behavior that has developed or suicidal ideation, self-medication, or exacerbation of an existing medical disorder should be assessed.

Diagnostic criteria for panic disorder without agoraphobia

Recurrent, unexpected panic attacks
And
At least one attack has been followed by at least 1 month of one (or more) of the following:
Persistent concern about experiencing more attacks
Worry about the meaning of the attack or its consequences (fear of losing control, having a heart attack, or "going crazy")
A significant behavioral change related to the attacks
And
Absence of agoraphobia
And
Direct physiological effects of a substance (drug abuse or medication) or general medical condition has been ruled out as a cause of the attacks
And
The panic attacks cannot be better accounted for by another mental disorder

II. Management
A. Patients should reduce or eliminate caffeine consumption, including coffee and tea, cold medications, analgesics, and beverages with added caffeine. Alcohol use is a particularly insidious problem because patients may use drinking to alleviate the panic.

Pharmacologic treatment of panic disorder

Drug	Initial dosage (mg/d)	Therapeutic dosage (mg/d)
SSRIs		
Fluoxetine (Prozac)	5-10	10-60
Fluvoxamine (LuVox)	25-50	25-300
Paroxetine (Paxil)	10-20	20-50
Sertraline (Zoloft)	25-50	50-200
Citalopram (Celexa)	10-20 mg qd	20-40
Benzodiazepines		
Alprazolam (Xanax)	0.5 in divided doses, tid-qid	1-4 in divided doses, tid-qid
Alprazolam XR (Xanax XR)	0.5 to 1 mg/day given once in the morning.	3-6 mg qAM
Clonazepam (Klonopin)	0.5 in divided doses, bid-tid	1-4 in divided doses, bid-tid
Diazepam (Valium)	2.0 in divided doses, bid-tid	2-20 in divided doses, bid
Lorazepam (Ativan)	0.5 in divided doses, bid-tid	1-4 in divided doses, bid-tid
TCAs		
Amitriptyline (Elavil)	10	10-300
Clomipramine (Anafranil)	25	25-300
Desipramine (Norpramin)	10	10-300
Imipramine (Tofranil)	10	10-300
Nortriptyline (Pamelor)	10	10-300
MAOIs		
Phenelzine (Nardil)	1510	15-90
Tranylcypromine (Parnate)		10-30

B. **Selective serotonin reuptake inhibitors (SSRIs)** are an effective, well-tolerated alternative to benzodiazepines and TCAs. SSRIs are superior to either imipramine or alprazolam. They lack the cardiac toxicity and anticholinergic effects of TCAs. Fluoxetine (Prozac), fluvoxamine (LuVox), paroxetine (Paxil), sertraline (Zoloft), and citalopram (Celexa) have shown efficacy for the treatment of panic disorder.

C. **Tricyclic antidepressants (TCAs)** have demonstrated efficacy in treating panic. They are, however, associated with a delayed onset of action and side effects--particularly orthostatic hypotension, anticholinergic effects, weight gain, and cardiac toxicity.

D. **Benzodiazepines**
   1. Clonazepam (Klonopin), alprazolam (Xanax), and lorazepam (Ativan), are effective in blocking panic attacks. Advantages include a rapid onset of therapeutic effect and a safe, favorable, side-effect profile. Among the drawbacks are the potential for abuse and dependency, worsening of depressive symptoms, withdrawal symptoms on abrupt discontinuation, anterograde amnesia, early relapse on discontinuation, and inter-dose rebound anxiety.
   2. Benzodiazepines are an appropriate first-line treatment only when rapid symptom relief is needed. The most common use for benzodiazepines is to stabilize severe initial symptoms until another treatment (eg, an SSRI or cognitive behavioral therapy) becomes effective.
   3. The starting dose of alprazolam is 0.5 mg bid. Approximately 70% of patients will experience a discontinuance reaction characterized by increased anxiety, agitation, and insomnia when alprazolam is tapered. Clonazepam's long duration of effect diminishes the need for multiple daily dosing. Initial symptoms of sedation and ataxia are usually transient.

E. **Monoamine oxidase inhibitors (MAOIs).** MAOIs such phenelzine sulfate (Nardil) may be the most effective agents for blocking panic attacks and for relieving the depression and concomitant social anxiety of panic disorder. Recommended doses range from 45-90 mg/d. MAOI use is limited by adverse effects such as orthostatic hypotension, weight gain, insomnia, risk of hypertensive crisis, and the need for dietary monitoring. MAOIs are often reserved for patients who do not respond to safer drugs.

F. **Beta-blockers** are useful in moderating heart rate and decreasing dry mouth and tremor; they are less effective in relieving subjective anxiety.

References: See page 294.

Insomnia

Insomnia is the perception by patients that their sleep is inadequate or abnormal. Insomnia may affect as many as 69% of adult primary care patients. The incidence of sleep problems increases with age. Younger persons are apt to have trouble falling asleep, whereas older persons tend to have prolonged awakenings during the night.

I. **Causes of insomnia**
   A. **Situational stress** concerning job loss or problems often disrupt sleep. Patients under stress may experience interference with sleep onset and early morning awakening. Attempting to sleep in a new place, changes in time zones, or changing bedtimes due to shift work may interfere with sleep.
   B. **Drugs associated with insomnia** include antihypertensives, caffeine, diuretics, oral contraceptives, phenytoin, selective serotonin reuptake inhibitors, protriptyline, corticosteroids, stimulants, theophylline, and thyroid hormone.
   C. **Psychiatric disorders.** Depression is a common cause of poor sleep, often characterized by early morning awakening. Associated findings in-

clude hopelessness, sadness, loss of appetite, and reduced enjoyment of formerly pleasurable activities. Anxiety disorders and substance abuse may cause insomnia.

D. **Medical disorders.** Prostatism, peptic ulcer, congestive heart failure, and chronic obstructive pulmonary disease may cause insomnia. Pain, nausea, dyspnea, cough, and gastroesophageal reflux may interfere with sleep.

E. **Obstructive sleep apnea syndrome**

1. This sleep disorder occurs in 5-15% of adults. It is characterized by recurrent discontinuation of breathing during sleep for at least 10 seconds. Abnormal oxygen saturation and sleep patterns result in excessive daytime fatigue and drowsiness. Loud snoring is typical. Overweight, middle-aged men are particularly predisposed. Weight loss can be helpful in obese patients.

2. Diagnosis is by polysomnography. Use of hypnotic agents is contraindicated since they increase the frequency and the severity of apneic episodes.

II. Clinical evaluation of insomnia

A. Evaluation should include a review of sleep habits, drug and alcohol consumption, medical, psychiatric, and neurologic illnesses, pain, sleep environment, and family history. The physical examination should exclude asthma or congestive heart failure, which may contribute to the patient's sleep problem.

B. **Sleep history.** The onset, frequency, duration, and severity of sleep complaints should be assessed. The progression of symptoms, fluctuations over time, and any possible precipitating events should be evaluated.

1. A sudden onset suggests that a change in sleep environment or a stressful life event may be responsible. Persistent insomnia is usually a consequence of medical, neurologic, or psychiatric disease; persistent insomnia can also result from primary sleep disorders, including restless leg syndrome.

2. The evaluation should determine if sleep difficulties involve initiation or maintenance of sleep.

3. Specific symptoms that occur around sleep onset should be sought, including paresthesia or other unpleasant sensations and uncontrollable limb movements of restless leg syndrome; eg, repeated awakenings, snoring, or cessation of breathing in sleep apnea syndromes should be sought; daytime fatigue, irritability, or lack of concentration should be evaluated.

4. Frequent awakenings may be seen when insomnia occurs secondary to drugs or underlying medical conditions; early morning awakenings frequently occur secondary to anxiety or depression.

5. The patient's functional status and mood during the daytime should be assessed. Episodes of unintentional sleep are suggestive of sleep apnea syndrome or narcolepsy.

C. **Alcohol and drug history.** The patient should be questioned about the use of drugs that can directly cause insomnia (eg, central nervous system stimulants, beta blockers, bronchodilators, corticosteroids), and about withdrawal of central nervous system depressant drugs (eg, sedatives, hypnotics, corticosteroids). Alcohol, caffeine, and tobacco consumption should also be documented, since they can adversely affect sleep.

D. **Psychiatric history.** Symptoms or history of depression, anxiety, psychosis, or unusually stressful life events. Sleep disorders that occur secondary to psychiatric illness respond in most cases to psychotherapeutic modalities; an additional cause of disturbed sleep or a primary sleep disorder should be suspected if insomnia complaints.

E. **Medical, neurologic, and family history.** A thorough history of medical and neurologic complaints and past illnesses should be obtained to detect potential causes of secondary insomnia. A family history of insomnia may suggest certain primary sleep disorders. A positive family history is found in about one-third of patients with idiopathic restless leg syndrome.

F. Physical examination. A careful physical examination may direct attention to medical disorders involving the respiratory, cardiovascular, gastrointestinal, endocrine, or neurologic systems. A wide variety of medical conditions or their treatment may result in insomnia.

Medical causes of insomnia
Congestive cardiac failure
Ischemic heart disease
Nocturnal angina
Chronic obstructive pulmonary disease (COPD)
Bronchial asthma including nocturnal asthma
Peptic ulcer disease
Reflux esophagitis
Rheumatic disorders
Lyme disease
Acquired immunodeficiency syndrome (AIDS)
Chronic fatigue syndrome

III. **Laboratory evaluation** may suggest an underlying medical diagnosis in patients with other suggestive historical or physical findings.
   A. **Polysomnography (PSG).** Formal sleep studies are rarely indicated in the initial evaluation of insomnia. PSG may be useful in the following situations:
      1. A sleep-related breathing disorder is suspected.
      2. Insomnia has been present for more than six months, and medical, neurologic, and psychiatric causes have been excluded.
      3. Insomnia has not responded to behavioral or pharmacologic treatment.
IV. **Pharmacologic management**
   A. Hypnotics are the primary drugs used in the management of insomnia. These drugs include the benzodiazepines and the benzodiazepine receptor agonists in the imidazopyridine or pyrazolopyrimidine classes.

Recommended dosages of hypnotic medications (elderly dosages are in parentheses)				
Benzodiazepine hypnotics	Recommended dose, mg	T_{max}	Elimination half-life	Receptor selectivity
Benzodiazepine receptor agonists				
Zolpidem (Ambien)	5-10 (5)	1.6	2.6	Yes
Zaleplon (Sonata)	5-10 (5)	1	1	Yes
Eszopiclone (Lunesta)	2-3 (1-2)	1	6	Yes
Hypnotic Medications				
Estazolam (ProSom)	1-2 (0.5-1)	2.7	17.1	No
Flurazepam (Dalmane)	15-30 (15)	1	47.0-100	No
Triazolam (Halcion)	0.250 (0.125)	1.2	2.6	No

Benzodiazepine hypnotics	Recom-mended dose, mg	T_{max}	Elimina-tion half-life	Receptor selectiv-ity
Temazepam (Resto-ril)	7.5-60 (7.5-20)	0.8	8.4	No
Quazepam (Doral)	7.5-15.0 (7.5)	2	73	No

    B. Zolpidem (Ambien) and zaleplon (Sonata) have the advantage of achieving hypnotic effects with less tolerance and fewer adverse effects.

    C. The safety profile of these benzodiazepines and benzodiazepine receptor agonists is good; lethal overdose is rare, except when benzodiazepines are taken with alcohol. Sedative effects may be enhanced when benzodiazepines are used in conjunction with other central nervous system depressants.

    D. Zolpidem (Ambien) is a benzodiazepine agonist with a short elimina-tion half-life that is effective in inducing sleep onset and promoting sleep maintenance. Zolpidem may be associated with greater residual impair-ment in memory and psychomotor performance than zaleplon.

    E. Zaleplon (Sonata) is a benzodiazepine receptor agonist that is rapidly absorbed (T_{MAX} = 1 hour) and has a short elimination half-life of 1 hour. Zaleplon does not impair memory or psychomotor functioning as at early as 2 hours after administration, or on morning awakening. Zaleplon does not cause residual impairment when the drug is given in the middle of the night. Zaleplon can be used at bedtime or after the patient has tried to fall asleep naturally.

    F. Eszopiclone (Lunesta) is a benzodiazepine receptor agonist with a half-life of 6 hours. It is approved for prolonged use; the use of the other agents is restricted to 35 days.

    G. Benzodiazepines with long half-lives, such as flurazepam (Dalmane), may be effective in promoting sleep onset and sustaining sleep. These drugs may have effects that extend beyond the desired sleep period, however, resulting in daytime sedation or functional impairment. Pa-tients with daytime anxiety may benefit from the residual anxiolytic effect of a long-acting benzodiazepine administered at bedtime. Benzodiazepines with intermediate half-lives, such as temazepam (Restoril), facilitate sleep onset and maintenance with less risk of daytime residual effects.

    H. Benzodiazepines with short half-lives, such as triazolam (Halcion), are effective in promoting the initiation of sleep but may not contribute to sleep maintenance.

    I. Sedating antidepressants are sometimes used as an alternative to benzodiazepines or benzodiazepine receptor agonists. Amitriptyline (Elavil), 25-50 mg at bedtime, or trazodone (Desyrel), 50-100 mg, are common choices.

References: See page 294.

Nicotine Dependence

Smoking causes approximately 430,000 smoking deaths each year, accounting for 19.5% of all deaths. Daily use of nicotine for several weeks results in physical dependence. Abrupt discontinuation of smoking leads to nicotine withdrawal within 24 hours. The symptoms include craving for nicotine, irritabil-ity, frustration, anger, anxiety, restlessness, difficulty in concentrating, and mood swings. Symptoms usually last about 4 weeks.

I. Drugs for treatment of nicotine dependance

A. Treatment with nicotine is the only method that produces significant withdrawal rates. Nicotine replacement comes in three forms: nicotine polacrilex gum (Nicorette), nicotine transdermal patches (Habitrol, Nicoderm, Nicotrol), and nicotine nasal spray (Nicotrol NS) and inhaler (Nicotrol). Nicotine patches provide steady-state nicotine levels, but do not provide a bolus of nicotine on demand as do sprays and gum.

B. Bupropion (Zyban) is an antidepressant shown to be effective in treating the craving for nicotine. The symptoms of nicotine craving and withdrawal are reduced with the use of bupropion, making it a useful adjunct to nicotine replacement systems.

Treatments for nicotine dependence

Drug	Dosage	Comments
Nicotine gum (Nicorette)	2- or 4-mg piece/30 min	Available OTC; poor compliance
Nicotine patch (Habitrol, Nicoderm CQ)	1 patch/d for 6-12 wk, then taper for 4 wk	Available OTC; local skin reactions
Nicotine nasal spray (Nicotrol NS)	1-2 doses/h for 6-8 wk	Rapid nicotine delivery; nasal irritation initially
Nicotine inhaler (Nicotrol Inhaler)	6-16 cartridges/d for 12 wk	Mimics smoking behavior; provides low doses of nicotine
Bupropion (Zyban)	150 mg/day for 3 d, then titrate to 300 mg	Treatment initiated 1 wk before quit day; contraindicated with seizures, anorexia, heavy alcohol use

C. Nicotine polacrilex (Nicorette) is available OTC. The patient should use 1-2 pieces per hour. A 2-mg dose is recommended for those who smoke fewer than 25 cigarettes per day, and 4 mg for heavier smokers. It is used for 6 weeks, followed by 6 weeks of tapering. Nicotine gum improves smoking cessation rates by about 40%-60%. Drawbacks include poor compliance and unpleasant taste.

D. Transdermal nicotine (Habitrol, Nicoderm, Nicotrol) doubles abstinence rates compared with placebo, The patch is available OTC and is easier to use than the gum. It provides a plateau level of nicotine at about half that of what a pack-a-day smoker would normally obtain. The higher dose should be used for 6-12 weeks followed by 4 weeks of tapering.

E. Nicotine nasal spray (Nicotrol NS) is available by prescription and is a good choice for patients who have not been able to quit with the gum or patch or for heavy smokers. It delivers a high level of nicotine, similar to smoking. Nicotine nasal spray doubles the rates of sustained abstinence. The spray is used 6-8 weeks, at 1-2 doses per hour (one puff in each nostril). Tapering over about 6 weeks. Side effects include nasal and throat irritation, headache, and eye watering.

F. Nicotine inhaler (Nicotrol Inhaler) delivers nicotine orally via inhalation from a plastic tube. It is available by prescription and has a success rate of 28%, similar to nicotine gum. The inhaler has the advantage of avoiding some of the adverse effects of nicotine gum, and its mode of delivery more closely resembles the act of smoking.

G. **Bupropion (Zyban)**
   1. Bupropion is appropriate for patients who have been unsuccessful using nicotine replacement. Bupropion reduces withdrawal symptoms and can be used in conjunction with nicotine replacement therapy. The treatment is associated with reduced weight gain. Bupropion is contraindicated with a history of seizures, anorexia, heavy alcohol use, or head trauma.
   2. Bupropion is started at a dose of 150 mg daily for 3 days and then increased to 300 mg daily for 2 weeks before the patient stops smoking. Bupropion is then continued for 3 months. When a nicotine patch is added to this regimen, the abstinence rates increase to 50% compared with 32% when only the patch is used.

References: See page 294.

Alcohol and Drug Addiction

The prevalence of alcohol disorders is 16-28%, and the prevalence of drug disorders is 7-9%. Alcoholism is characterized by impaired control over drinking, preoccupation with alcohol, use of alcohol despite adverse consequences, and distortions in thinking (denial). Substance abuse is a pattern of misuse during which the patient maintains control. Addiction or substance dependence is a pattern of misuse during which the patient has lost control.

I. **Clinical assessment of alcohol use and abuse**
   A. The amount and frequency of alcohol use and other drug use in the past month, week, and day should be determined. Whether the patient ever consumes five or more drinks at a time (binge drinking) and previous abuse of alcohol or other drugs should be assessed.
   B. Effects of the alcohol or drug use on the patient's life may include problems with health, family, job or financial status or with the legal system. History of blackouts, motor vehicle crashes, and the effect of alcohol use on family members or friends should be evaluated.

Clinical Clues to Alcohol and Drug Disorders	
Social history Arrest for driving under the influence Loss of job or sent home from work for alcohol- or drug-related reasons Domestic violence Child abuse/neglect	Family instability (divorce, separation) Frequent, unplanned absences Personal isolation Problems at work/school Mood swings
Medical history History of addiction to any drug Withdrawal syndrome Depression Anxiety disorder Recurrent pancreatitis Recurrent hepatitis Hepatomegaly Peripheral neuropathy Myocardial infarction at less than age 30 (cocaine) Blood alcohol level greater than 300 mg per dL or greater than 100 mg per dL	Alcohol smell on breath or intoxicated during office visit Tremor Mild hypertension Estrogen-mediated signs (telangiectasias, spider angiomas, palmar erythema, muscle atrophy) Gastrointestinal complaints Sleep disturbances Eating disorders Sexual dysfunction

DSM-IV Diagnostic Criteria for Substance Dependence

A maladaptive pattern of substance use leading to clinically significant impairment or distress as manifested by 3 or more of the following occurring at any time during the same 12-month period.

Tolerance, as defined by one of the following:
- A need for markedly increased amounts of the substance to achieve intoxication of the desired effect.
- Markedly diminished effect with continued use of the same amount of the substance.

Withdrawal, as manifested by one of the following:
- The characteristic withdrawal syndrome for the substance.
- The same, or a closely related, substance is taken to relieve or avoid withdrawal symptoms.
- The substance is often taken in larger amounts or over a longer period than was intended.
- There is a persistent desire or unsuccessful efforts to cut down or control substance use.
- A great deal of time is spent in activities necessary to obtain the substance, use the substance, or recover from its effects.
- Important social, occupational, or recreational activities are given up or reduced because of substance use.
- Substance use is continued despite knowledge of having a persistent or recurrent physical or psychologic problem that is likely caused or exacerbated by the substance.

II. **Laboratory screening**
   A. **Mean corpuscular volume.** An elevated mean corpuscular volume (MCV) level may result from folic acid deficiency, advanced alcoholic liver disease, or the toxic effect of alcohol on red blood cells. MCV has poor sensitivity for predicting addiction.
   B. **Gamma-glutamyltransferase.** The sensitivity of GGT for predicting alcohol addiction is higher than that of MCV, but its specificity is low.
   C. **Other liver function test** results may be elevated because of heavy alcohol consumption, including aspartate aminotransferase (AST) and alanine aminotransferase (ALT). These markers have low sensitivity and specificity. An AST/ALT ratio greater than 2:1 is highly suggestive of alcohol-related liver disease.
   D. **Carbohydrate-deficient transferrin (CDT).** Consumption of 4 to 7 drinks daily for at least 1 week results in a decrease in the carbohydrate content of transferrin. The sensitivity and specificity of CDT are high.
III. **Alcohol intoxication.** Support is the main treatment for alcohol intoxication. Respiratory depression is frequently the most serious outcome. Unconscious patients should receive thiamine intravenously before receiving glucose.
IV. **Alcohol withdrawal.** Treatment consists of four doses of chlordiazepoxide (Librium), 50 mg every 6 hours, followed by 3 doses of 50 mg every 8 hours, followed by 2 doses of 50 mg every 12 hours, and finally 1 dose of 50 mg at bedtime.

Signs and Symptoms of Alcohol Withdrawal

Withdrawal is characterized by the development of a combination of any of the following signs and symptoms several hours after stopping a prolonged period of heavy drinking:

1. Autonomic hyperactivity: diaphoresis, tachycardia, elevated blood pressure
2. Tremor
3. Insomnia
4. Nausea or vomiting
5. Transient visual, tactile, or auditory hallucinations or illusions
6. Psychomotor agitation
7. Anxiety
8. Generalized seizure activity

Management of Alcohol Withdrawal

Clinical Disorder	Mild/Moderate AWS, able to take oral	Mild/Moderate AWS, unable to take oral	Severe AWS
Adrenergic Hyper-activity	Lorazepam (Ativan) 2 mg po q2h or Chlordiazepoxide (Librium) 25-100 mg po q6h	Lorazepam 1-2 mg IM/IV q1-2h as needed	Lorazepam 1-2 mg IV q 5-10 min
Dehydration	Water or juice po	NS 1 liter bolus, then D5NS 150-200 mL/h	Aggressive hydration with NS /D5NS
Nutritional Deficiency	Thiamine 100 mg po Multivitamins Folate 1 mg po	Thiamine 100 mg IV Multivitamins 1 amp in first liter of IV fluids Folate 1 mg IV in first liter of IV fluids	Thiamine 100 mg IV Multivitamins 1 amp in first liter of IV fluids Folate 1 mg IV in first liter of IV fluids
Hypoglycemia	High fructose solution po	25 mL D50 IV (repeat as necessary)	25 mL D50 IV (repeat as necessary)
Hyperthermia			Cooling blankets
Seizures	Lorazepam (Ativan) 2 mg IV	Lorazepam 2 mg IV	Lorazepam 2 mg IV

V. Sedative-hypnotic withdrawal. Establishment of physical dependence usually requires daily use of therapeutic doses of these drugs for 6 months or higher doses for 3 months. Treatment of withdrawal from sedative-hypnotics is similar to that of withdrawal from alcohol; chlordiazepoxide (Librium) and lorazepam (Ativan) are the drugs of choice.

VI. Maintenance treatment
   A. Twelve-step programs make a significant contribution to recovery. Alcoholics Anonymous (AA) is the root of 12-step programs.
   B. Drugs for treatment of alcohol addiction
   1. **Disulfiram** inhibits aldehyde dehydrogenase. On ingesting alcohol, patients taking disulfiram experience flushing of the skin, palpitations, decreased blood pressure, nausea, vomiting, shortness of breath, blurred vision, and confusion. Death has been reported. Side effects include drowsiness, lethargy, peripheral neuropathy, hepatotoxicity, and hypertension. The usual dose is 250 to 500 mg daily.
   2. **Naltrexone,** an opioid antagonist, reduces drinking. It has diminished effectiveness over time and does not reduce relapse rates.
   3. **Serotonergic drugs** reduce drinking in heavy-drinking, nondepressed alcoholic patients, but only 15% to 20% from pretreatment levels.

4. **Acamprosate (calcium acetylhomotaurinate)** reduces the craving for alcohol. Acamprosate appears to result in more frequent and longer-lasting periods of abstinence than does naltrexone.

VII.   **Opiates**

Signs and Symptoms of Opiate Withdrawal

1. Mild elevation of pulse and respiratory rates, blood pressure, and temperature
2. Piloerection (gooseflesh)
3. Dysphoric mood and drug craving
4. Lacrimation and/or rhinorrhea
5. Mydriasis, yawning, and diaphoresis
6. Anorexia, abdominal cramps, vomiting, and diarrhea
7. Insomnia
8. Weakness

Agents Used to Treat Opiate Withdrawal

Methadone (Dolophine) is a pure opioid agonist restricted to inpatient treatment or specialized outpatient drug treatment programs. Treatment is a 15- to 20-mg daily dose for 2 to 3 days, followed by a 10 to 15 percent reduction in daily dose.

Clonidine (Catapres) is an alpha-adrenergic blocker. One 0.2-mg dose every 4 hours to relieve symptoms of withdrawal may be effective. It may be continued for 10 to 14 days, followed by tapering.

Buprenorphine (Buprenex) is a partial mu-receptor agonist which can be administered sublingually in doses of 2, 4, or 8 mg every 4 hours for the management of opiate withdrawal symptoms.

Naltrexone (ReVia, Trexan)/clonidine involves pretreatment with 0.2 to 0.3 mg of clonidine, followed by 12.5 mg of naltrexone (a pure opioid antagonist). Naltrexone is increased to 25 mg on day 2, 50 mg on day 3, and 100 mg on day 4, with clonidine doses of 0.1 to 0.3 mg 3 times daily.

VIII. Stimulant Drugs

Signs and Symptoms of Cocaine or Stimulant Withdrawal

1. Dysphoric mood
2. Fatigue, malaise
3. Vivid, unpleasant dreams
4. Sleep disturbance
5. Increased appetite
6. Psychomotor retardation or agitation

A. Stimulant withdrawal is treated with bromocriptine (Parlodel). This drug reduces stimulant craving and withdrawal symptoms. Bromocriptine dosage is 0.625 to 2.5 mg taken orally three times daily.
B. An alternative protocol uses desipramine to reduce the stimulant craving and postwithdrawal symptoms. Desipramine may be used alone or with bromocriptine. The initial dosage of desipramine is 50 mg per day taken orally. This dosage is increased until a dosage of 150 to 200 mg is achieved. Paranoia or combativeness is treated with lorazepam, 2-mg IM.

References

References may be obtained at www.ccspublishing.com.

Index

Order Form

Current Clinical Strategies books can also be purchased at all medical bookstores

Title	Book	CD
MicrobiologyFlash with Immunology Review Flashcards	$49.95	
NCLEX-RN-Flash Board Review Flashcards	$49.95	
BoardWiz 1 USMLE Step 1 Board Review Flashcards	$49.95	
BoardWiz 2 USMLE Step 2 Board Review Flashcards	$49.95	
Treatment Guidelines in Medicine, 2010 Edition	$19.95	$36.95
Psychiatry History Taking, Third Edition	$12.95	$28.95
Psychiatry, 2010 Edition	$12.95	$28.95
Anesthesiology, 2008 Edition	$16.95	$28.95
Medicine, 2009 Edition	$16.95	$28.95
Pediatric Treatment Guidelines, 2007 Edition	$19.95	$29.95
Physician's Drug Manual	$9.95	$28.95
Surgery, Sixth Edition	$12.95	$28.95
Gynecology and Obstetrics, 2008 Edition	$16.95	$30.95
Pediatrics, 2007 Edition	$12.95	$28.95
Family Medicine, 2008 Edition	$26.95	$46.95
History and Physical Examination in Medicine, Tenth Edition	$14.95	$28.95
Outpatient and Primary Care Medicine, 2010 Edition	$16.95	$28.95
Critical Care Medicine, 2007 Edition	$16.95	$32.95
Handbook of Psychiatric Drugs, 2008 Edition	$14.95	$28.95
Pediatric History and Physical Examination, Fourth Edition	$12.95	$28.95
Current Clinical Strategies CD-ROM Collection for iPhone, Palm, Pocket PC, Windows, and Macintosh		$59.95

CD-ROMs are compatible with iPhone, Palm, Pocket PC, Windows and Macintosh.

Quantity	Title	Amount

Order by Fax: 800-965-9420 or 909-744-8071
Internet Orders: http://www.ccspublishing.com/ccs
Mail Orders:
    Current Clinical Strategies Publishing
    PO Box 1753
    Blue Jay, CA 92317

Credit Card Number: _____

Exp: ____/____

Shipping charge: $6.00 per order. International shipping $10.00

Signature: _____

Phone Number: (_____)_____

Name and Address (please print):

_____

_____

_____

_____